Fit to Be Tied

Critical Issues in Health and Medicine

Edited by Rima D. Apple, University of Wisconsin–Madison,
and Janet Golden, Rutgers University, Camden

Growing criticism of the U.S. health care system is coming from consumers, politicians, the media, activists, and health care professionals. Critical Issues in Health and Medicine is a collection of books that explores these contemporary dilemmas from a variety of perspectives, among them political, legal, historical, sociological, and comparative, and with attention to crucial dimensions such as race, gender, ethnicity, sexuality, and culture.

For a list of titles in the series, see the last page of the book.

Fit to Be Tied

Sterilization and Reproductive Rights in America, 1950–1980

Rebecca M. Kluchin

Rutgers University Press

New Brunswick, New Jersey, and London

First paperback printing, 2011

Library of Congress Cataloging-in-Publication Data

Kluchin, Rebecca M. (Rebecca Marie)
    Fit to be tied : sterilization and reproductive rights in America, 1950–1980 / Rebecca M. Kluchin.
        p. cm. — (Critical issues in health and medicine)
    Rev. ed. of thesis: Fit to be tied? : sterilization and reproductive rights in America, 1960–1984 / by Rebecca M. Kluchin. c2004.
    Includes bibliographical references and index.
    ISBN 978-0-8135-4527-1 (hardcover : alk. paper)
    ISBN 978-0-8135-4999-6 (pbk. : alk. paper)
    1. Sterilization (Birth control)—United States—History—20th century.   2. Birth control—Government policy—United States—History—20th century.   3. Reproductive rights—United States—History—20th century.   I. Title.   II. Series.
    [DNLM: 1. Sterilization, Reproductive—history—United States.   2.   Family Planning Policy—history—United States.   3. Socioeconomic Factors—United States.   4. Sterilization, Involuntary—legislation & jurisprudence—United States.   5. Women's Rights—history—United States. WP 11 AA1 K66f 2009]
    HQ766.5.U5K55   2009
    363.9'7—dc22   2008036418

A British Cataloging-in-Publication record for this book is available from the British Library.

Visit our Web site: http://rutgerspress.rutgers.edu

Manufactured in the United States of America

For my mother, Judith Allen

Contents

Acknowledgments

Writing is often described as a solitary task, but in many ways, this book has been a collective project. I am grateful for the financial support I received from the Woodrow Wilson National Fellowship Foundation; the Center for Africanamerican Urban Studies and the Economy (CAUSE) at Carnegie Mellon University; Carnegie Mellon University Graduate Programs Office; California State University, Sacramento; the Rockefeller Archive Center; the Smith College Archives; the Schlesinger Library on the History of Women in America; and the University of Minnesota Social Welfare History Archives.

I benefited from the knowledge and assistance of archivists at the Schlesinger Library; the Sophia Smith Collection at Smith College; the Rockefeller Archive Center; the Seeley G. Mudd Manuscript Library at Princeton University; the Barco Law Library at the University of Pittsburgh; the Hillman Library at the University of Pittsburgh; the Archives and Special Collections Department at Northeastern University; the California Ethnic and Multicultural Archives at the University of California, Santa Barbara; Stanford University Department of Special Collections; University of California, Los Angeles, Chicano Studies Research Center Library; and the Charles Deering McCormick Library of Special Collections at Northwestern University. I want to extend a special thank-you to David Klaassen and Linnea Anderson at the University of Minnesota Social Welfare History Archives for working closely with me to locate important documents within the Association for Voluntary Sterilization records as well as for helping me to gain access to sealed materials. I would also like to thank Sue Collins at Carnegie Mellon's Hunt Library for serving as an indispensable resource during the early stages of this project.

I received incredible support from my teachers and colleagues at Carnegie Mellon University. Tera Hunter read drafts of this manuscript with great care, lent her sharp insight, and offered encouragement. Elizabeth Siegel Watkins has been a friend and mentor since the beginning, and I am grateful for the guidance and inspiration she provided. Judith Schacter, Katherine Lynch, Wendy Goldman, David Hounshell, and Scott Sandage taught me to think critically and ask difficult questions. Friends and colleagues in Pittsburgh read and commented on portions of the manuscript and generously contributed their thoughts. Many thanks to Asif Siddiqi, Robin Dearmon Jenkins, Jessie Ramey, Lisa Johnson, Jim Longhurst, Steve Burnett, Glen Asner, Carl Zimring, Jen Potter, and Jeff Suzik. Trent and Jennifer Alexander, Kara Allen, my sister Abby Kluchin, and Abby's friends Adrienne Fowler and Mara Gustafson put me up and kept me fed when I traveled to the archives.

I am lucky to be surrounded by thoughtful colleagues in the History Department at California State University, Sacramento. Christopher Castaneda, Michael Vann, Patrick Ettinger, Chloe Burke, Shirley Ann Wilson Moore, Jennifer Terry, Erika Quinn, and Julie Cahill have been especially kind and supportive. Lee Simpson, Katerina Lagos, and Mona Siegel have become close friends as well as colleagues. They keep me smiling, engaged, and eager to come to work each day. Lee also read the manuscript in its entirety with her usual intensity at a critical moment in the revision process. I benefited from the insight of scholars outside of my department who took time to work through ideas with me and pushed me to think more critically. This book is better because of contributions by Adele Clarke, Dominique Tobbell, Naomi Rogers, Susan Smith, Judith Houck, Susan Reverby, Deborah Levine, Lisa Levenstein, Miroslava Chávez-Garcia, Sally Torpy, and Robyn Spencer. I am very grateful to Wendy Kline for her continued support and friendship. Not only did she kept me on track with our weekly check-ins, but she also offered kind words when I felt discouraged, cheered loudly when I met deadlines, and made all the conferences we attended together so much fun. Douglas Dunham and Robert Kluchin tutored me in constitutional law and offered important last-minute advice on class action claims. Estelle Carol, Bob Simpson, Katherine Mallin, Pat Rush, Coral Norris, Jenny Knauss, Lauren Crawford, Laura McAlpine, and Cindy Zucker shared their memories and records of feminist and reproductive rights activism in Chicago during the 1960s and 1970s.

It was a pleasure to work with the staff at Rutgers University Press, especially Doreen Valentine, who helped me fine-tune my ideas and language, and series editors Rima Apple and Janet Golden. I also appreciate the keen eye of copyeditor Robert Burchfield and the external reader's thoughtful review.

From 1999 to 2003, I had the privilege of working at Allegheny Reproductive Health Center (ARHC). The counselors, lab technician, nurses, anesthetists, and administrators shared their personal experiences with abortion and sterilization with me and allowed me to observe their work. The doctors answered my questions about medical research and technology and shared their thoughts about the ethics of sterilization. The staff at ARHC provide the type of patient-centered health care premised upon compassion and respect that we should all have the luxury of expecting from our health care providers. I have deep affection and great admiration for Claire, Renny, Darlene, Ronnie, Jackie, Erica, Dr. Turner, Dr. Thompson, and the late Dr. Kisner.

My greatest debt is to my friends and family, who sustained and nurtured me throughout this process. Danielle Pener and Jeremy Shoenig, Claire Keyes, Jennifer DiMercurio, and Bobbi Little cultivated my nonhistorical interests with provocative conversations, delicious meals, and long rides. David Hoffman, Ruth Callaghan, Christina Neff, Fung Chin, and Mei Chin form my extended family in Chicago. Their love and support have been a constant throughout my life, and I am pleased to (finally) be able to share this book with them. My grandfather, Ben Kluchin, died just before this book was published. The many stories he told reminded me of the links between past and present, and reinforced the importance of chronicling historical events. I am deeply saddened that I cannot share the stories in this book with him. Throughout the research, writing, and revision process, my sister Abby acted as a sounding board, editor, friend, and confidant. Our conversations—especially the silly ones—revitalized me when I needed to escape the world of sterilization. My parents, Judith Allen and Robert Kluchin, bore witness to this project from its inception through its conclusion. My father spent hours with me on the phone talking through my interpretations of sterilization-related lawsuits and helping me hone my use of legal sources. These conversations were the most enjoyable part of the research process; I learned as much about him as I did the law. This book is about motherhood: who gets to define what a mother should do and be and what happens when public ideas about motherhood infringe upon private lives. My interest in this topic grew out of my love, respect, and admiration for my own mother, who taught me to look critically at social norms and to value reproductive labor. This book is dedicated to her. Finally, I owe great thanks to my husband, Bryan Warhold, who graciously lived with this project for the last five years. He distracted me when I needed breaks, endured my foul moods when my writing and revisions stalled, but, most important, made me laugh and feel loved.

Fit to Be Tied

Introduction

The 1960s ushered in a revolution in American contraceptive practice. The introduction of the birth control pill (the Pill) in 1960 and the redesign and return of the intrauterine device (IUD) in 1964 offered women contraception that was nearly 100 percent effective. No longer forced to rely upon messy diaphragms, jellies, and condoms with high failure rates, the IUD and the Pill offered women reliable birth control that did not interfere with the sex act. Contraceptive sterilization—tubal ligation and vasectomy—offered the same benefits, and between 1965 and 1975 this surgery gained public and medical acceptance as a legitimate and cost-effective method of birth control. By 1975, 7.9 million Americans had undergone sterilization, and sterilization had become the most popular method of contraception used by married couples.[1]

Before it became a popular method of birth control, sterilization was a tool of eugenics, the science of racial betterment that developed in America around the turn of the twentieth century. Most early eugenicists endorsed a rather crude notion of biological determinism that deemed mental, physical, and behavioral "defects" to be genetic and unalterable. Eugenicists believed poverty, criminality, illegitimacy, epilepsy, feeblemindedness, and alcoholism (among others) were inherited traits that could not be altered. Concerned about the quality of American citizens during a period of mass eastern and southern European immigration, industrialization, and urbanization, eugenicists sought to control the quality and quantity of the American population in order to prevent the country from being overrun by the "unfit." By emphasizing the "natural" aptitude of white, native-born Americans, eugenicists sought to preserve this group's social, economic, and political power. Biological determinism naturalized racial and ethnic differences and secured middle- and upper-class white men's position at the top of the social hierarchy. Eugenicists encouraged the reproduction of "fit" citizens, defined as those who were native-born, white, and middle class and who shared family histories free from "defects." They discouraged the reproduction of "unfit" citizens—those with histories filled with "destructive" traits, who were not white (eastern and southern European immigrants were considered not white), and whose reproduction eugenicists defined as costly and harmful. To prevent the reproduction of the "unfit," eugenicists first segregated them from the rest of the population. Eugenicists later came to favor the more cost-effective "solution" of sterilization (via tubal ligation and vasectomy). Unable to reproduce, the logic went, the negative impact of "unfit" individuals could be tempered over time.

Eugenicists were especially concerned about the costs associated with caring for people who were poor, people with disabilities, criminals, and women who bore children out of wedlock. Biological determinism ensured that these groups would inevitably bear children afflicted with the same defects, and the state would be forced to fund their care. Sterilization prevented the "unfit" from reproducing and eliminated the financial burdens that future generations of "unfit" Americans would undoubtedly generate for the government and taxpayers. Responding to such concerns, states began to enact involuntary sterilization laws, and in 1927 the Supreme Court validated states' right to sterilize their "unfit" citizens. By 1941, 38,087 Americans had been sterilized under eugenic statutes.[2]

Rates of eugenic sterilization fell during World War II, and the formal eugenics movement concluded by the end of the baby boom, but eugenicists' preoccupation with reproductive "fitness"—a term used to describe the relative worth of a person's genetic and cultural abilities—continued on in American culture, society, medicine, and law.[3] Reproductive fitness evaluates the quality of a given individual and assigns a value to her or his reproduction. Eugenicists used race, class, ethnicity, intelligence, physical well-being, mental health, and sexual behavior as indicators of reproductive fitness. In the first half of the twentieth century, a white native-born middle-class woman with no family history of crime, illegitimacy, alcoholism, or other "defects" would be deemed "fit" to reproduce, and encouraged to do so in defense of the white race. A poor eastern European immigrant woman, in contrast, would be deemed "unfit" on the grounds of her ethnicity and poverty. If she bore a child out of wedlock or transgressed other sexual boundaries, her reproductive fitness would decline even further. Eugenicists considered "fit" women's reproduction to be productive, healthy, and beneficial to the nation. They viewed "unfit" women's reproduction as destructive, unhealthy, and debilitating because the children "unfit" women bore were tainted by inherent defects that would cause them to become dependent upon the state for assistance. Eugenicists focused more on women than men because of women's childbearing capabilities.[4]

Ideas of reproductive fitness are historically specific; they shape and reflect cultural values and social tensions—especially those related to race and gender—and they influence public policy and medical practice. *Fit to Be Tied* examines these changing principles in the second half of the twentieth century, the sterilization trends they inspired, and the public policies they shaped. In the 1950s, 1960s, and 1970s, standards of reproductive fitness shifted in response to contemporary social anxieties, including blacks' demands for racial equality, rising rates of Mexican and Puerto Rican immigration, the development of federal antipoverty programs, the expansion of welfare, and fears of overpopulation. Eugenics faded from public view by the end of the baby boom, but did not disappear from American society, culture, or politics. Instead, it was replaced by neo-eugenics. Neo-eugenics refers to the ideas, practices, and policies that continued some legacies of eugenics in the post–baby boom years but that also differ significantly. Neo-eugenics was not a formal movement, but it had a wide range of adherents, including scientists, physicians, politicians, and social conservatives, who rested their social critiques on neo-eugenic standards of reproductive fitness. Like eugenicists, neo-eugenicists believed that poverty, criminality, illegitimacy, and other "defects" were reproduced, but neo-eugenicists believed that culture rather than genes constituted the method of transmission. Both eugenicists and neo-eugenicists pointed to the traits above as "symptoms" of a lack of reproductive fitness, but they associated these "defects" with different racial and ethnic groups than earlier eugenicists had targeted. Eugenicists focused on preserving the white race; they worried that eastern and southern European immigrants could "pass" as white and "dilute" the genetic makeup of native-born whites, dragging the country down in the process. By the 1950s, though, these immigrant groups had assimilated, and immigration restrictions passed in 1921 and 1924 prevented additional influxes. Americans in the 1950s, 1960s, and 1970s confronted new "threats" to white power and privilege: the civil rights, Black Power, Chicano/a rights, and Native American rights movements. As blacks, Chicanos/as, Native Americans, and other minorities demanded an end to segregation and racial discrimination, as well as equal rights under the law, they challenged white power structures and became the target of neo-eugenicists as a result. Some whites in power used ideas of racial difference to defend their positions of privilege. Neo-eugenics supplied such rationales.

Those who adhered to neo-eugenic ideas expressed specific concern about the expansion of welfare and the inclusion of people of color in these programs, at once continuing the eugenic preoccupation with the costs associated with caring for the "unfit," but also responding to specific concerns about America's post–World War II welfare system. Eugenicists complained about the cost of caring for criminals and individuals admitted to mental institutions. Neo-eugenicists took issue with an expanding welfare system, established during the Great Depression in the 1930s and strengthened in the 1960s under the Great Society. Conservative white middle-class Americans expressed anger at the "unworthy" poor on the public dole, especially as unwed, nonwhite mothers gained access to government assistance, and they drew upon neo-eugenic principles to support their complaints. They developed stereotypes like the "welfare queen" to denigrate poor women who received assistance and to devalue their reproductive labor. These offensive stereotypes were premised upon the notion that "defective" traits like poverty and illegitimacy were "bred" through culture (rather than genes). Why should we help "unworthy" women raise their families when their children will only create more social problems, neo-eugenicists asked. Why should we fund the reproduction of social ills? Viewed through this framework, the welfare system enabled "unfit" Americans to continue their "destructive" lifestyles at the expense of decent white middle-class taxpayers.

Sterilization once again offered a "solution" to the cycle of dependency. If "unfit" Americans remained destined to reproduce their defects, then sterilization continued to offer a cost-effective method of preventing this threat from materializing. Here, biological and environmental determinism blurred together in neo-eugenic thought. Some advocates of sterilization held on to older, traditional eugenic ideas of biological determinism, but most recognized the interrelation between environment and genes in shaping behavior, consistent with contemporary theories about the nature-nurture debate. Neo-eugenic physicians, academics, and policy makers advocated sterilization of the "unfit" as a way to prevent their reproduction and save taxpayers and the government money. Sterilization constituted a biological solution to what neo-eugenicists characterized as a cultural phenomenon. Neo-eugenicists did not view this as inconsistent. By preventing poor women of color, especially single mothers, from bearing children, neo-eugenicists sought to preclude them from creating families that these women would predictably endow with the destructive values they embodied. Neo-eugenicists recognized the role of the environment in shaping behavior, but they argued that the most effective means of preventing the cultural transmission of defects was to surgically prevent the "unfit" from bearing children in the first place. Thwarting harmful reproductive behavior required surgical intervention. The legislators who proposed bills designed to criminalize illegitimacy among welfare recipients and to punish offenders with sterilization and the doctors who sterilized poor women without their knowledge or informed consent did not view their actions as violations of women's reproductive rights. In their minds, women on welfare relinquished these rights as a condition of receiving aid. They believed that those who accepted government assistance should submit to government oversight and conform to mainstream, white middle-class values and gender roles. The women they targeted disagreed.

Neo-eugenics lacked the formality of eugenics, but at least one older organization bridged the movements. The Association for Voluntary Sterilization (AVS) placed itself at the forefront of the transition from eugenics to neo-eugenics. Cognizant that both science and society had moved beyond traditional eugenics, the AVS changed its ideology, its goals, and to some extent its membership in an effort to remain relevant. Capitalizing on contemporary social anxieties of the immediate postwar era, including concerns about Communism, overpopulation, and the expansion of welfare, the former eugenics group reinvented itself in the 1950s as a voluntary sterilization organization committed to the use of sterilization as a technological "solution" to contemporary social "problems" like single motherhood, poverty, overpopulation, and criminality—symptoms of a lack of reproductive fitness. The AVS refocused itself on a central goal: make sterilization available and accessible to all Americans and encourage the "unfit" to choose permanent contraception.

The organization's sterilization agenda affected the reproductive decisions of both "fit" and "unfit" Americans. The AVS developed popular rationales for contraceptive sterilization (tubal ligation and vasectomy) of the "unfit" in the 1950s that "fit" women and men in the 1960s and 1970s seized upon as they began to search for alternatives to the Pill and the IUD. Initially, the AVS focused on making tubal ligation and vasectomy available to the "unfit." It received considerable support from the population control movement, which emerged in the wake of World War II. Neither group considered sterilization an appropriate surgery for "fit" Americans, especially for "fit" women during the baby boom. But in the late 1960s and early 1970s, "fit" women began to look toward contraceptive sterilization as an alternative to the Pill and the IUD after medical concerns about the safety of these technologies arose. Many women eager to undergo tubal ligation found their efforts to obtain the surgery stymied by restrictive hospital policies, enacted during the baby boom to promote "fit" women's reproduction. The AVS smelled an opportunity. If the organization could help "fit" women overturn barriers to tubal ligation, it could expand all Americans' access to the surgery and thereby accomplish its goal of transforming sterilization from a eugenic procedure associated with "defectives" to an acceptable method of birth control used by all Americans, including those it deemed "unfit" on the ground of their poverty, race, and illegitimacy. By the late 1960s and early 1970s, fears of overpopulation diminished the emphasis on "fit" women's reproduction, which in turn reduced physicians' resistance to these women's efforts to terminate their fertility. Building on recent Supreme Court decisions legalizing birth control (and later abortion), the AVS adopted the rhetoric of reproductive rights and inaugurated a campaign to overturn hospital restrictions that also involved Zero Population Growth (ZPG), a population control organization, and the American Civil Liberties Union (ACLU). Of the three organizations, only the ACLU remained free of neo-eugenic motives. Plaintiffs' determination and racial privilege helped to make this campaign a success.

Florence Caffarelli was one of the first plaintiffs to file suit against a hospital that refused her request for surgery. In 1971, this white working-class housewife petitioned the Peekskill Community Hospital in Peekskill, New York, for a tubal ligation. The twenty-six-year-old mother of three could not take birth control pills because of the appearance of a breast tumor. She had conceived her third child while using an IUD, which had caused her to cramp and bleed uncomfortably. Caffarelli's local hospital denied her request, citing its policy of performing sterilization only in life-threatening situations.[5] It also pointed to the ambiguous legal status of the procedure. Like the majority of states, New York did not have a law governing contraceptive sterilization. As such, the procedure was not explicitly legal, nor was it illegal, like abortion. According to her lawyers, the Peekskill Community Hospital told Caffarelli that it would "not permit any such operation unless and until the Legislature authorizes it or a court directs it."[6] Caffarelli responded by filing a lawsuit against the hospital. She won access to the surgery, as did other women that the AVS, ZPG, and the ACLU assisted, and as a result, rates of tubal ligation rose steadily through the 1970s. Unfortunately, this success had an unexpected consequence for "unfit" women: it hid the emergence of a new trend in forced sterilization.

Region and race intersected to create distinct trends of forced sterilization in the second half of the twentieth century. In the 1950s, black women in the South became targets of forced sterilization via hysterectomy, commonly referred to by women as "Mississippi appendectomies," because women entered hospitals to have abdominal surgery and left, unknowingly, without their uteruses. The practice became widespread in communities entrenched in civil rights struggles.

Physicians, social workers, and members of state eugenics boards concerned about the rising costs of welfare also exploited existing eugenic laws to sterilize poor black women with the specific intention of reducing the number of blacks eligible to receive public assistance. Forced sterilization practices changed and spread in the late 1960s and early 1970s through newly established federal family planning programs. Increasingly, poor women of color entered hospitals for labor and delivery, where the neo-eugenic physicians who treated them forced them to undergo tubal ligation. Black women remained the targets of such physicians in the South, while women of color in other regions came under increasing scrutiny. As concerns about Mexican immigration increased in California and other border states and as these states became embroiled in contentious debates about immigrants' right to government aid, Mexican and Mexican American women were subjected to forced sterilization in public hospitals. In New York City and to a lesser extent Chicago, physicians pressured Puerto Rican women to undergo surgery when these cities experienced rising rates of immigration. On reservations, Native American women became targets of physicians employed by the Indian Health Service (IHS) who believed that restricting these women's reproduction would reduce their poverty and their dependence on government assistance. Between 1970 and 1976, IHS hospitals and their affiliates sterilized between 25 and 42 percent of all Native American women of childbearing age.[7] This book chronicles the changes in forced sterilization practices in the second half of the twentieth century, focusing especially on the ways in which neo-eugenic physicians, social workers, judges, and lawmakers employed the surgery in defense of racial hierarchies specific to their geographic regions. It is equally concerned with the ways in which women contested these efforts and challenged the neo-eugenic philosophies guiding forced sterilization.

Born in Fort Worth, Texas, and of Mexican heritage, Elena Orozco was one of ten plaintiffs who filed suit against administrators and physicians at a Los Angeles hospital in 1975 for sterilizing them against their will and without their informed consent. On July 11, 1972, Orozco was permanently sterilized without her informed consent at the University of Southern California, Los Angeles County Medical Center. Orozco entered the hospital one day earlier to deliver her sixth child. She had been receiving prenatal care at an outpatient clinic affiliated with the hospital, where the doctors who monitored her pregnancy repeatedly pressured her to undergo tubal ligation upon delivery. She refused their requests, which infuriated one doctor so much he shouted at her. When Orozco arrived at the Medical Center in labor, she learned that she was scheduled for a tubal ligation upon delivery. According to her lawyers, Orozco "indicated that she did not wish to have her tubes tied at that time." Despite her insistence, several doctors pressured her to reconsider and suggested that future cesarean sections—Orozco bore all six of her children via cesarean—would constitute a health risk. They explained the risks of tubal ligation but not the permanence of the procedure. She resisted their requests for a while. Then, in heavy labor, feeling uncomfortable with the number of doctors and nurses surrounding her while she lay on an examination table exposed from the waist down, and concerned that her resistance might jeopardize her delivery, Orozco relented and signed the consent form. She did so under the mistaken impression that the surgery was reversible. When she signed the form, Orozco believed that her tubes could be untied, not that they would be severed and ligated. Neither she nor her husband thought that they had completed their family. Unlike Florence Caffarelli, Orozco and her fellow plaintiffs lost their suit when the judge ruled their loss of fertility to be an unfortunate result of the Spanish-speaking plaintiffs' "inability to communicate clearly."[8]

Historically, women's access to contraception has been determined by their race, ethnicity, and class status. The contradictory trends of sterilization in the baby boom and post–baby boom years follow this pattern and illuminate the extent to which neo-eugenic notions of reproductive fitness influenced family planning policy and medical practice in the second half of the twentieth century. White women of different socioeconomic classes struggled to obtain contraceptive sterilization while poor women, predominantly women of color, struggled to resist coercive sterilization. Restrictive, pronatalist hospital policies prevented "fit" women from choosing voluntary sterilization at the same time that physicians, nurses, and social workers pushed sterilization on "unfit" women. The creation of a comprehensive federal family planning system in 1970 promoted this practice by paying for poor women to be treated by medical personnel who believed that they had the right to make reproductive decisions for their patients. Increasingly, when poor women entered hospitals to give birth, they confronted physicians adamant about their "need" for sterilization. Physicians recorded forced sterilizations as voluntary, making the forced surgeries appear to be part of the rising rate of tubal ligation. *Fit to Be Tied* reveals the intimate connections between the histories of voluntary and involuntary sterilization in America in the second half of the twentieth century, both in terms of the contradictory trends that developed and women's resistance to these trends.

Eugenics and neo-eugenics centered on the premise that motherhood was a social act to be regulated by experts and laws. The social engineers behind these philosophies viewed reproduction as a choice that held important social ramifications; as such, they believed that reproductive decisions should be made by experts and governed by the state, as men and especially women could not be trusted to make responsible reproductive decisions. Second-wave feminists rejected these assumptions through their demands for unrestricted access to contraception and abortion. "Fit" women denied access to sterilization and "unfit" women forcibly sterilized did the same by filing lawsuits in defense of their reproductive rights. In these suits, women insisted that they possessed the fundamental right to determine the terms and conditions of their reproductive decisions. When this right was violated—either by a restriction that prevented a woman from obtaining tubal ligation or by a physician who operated on a woman without her informed consent—women used the courts to protest. When victims of forced sterilization demanded damages for the loss of their fertility, they challenged the neo-eugenic sentiments behind their sterilization, affirmed the value of their reproduction, and defended their reproductive rights.

The lawsuits examined here show that sterilization, not abortion, topped many women's lists of reproductive concerns. The contemporary abortion debate has dominated public perceptions of reproductive rights in the 1970s, 1980s, and 1990s, but it did not occur within a vacuum, nor did it define the reproductive politics of all American women. Abortion politics shaped women's sterilization experiences to some extent. In the era before *Roe v. Wade*, women chose voluntary sterilization to ensure that they would not have to make a decision about whether to have an abortion. Many of these women had experienced an unplanned pregnancy (often while using temporary and unreliable methods of birth control), and this caused them to seek permanent contraception in order to avoid a similar situation. But the right to legal abortion held little significance for sterilization abuse victims who could never become pregnant again. Abortion debates center on two questions: when does life begin, and who gets to decide if and when a pregnancy should be terminated? Sterilization debates revolved around another version of the second question: who gets to make sterilization decisions and why? At its core, this book is about the reproductive choices available to women and the extent to which notions of reproductive fitness determine what these choices will be and who has the power to make them. This is a book about power struggles, the contested margins between private choices and public policies, and the ways in which race, class, and gender determine these boundaries.

Chapter 1

From Eugenics to Neo-eugenics

Eugenics developed in America at the turn of the twentieth century as a response to cultural, social, and political anxieties specific to the era. As the decades advanced and the country experienced a massive depression and two world wars, eugenic ideas and practices evolved as well. Positive eugenics, or the encouragement of "fit" women's reproduction, experienced a revival during the baby boom, but only a few eugenically driven institutions, notably Paul Popenoe's American Institute of Family Relations (AIFR), supported this trend. Popenoe's emphasis on "fit" women's reproduction did not replace previous efforts to quell the reproduction of "unfit" individuals through compulsory sterilization laws, immigration quotas, and antimiscegenation legislation. These practices continued to some extent in the second half of the twentieth century; but with the exception of the Association for Voluntary Sterilization (AVS), the American Eugenics Society (AES), and the Pioneer Fund, few of the older, traditional eugenics laboratories and organizations remained intact after World War II, and the number of compulsory surgeries declined significantly after the war.[1] By the 1960s, the formal eugenics movement had crumbled, but eugenic ideas and practices remained embedded in American society, culture, and politics.

The eugenicists and eugenic organizations that remained in existence after World War II continued to revise their standards of reproductive fitness to reflect contemporary social concerns about welfare, overpopulation, civil rights, Mexican immigration, and the sexual revolution. These standards were both similar to those advanced by eugenicists in the first half of the century and at the same time distinct from these earlier ideas because they responded to very historically specific concerns and trends. Not quite eugenic anymore, these new ideas and practices of social engineering are best described as neo-eugenic.

Neo-eugenic physicians, social workers, and politicians capitalized on the changing use of sterilization to put these new politics into practice. Between roughly 1965 and 1975, sterilization was transformed from a eugenic procedure to one of the most popular methods of contraception in America. In 1965, roughly 13 percent of all married couples had undergone sterilization for contraceptive purposes. The percentage increased to about 18 percent by 1970 and soared to about 29 percent in 1973. By 1975, 7.9 million Americans had undergone sterilization, and sterilization had become the most popular method of contraception used by married couples.[2] The AVS in particular strove to make contraceptive sterilization—tubal ligation or vasectomy undertaken solely for birth control purposes—acceptable to physicians and available to the public, especially the poor, with the hope that access to the surgery would prompt "unfit" citizens to choose permanent contraception.

The AVS stood at the forefront of the transition between eugenics and neo-eugenics and at the head of the campaign to legitimize contraceptive sterilization among physicians and the public. Not only did the organization persist in the postwar era after most of its contemporaries had disbanded, but it was the vanguard of a new movement to legitimize contraceptive sterilization and, in this way, deliberately and publicly strove to modify popular standards of reproductive fitness and to transform medical practice and public policy to accommodate these changes. In the 1950s and 1960s, the former eugenic organization repackaged its efforts to improve the reproductive fitness of Americans in order to reflect postwar and post–baby boom social trends and concerns. The AVS's campaign to legitimize voluntary sterilization set it apart from the AIFR, the AES, and the Pioneer Fund and makes it an appropriate lens through which to view the transition from eugenics to neo-eugenics.

A Brief History of Eugenics

Eugenics is the ideology and practice of selective breeding that encourages the reproduction of individuals deemed fit (positive eugenics) and discourages the reproduction of individuals deemed unfit (negative eugenics). Definitions of fitness have changed over time; however, American eugenicists have consistently measured reproductive fitness according to economic status, race, ethnicity, criminality, illegitimacy, intelligence, and sexual deviance.[3]

The English scientist Francis Galton first developed the concept of eugenics in 1869, although he officially coined the term in 1883. In his 1869 publication *Hereditary Genius*, Galton argued that behavior and talent, like physical attributes, were hereditary traits. His study found that reputable families graced with money, education, and opportunity produced more economically and socially privileged children than their lower-class, uneducated counterparts. Galton attributed the success of children from reputable families to their heredity rather than to their social and economic privileges, and this led him to conclude that nature endowed certain individuals with stronger attributes than others. According to Galton, biology, not environment, governed social and economic inequalities. His thesis, that hereditary traits were fixed and unalterable, gained prominence, in part because it drew upon the discoveries of Charles Darwin, August Weissman, and Gregor Mendel, but also because when put into practice through segregation and sterilization of the "unfit," it offered "scientific" solutions to social problems that soothed white middle-class anxieties.[4]

Eugenics became popular in America around 1900, as the country underwent fundamental changes that threatened to upset established racial, gender, and economic hierarchies. In the first two decades of the twentieth century, immigration, industrialization, woman suffrage, the birth control movement, World War I, massive labor unrest, and the Great Migration collided to create an atmosphere rife with social conflict and disorder. Feeling besieged by the rapid transformations to the world as they knew it, many white middle-class men and women seized upon eugenics as a strategy to exert their racial and economic authority and protect their privileged positions in American society. The science and politics of eugenics were enmeshed; those who studied eugenics intended for their research to have immediate social implications, and those who campaigned for an end to foreign immigration and the institutionalization (and later sterilization) of "feebleminded" persons used scientific research to justify their claims. The "scientific" basis of eugenics appealed to Progressive Era reformers who championed rational solutions to social problems, and the malleability of eugenics allowed a diverse group of experts to draw upon this "science" to advance their social agendas.[5]

Between 1910 and 1930, eugenicists established research centers like the Eugenics Records Office (ERO) at Cold Springs Harbor, New York, where they collected evidence and conducted studies to support their claims of fixed genetic traits. Wealthy philanthropists like the Rockefellers, Carnegies, Kelloggs, and Mrs. E. H. Harriman endowed these research centers, which trained young scholars and served as clearinghouses for the national eugenics movement. Based on the 1900 rediscovery of Mendel's laws of segregation and independent assortment, researchers at the ERO and other institutions identified "definitive" links between hereditary defects and epilepsy, alcoholism, prostitution, criminality, illegitimacy, and sexual promiscuity. They also compiled histories of

Indiana passed the first eugenic statute in 1907, and this law inaugurated a new legislative trend. Between 1905 and 1922, eighteen state legislatures passed thirty bills authorizing the involuntary sterilization of institutionalized persons (although by 1922 only fifteen states actually had active eugenics laws on their books because of governors' vetoes). Several states, most notably California, proved so zealous in their attempts to contain "feebleminded" women that they enacted two or more sterilization statutes.[12]

But despite lawmakers' enthusiasm for sterilization legislation, states only tentatively applied the new laws in the years leading up to World War I. Only 1,422 institutionalized persons were sterilized nationwide between 1907 and 1914. The relatively small number of eugenic sterilizations reflected physicians' and institutional superintendents' preference for segregation over sterilization in the prewar period.[13] Not until the war ended and the "girl problem" became pronounced did most eugenicists turn to sterilization as a "solution" to feeblemindedness.

Critics of eugenic sterilization included social scientists and victims and their advocates. Sociologists and anthropologists like Lester Ward and Franz Boas condemned the practice of forced sterilization in their research. Victims and their advocates challenged eight sterilization laws in court between 1912 and 1921, seven of which were struck down. Judges ruled that the laws violated the right to due process and equal protection under the law.[14]

Undeterred, eugenicists mounted a second battle for compulsory sterilization. In 1923, Oregon, Montana, Delaware, and Michigan adopted new compulsory sterilization statutes that complied with the court rulings. Virginia passed similar legislation in 1924, and seven more states followed suit in 1925.[15] These new laws included procedural safeguards like mandatory hearings, jury trials, and appeals processes that satisfied opponents' due process claims. Opponents again challenged the constitutionality of these new statutes, but this time failed. In 1927, the Supreme Court upheld Virginia's sterilization statute eight to one in the landmark decision *Buck v. Bell*.

Buck v. Bell illustrates the ways in which eugenicists exploited sterilization to control the reproduction of women who transgressed middle-class sexual boundaries, either intentionally or as victims of sexual assault. On January 23, 1924, J. T. and Alice Dobbs committed their adopted daughter, seventeen-year-old Carrie Buck, to the State Colony for Epileptics and the Feeble-Minded in Lynchburg, Virginia. The illegitimate daughter of an allegedly feebleminded mother, Buck had become pregnant out of wedlock, and the Dobbses read her socially unacceptable condition as proof of her lack of reproductive fitness. The institution's superintendent, Dr. A. S. Priddy, petitioned the state to sterilize Buck on the basis of her sexual immorality, "evidenced" by her illegitimate pregnancy and her family history of feeblemindedness. State officials used Buck's case to test the constitutionality of Virginia's new eugenics code. They presented the court with an enormous amount of "scientific" evidence that "proved" Buck's mental incompetence, but none that was based upon any actual examination of the plaintiff.[16]

Privileging the state's interest in the reproduction of its citizens over citizens' right to reproductive autonomy, in *Buck v. Bell* (1927) the Supreme Court held that Virginia's eugenic law did not treat institutionalized individuals differently from noninstitutionalized persons, as Buck charged. Exhibiting clear eugenic propensities, Justice Oliver Wendell Holmes wrote for the majority: "It is better for all the world, if instead of waiting to execute degenerate offspring for crime, or to let them starve for their imbecility, society can prevent those who are manifestly unfit from continuing their kind." He concluded with the now infamous declaration, "three generations of imbeciles are enough."[17] Carrie Buck was sterilized on October 19, 1927, and the Virginia statute became a model law. Thirty states adopted similar eugenic statutes by 1942, up from seventeen in 1927.[18]

Buck v. Bell validated the logic of eugenics and formalized the discriminatory philosophy into public policy. But in the early 1980s, several scholars, most famously Stephen Jay Gould, reexamined Buck's files and concluded that "her case was never about mental deficiency; it was always a matter of sexual morality and social deviance."[19] Carrie Buck was not a promiscuous woman. She was a rape victim who had been violated by a relative of her adopted family, but whose family refused to recognize her victimization. Family members interpreted her pregnancy as evidence of feeblemindedness and inherent immorality, and in this way transferred the social stigma of unwed motherhood from the family to Buck as an individual woman. Rather than punish the rapist for his violence against Buck, her family and the state of Virginia punished the victim with institutionalization and sterilization. Carrie Buck was one of thousands of American women whose legal rights and reproductive autonomy were violated when society refused to recognize their victimization.

Sterilization rates skyrocketed in the years following *Buck v Bell*. Only 3,233 people had been sterilized in the United States as of 1920, but this number shot up to 12,145 by 1931 and to 38,087 ten years later.[20] Before the Supreme Court legalized eugenic sterilization, states performed a few hundred eugenic sterilizations annually. After the landmark decision, states sterilized between 2,000 and 3,000 people each year. California led the nation in eugenic sterilizations, performing more than half of all surgeries. The "success" of California sterilization programs caught the attention of scientists and politicians in Nazi Germany, who used California's legislation as a model for their own sterilization codes.[21]

Eugenicists sterilized women and men for different reasons. They sterilized women to control their sexuality; they sterilized men to punish their criminal behavior and treat their aggression. Between 1907 (when Indiana passed the first eugenic law) and 1928, eugenicists sterilized men to a slightly greater extent than they did women. But the number of female sterilizations soon overtook those of male sterilizations as the "girl problem" grew and as eugenicists' faith in segregation waned. Women accounted for 42 percent of sterilizations between 1907 and 1920, but 58 percent of all sterilizations between 1920 and 1940. By 1961, 61 percent of the 62,162 total eugenic sterilizations performed in the United States involved women.[22]

Institutional difficulties caused by economic instability coupled with successful lawsuits filed by male criminals caused the shift from male to female sterilization to occur. In the 1920s and 1930s, institutional superintendents confronted overcrowded conditions and increasing patient loads while simultaneously experiencing funding cuts, especially during the Depression years. Without the resources to house, much less treat, the increasing numbers of patients under their care, superintendents "offered" inmates their freedom in exchange for their fertility, often times making women's release contingent upon "consent" to surgery. Superintendents defended this quid pro quo by arguing that sterilization liberated women from institutionalization while simultaneously protecting society against the cost of feebleminded women's "destructive" behavior.[23] The quid pro quo, sterilization for release, affected women far more than men because it was devised as a solution to a specific problem with female institutionalization.

Part of the reason that sterilization was presented as a "solution" to institutional overcrowding was that eugenicists held women more accountable than men for the reproduction of "defectives" because women bore children. As such, women became the primary targets of social engineers struggling to regulate the birth rate and "protect" white racial health. Gender associations regarding reproduction shaped the shift from male to female sterilization in another way. The first series of sterilization lawsuits filed late in the second decade of the twentieth century challenged the link between heredity and criminality and eliminated punitive male sterilization.[24] Rather than conclude that if heredity did not cause criminality, it therefore also did not cause illegitimacy and poverty (the primary symptoms of female feeblemindedness), eugenicists instead redoubled their efforts to sterilize "delinquent" women. This reinforced and reflected their association of transmission of "defective" genetic material with women far more than men.

The rate of female sterilization rose during the 1930s because, for several reasons, women could not capitalize on the precedents set by male criminals to escape sterilization. First, men charged the state with cruel and unusual punishment, but women could not bring these charges against the government because they had not been convicted of a crime; they were "guilty" of sexual "delinquency," subjected to institutionalization but not incarceration. Second, the safeguards the courts mandated to satisfy the due process clause offered little protection for women who lacked the legal autonomy to override the substituted consent of their husbands and fathers. Finally, improvements in the technology of tubal ligation between 1910 and 1920, developed during a decade when physicians began to question the "therapeutic" effects of vasectomy and castration, also encouraged female sterilization. The intersection of these factors caused the number of female sterilizations to rise in the 1930s.[25]

Eugenics came under heavy criticism in the 1930s from the Catholic Church, social scientists, and geneticists. The first two groups had begun their protests after 1910, and the latter, whose nascent field began in the 1930s, joined the chorus two decades later to provide evidence that disputed and disproved of the "scientific" premises of eugenics. Geneticists exposed the simplicity and inaccuracy of biological determinism, and social scientists, who had recently achieved some progress in arguing for the nurture component of the nature–nurture debate, forced eugenicists to recognize the role of environment in human development. Despite these enormous setbacks, eugenics did not collapse, as some scholars have suspected. Instead, eugenicists survived scientific rebukes in the 1930s by expanding their notion of heredity to include environmental factors.[26] Eugenicists' shift from biological to environmental determinism in the 1930s ushered in new rationales for race betterment that drove the movement through the 1950s and subsequently became the intellectual basis for neo-eugenics.

As part of their recovery and survival strategy, Depression-era eugenicists transformed the private act of reproduction into a public health issue, urging "unfit" Americans to submit to sterilization in order to preserve the American family and the nation. In this context, motherhood became a political, rather than personal, choice. Shaping the discussion to emphasize the regulation of motherhood, eugenicists downplayed their continuing intentions to control the quality of American citizens and preserve white racial health. By the end of the 1930s, eugenicists moved away from the negative practices of the previous decade and undertook a positive eugenics campaign based upon a "doctrine of reproductive morality" that attempted to push "fit" women back into the private roles of wife and mother and teach them to make reproductive decisions that advanced the interests of the white middle class. Eugenicists prompted a gendered separation of spheres that they believed to be essential to a healthy society. Their campaign was consistent with the post–World War II discourse of returning women back to their "natural" place, the home, after years of wartime factory labor. The positive eugenics that developed during the Depression and World War II culminated in the baby boom of the 1950s.[27]

In 1942, the Supreme Court struck down Oklahoma's Habitual Criminal Sterilization Act in *Skinner v. Oklahoma.* The High Court declared the Oklahoma law unconstitutional on the grounds that it violated the equal protection clause of the Fourteenth Amendment; the statute exempted some convicted felons from punitive sterilization but not others, and as such, was not applied to all felons equally. The *Skinner* decision received little public attention at the time because it did not affect existing state eugenics statutes, although it is likely that it deterred other states from enacting similar laws that punished criminals with sterilization. *Skinner* bears significance, though, for in its ruling the High Court held the right to bear children to be fundamental, and this claim shaped post–baby boom contraception and abortion policies, which provided the precedents used by women seeking to overturn restrictions on voluntary sterilization.[28]

Skinner was decided during World War II, when the number of sterilizations performed fell far below their prewar levels. In part the decline was a response to denunciations of the "science" of eugenics by geneticists, social scientists, and the Catholic Church, but the decrease was also largely caused by the war—specifically, the lack of medical personnel available to perform the surgery. Many surgeons left to fight in World War II, and those doctors who remained at home struggled to keep up with the demand for their services. Sterilization ceased to be a top priority for most medical professionals during the war.[29] Eugenic sterilization rates did not rebound to their prewar levels, but forced sterilization did not end at midcentury. Instead, neo-eugenic physicians, social workers, and politicians adopted new methods of coercion in the 1950s, 1960s, and 1970s.

Continuity and Changes in Eugenic Ideas and Practices

The term "neo-eugenics" refers to the ideas, practices, and policies that continued the legacies of eugenics in the post–baby boom years but that did so in historically specific ways, in response to contemporary social anxieties, including blacks' demands for racial equality, Mexican immigration, antipoverty programs, the expansion of welfare, and fears of overpopulation. The politics and ideas that led to the legitimization of contraceptive sterilization were at once deeply rooted in the formal eugenics movement and at the same time a product of post–baby boom social conflicts, concerns, and debates. Enough distinctions existed between the ideas and practices of racial betterment in the first and second halves of the twentieth century to warrant a change of terminology.

Eugenics and neo-eugenics shared some similar traits. Adherents to both concepts believed that poverty, criminality, and illegitimacy were reproduced. They also interpreted these traits to be "symptoms" of a lack of reproductive fitness. Similarly, individuals subscribing to eugenic and neo-eugenic policies held that "unfit" individuals should not be allowed to reproduce because their reproduction was costly and burdensome to the American taxpayer, who would have to support "irresponsible" behavior by funding mental institutions and welfare services. Neo-eugenics was as malleable as its predecessor; a wide range of individuals with varying politics and professional affiliations could use theories of reproductive fitness to support their causes.

But eugenics and neo-eugenics differ in significant ways, and many of these differences reflect the unique historical eras in which these movements developed and grew. Eugenicists and neo-eugenicists understood the transmission of "defective" traits differently. Eugenicists began with a firm belief in biological determinism, and as the nature-nurture debate shifted to increasingly emphasize the role of environment in shaping behavior in the 1930s, some began to include environment in their theories of "defects." Neo-eugenicists began with the acceptance of environmental determinism; the ideology emerged after this shift had occurred. As they confronted the civil rights movement, an expansion of the welfare system, and the inclusion of people of color into federal programs, politicians, physicians, and other citizens who endorsed this idea increasingly argued that "defects" like poverty and illegitimacy were transmitted via culture instead of genes. Many opposed welfare reforms because they believed that these programs encouraged the reproduction of such "social problems."[30]

Racial politics at midcentury differed from those fifty years earlier, which contributed to the unique features of neo-eugenics. At the turn of the twentieth century, eugenicists feared that nonnative-born white immigrants (especially poor immigrants) would "pass" for "normal," "mate" with native-born whites, and dilute the genes of the white race. White immigrant women who challenged sexual mores and who transgressed social and sexual boundaries thus became eugenicists' primary targets. But by the 1950s, white eastern European immigrants generally had assimilated. On a national level, white racial anxieties in this era centered on blacks' demands for racial equality, and as the 1960s and 1970s approached, their concerns came to include Mexican immigration and the Chicano/a movement—although Californians had been debating these issues for decades.[31] When neo-eugenic individuals and institutions became involved in forced sterilization, they rarely targeted white women. Instead, they targeted poor women of color, who became labeled by conservative social critics as "welfare queens" and "pregnant pilgrims," the latter referring to pregnant

Mexican women who traveled to the United States to give birth to citizens who could receive government assistance.

One more critical distinction between eugenics and neo-eugenics involves institutional structures. Eugenics was a formal movement, with research centers, scholarly journals, political lobbies, and established organizations. Neo-eugenics never achieved the formal institutional status of its predecessor, and in fact, informality was one of its signature traits. The policies and practices of neo-eugenics tended to result from personal collaborations rather than organization efforts. For example, social workers teamed with physicians to identify "unfit" individuals who "needed" sterilization, and doctors and nurses collaborated to "persuade" pregnant patients to accept sterilization with delivery—often while patients were in labor.

Only a few organizations survived the transition between eugenics and neo-eugenics, and the AVS stands out among them because it adapted its goals so effectively to the new political, social, and cultural environment of the baby boom and post–baby boom years. The AES, in contrast, kept its name until 1973 (when it became the Society for the Study of Social Biology), signaling its adherence to more traditional eugenic ideas.[32] The AIFR played a critical role in promoting eugenically determined marriage choices and distinct gender roles for both sexes from the 1930s through the 1960s, but it did not become involved with the practice of contraceptive sterilization, and thus did not have the influence that the AVS did on post–baby boom contraceptive behavior or family planning practices. More than the AES or the AIFR, the AVS shifted its politics to both shape and reflect changing social anxieties of the new era. Its willingness to conform to new trends allowed it to influence public debates about welfare, family planning, and women's reproductive rights and to promote its standards of reproductive fitness in medicine, popular culture, and the courts. This flexibility enabled the AVS to usher changing standards of reproductive fitness into popular culture and to incorporate these changes in medical practice and public policy. Through its campaign to promote voluntary sterilization as a scientific solution to major social problems of the era, the AVS contributed to national dialogues about overpopulation, contraception, antipoverty measures, and reproductive freedom.

The Status of Sterilization in the 1950s and 1960s

The AVS's transition from a eugenic to neo-eugenic organization centered on its campaign to legitimize contraceptive sterilization and to make the surgery accessible to the general public. Contraceptive sterilization existed on the margins of medical practice in the 1950s and 1960s. Nationally, enthusiasm for eugenic surgeries declined during World War II, and such surgeries did not rebound to their original levels during the postwar years, although a few states continued to actively employ their eugenic codes during the 1940s. During the 1950s, hospitals established restrictive sterilization policies designed to deter women from undergoing contraceptive sterilization in an effort to support contemporary pronatalist sentiment. The most popular hospital restriction was the 120 rule, which deemed only those women whose age and parity (number of children) multiplied together reached or exceeded the number 120 to be appropriate surgical candidates. For example, a thirty-year-old woman needed to have at least four children in order to undergo surgery. While the 120 rule served as a popular model, many hospitals adopted a 150 or 175 rule in order to protect themselves against potential litigation. Age/parity restrictions significantly and immediately reduced the number of sterilizations performed at a given hospital. Grace Hospital in Detroit, for example, established a sterilization committee in 1950 to review applications for surgery and enforce its new policy. Before the restrictions took effect, the hospital sterilization rate was 3.4 percent of all deliveries. After the committee implemented an age/parity policy, the rate of sterilization fell to 0.9 percent of all deliveries.[33]

Although they did not openly target white women, hospital restrictions disproportionately affected white women, the group most celebrated by postwar pronatalism. Differential rates of sterilization between black and white women suggested this, as black women underwent sterilization at a considerably higher rate than white women and do not appear to have formally complained about their inability to obtain this service. In 1965, 14 percent of black women had undergone surgical sterilization as opposed to only 6 percent of white women. Five years later, both groups of women had increased their use of contraceptive sterilization, but the racial differential remained significant, with 20 percent of black women reporting sterilization as opposed to only 9 percent of white women. In part, age/parity policies disproportionately affected white women because white women bore fewer children than black women, and thus more black than white women met the qualifications for sterilization under these restrictive policies.[34]

But other evidence suggests that the policies also specifically targeted southern black women. It seems as though southern physicians—the first in the country to perform unlawful forced sterilizations on "healthy" women in the late 1950s—chose not to develop age/parity policies limiting the number of hospital sterilizations that could be performed so that they could continue to forcibly sterilize poor black women in the region. Indeed, only white women outside the South complained that they had been denied voluntary sterilization.

The voices of black women across the region were conspicuously silent in this regard, as were the voices of southern white women.

In response to white women's complaints about being denied access to voluntary sterilization, the American Civil Liberties Union (ACLU), Zero Population Growth (ZPG), and the AVS launched a national legal campaign in 1971 to overturn restrictive hospital policies. None of the organizations appear to have received complaints from black women, and white women were plaintiffs in all of the lawsuits filed. (Not all complaints resulted in lawsuits. Often the threat of a lawsuit was sufficient to push a hospital to revise its policy.) The ACLU also represented women who had been forcibly sterilized, the majority of whom were women of color. Not only did the ACLU represent victims of forced sterilization, but it also actively pursued civil rights litigation at this time.[35] It is reasonable to assume that the ACLU would have received complaints from black women denied voluntary sterilization had they existed. It is likely that these complaints did not surface because southern black women did not have difficulty accessing contraceptive sterilization.

The ACLU, the AVS, and ZPG received complaints from white women residing in the Northeast, West, and Midwest, but not the South, which suggests that contraceptive sterilization was more available to women—black and white—in the South than in other regions. Demographic data indicates that the percentage of southern white women who had been sterilized was noticeably higher in 1965 and 1970 than it was for white women in the Northeast, West, and Midwest in the same years.[36] This implies that southern hospitals did not institute as many barriers to voluntary sterilization as hospitals in other regions did. Given the coercive sterilization directed against southern black women at this time (discussed in chapter 3), it is likely that hospitals and physicians loosened restrictions in order to advance their neo-eugenic agendas.

Sterilization restrictions promoted pronatalism by denying women access to contraception that held the potential to liberate them from their "natural" role of mother. Historically, American physicians and politicians have expended considerable energy regulating the sexual behavior of women but ignoring the actions of their male partners. In a typical double standard, hospital administrators restricted access to tubal ligation but not to vasectomy. The American College of Obstetricians and Gynecologists (ACOG) and the American Medical Association (AMA) endorsed the 120 rule, but the American Urological Association remained noticeably silent on vasectomy.[37] Age/parity restrictions functioned as a form of social control, as a means of pushing the "fit" women who ventured into the paid labor force in increasing numbers after the war back into the home and into their "rightful" roles as full-time mothers and wives.

Hospitals established and doctors endorsed policies like the 120 rule around the same time they established abortion boards to reduce the number of procedures performed and enforce popular pronatalism. During a period when motherhood for white middle-class women (who pioneer contraceptive trends) was supposed to be synonymous with womanhood, ending one's fertility challenged powerful and dominant social norms. This was made clear by women's experiences with hospital abortion boards. In order to obtain a legal abortion, women had to have one or two psychiatrists diagnose them as mentally unsound, suicidal, depressed, anxious, and, as a result, unable to successfully carry a pregnancy to term and to raise a healthy child. To obtain a therapeutic abortion, women had to renounce their ability to fulfill contemporary gender norms and pay experts to declare them mentally unfit to mother. (Of course, this required financial resources, making therapeutic abortion far more accessible to women with means than those without.[38]) Some hospitals conditioned patients' receipt of contraceptive sterilization on the same terms, while others paired therapeutic abortion with sterilization to ensure that "unfit" women could no longer reproduce.

Medical and public health journals rarely discussed elective or therapeutic sterilization during the 1950s. The *Journal of the American Medical Association* published only two articles on contraceptive sterilization between 1950 and 1960, and the *American Journal of Obstetrics and Gynecology* published only one. The few other scattered articles published in regional or state medical journals reflect a slow liberalizing of physicians' attitudes toward contraceptive sterilization, one that would not really become visible until the late 1960s, when the Pill scare caused women's demands for the surgery to increase and when the AVS's campaign to legitimize voluntary sterilization intensified. The articles published in the 1950s and early 1960s insisted on medical indication for contraceptive sterilization. Most focused on female surgery.[39]

The few physicians discussing sterilization publicly in these years disagreed about what constituted a compelling reason for sterilization among generally healthy patients. Some physicians saw the procedure as an option for married women who had undergone three or more cesarean sections as well as women diagnosed with multiparity (or many children), although they did not agree on the number of pregnancies required for this diagnosis.[40] For the most part, in the 1950s physicians distinguished between eugenic surgeries of "hereditary defectives" and contraceptive surgeries performed on "normal" patients with medical problems. A review of the literature on "normal" female patients indicates that some physicians considered socioeconomic forces and patient demand to be indications for surgery when deciding whether to operate. Three physicians provided evidence of this trend in a 1954 article published in

Medical Records and Annals. "We are today confronted with this problem of being repeatedly asked by our patients that elective sterilization be done," they wrote, indicating that physicians' evolving attitudes constituted a response to female patients' requests. Perhaps even more telling of these physicians' evolving attitudes was their willingness to connect women's desire to limit their family size with women's efforts to gain financial stability. "It seems only proper and fair," the doctors explained, "that a woman should have the right to determine whether or not she cared to expose herself to pregnancy. Her social and economic factors play a very definite role."[41] These doctors assumed a liberal perspective on the issue. Dr. Lyle Bachman took a conservative approach when he disagreed with this assessment in a 1954 article published in the *Hawaii Medical Journal.* Here he argued that "social factors" were "occasionally valid" indications for surgery, but "economic conditions never are."[42] Another doctor reiterated this position in a popular periodical with a white middle-class audience. In 1959, Goodrich C. Schauffler tackled the issue of contraceptive sterilization in his *Ladies' Home Journal* advice column, "Tell Me Doctor . . . ," in which he declared that "no conscientious surgeon wants to sterilize a woman during her reproductive years for any but compelling reasons."[43]

Bachman's essay on female sterilization epitomizes conservative pronatalist ideas of the era. He argued that "depriving a woman of the power of reproduction is depriving her of one of her basic property rights," that is, the right to reproduce. On this point, many women, especially those involved in the feminist movement of the next decade, would have agreed. But Bachman reflected 1950s patriarchal values when he insisted that husbands, not wives, held the ultimate authority on this subject. A married woman is "the property of her husband," he declared. Following this logic, he held that a physician asked to perform a female sterilization must obtain the consent of both spouses, and if a husband refused his wife's request for surgery, then her physician was legally bound to refuse to perform the procedure.[44]

The ambiguous legal status of contraceptive sterilization compounded physicians' reticence to embrace it as a viable contraceptive option for their healthy patients and possibly quieted public discussion of the surgery because state laws only governed eugenic sterilization. Eugenic statutes remained on the books in most states during the baby boom years, although with a few exceptions, they received little use.[45] Eugenic sterilization laws involved the involuntary sterilization of "defectives"; they did not apply to healthy citizens, although some women manipulated local public health systems to obtain eugenic sterilizations for contraceptive purposes. Such laws had been upheld by the Supreme Court in 1927, but laws related to contraceptive sterilization did not exist in forty-seven of the fifty states. The remaining three states, Connecticut, Kansas, and Utah, criminalized contraceptive sterilization.[46] With these exceptions, the surgery existed in legal limbo in the states. Legislators remained silent on the issue, neither declaring the surgery to be legal or illegal. Understandably, such ambiguity made physicians reticent to perform the surgery, especially in the years before *Roe v. Wade* (1973) legalized abortion in the first two trimesters. A 1954 article published in the *Western Journal of Surgery, Obstetrics and Gynecology* reflected physicians' fear of litigation. In this article, two doctors cautioned their colleagues to sterilize only the "sick" patient, that is, the patient with a medical indication for surgery. "Sterilization for the husband according to his wish, for an indication in the wife, is a voluntary procedure, and may lead to a legal suit for mutilation," they wrote. "We are of the definite opinion that the patient with the indication should be sterilized, and not the mate."[47]

In 1962, Virginia became the first state to explicitly legalize contraceptive sterilization, and in 1963 North Carolina followed with a similar statute. But these states were exceptions to the general trend of confusion. Given steriliza-tion's ambiguous legal status, medical societies and journals instructed physi-cians to proceed with caution. In 1958, the *Journal of the American Medical Association* told its readers to treat contraceptive sterilization as they would abortion, as a criminal procedure. "The same public policy that underlies laws to prevent . . . criminal abortion applies to operations that produce sterility, even though that policy is in only a few states expressed by statute," it main-tained.[48] The legal counsel for the California Medical Association told *Medical World News* that although he had "not found any cases instituted against physi-cians charging mayhem for the performance of a sterilization," he believed that "until the law is settled, a physician should not perform such an operation except when it is therapeutically indicated." Failure to comply with this warn-ing could "subject him [the doctor] to either civil or criminal liability, or both."[49] Given this guidance in the medical literature, it is little wonder that many physicians shied away from contraceptive sterilization in this era.

The Evolution of the AVS

In the 1950s and 1960s, the AVS endeavored to transform medical attitudes and public perceptions of contraceptive sterilization. But in its early years, the organization maintained a traditional eugenics agenda. The AVS originated in 1937 as the Sterilization League of New Jersey. For more than ten years, founder Marion Olden and her colleagues labored to pressure New Jersey and the nation to promote white racial hygiene through compulsory sterilization. The league lobbied the New Jersey legislature to pass a eugenic statute that would serve as a national model, published pamphlets promoting eugenic sterilization, and pressured professional organizations and social clubs to support its proposed legislation.[50] The Sterilization League of New Jersey was one of only a few eugenics organizations to survive beyond World War II. Its successful navigation of the postwar era rested upon its willingness to alter its message to conform to contemporary scientific and social trends.

This transition, from a state-based eugenic organization dedicated to the passage of restrictive sterilization laws to a national organization committed to promoting voluntary sterilization through the education of experts and the lay public as well as to the provision of sterilization referrals and services, occurred incrementally, and the organization's progress can be tracked via its multiple name changes. In 1943, the Sterilization League of New Jersey renamed itself Birthright Inc. and adopted the slogan, "It is the birthright of every child born in American to have a sound mind in a sound body."[51] At this time, the group expanded from the state to the national level and worked to pass a model bill in New Jersey and to rally support for compulsory sterilization among social workers and medical professionals. In 1950, the organization changed its name again, this time to the Human Betterment Association of America (HBAA). In a 1979 speech recalling the history of the AVS, former president H. Curtis Wood explained this change as falling into step with new medical practices. Members "broadened our sights to include the philosophy that fertility control could make a significant contribution to solving many of our medical, social and economic problems," he declared.[52] During the golden age of science and medicine, the organization promoted sterilization as a technological solution to social problems akin to other major medical and scientific advancements of the era and harnessed the endorsement of experts in these respected fields.

The AVS did this by expanding its criteria for sterilization in the immediate post–World War II years. As discussed earlier, eugenicists survived scientific rebukes in the 1930s by expanding their notion of heredity to include environmental factors. If environment could determine reproductive fitness, eugenicists reasoned, then socioeconomic factors should also be considered valid indications for sterilization. "Regardless of how much of a defective's condition may be due to heredity or to environment," the Sterilization League of New Jersey declared, "such persons make poor parents." Ironically, by appropriating their opponents' criticisms, league members found themselves able to expand their target population of "unfit" Americans to include individuals deemed defective for socioeconomic reasons. Compulsory sterilization laws authorized only the sterilization of a small population, and after World War II many states either had ceased to employ these statutes or significantly reduced their use.[53] Ridding the country of "defectives" would take multiple generations by means of the traditional approach—too long in the AVS's estimate. Further, eugenic laws could not reach many poor families, whose numbers caused increasing concern among AVS members as the baby boom began and population controllers began to sound the alarm.[54]

In the immediate postwar years, AVS member and physician H. Curtis Wood became concerned that a real decline in intelligence was occurring, very slowly, among the general population. Compulsory sterilization of the more traditional sort could not possibly reach such a large group. Committed to the belief that poor families produced children with low IQs and that sterilization could hold this "production" in check, Wood began to craft a new agenda that involved voluntary sterilization of the socioeconomic "unfit." Group members moved with Wood, in part because they realized that their earlier efforts, as Birthright, to legislate compulsory sterilization had failed.[55]

The AVS understood that compulsory sterilization of those deemed "unfit" to reproduce for socioeconomic reasons could never gain public acceptance; the target population was simply too large. But AVS leaders believed that they could persuade Americans that voluntary sterilization held the potential to resolve contemporary social problems, specifically those related to poverty, unwed motherhood, and dependence on welfare. They therefore abandoned their emphasis on eugenic sterilizations and readjusted their agenda to focus instead on voluntary sterilization for socioeconomic purposes. Their new goal was to convince the poor and "unfit" to voluntarily terminate their fertility; their agenda became less about preventing the "unfit" from reproducing and more about helping the "unfit" poor to limit their family size and improve the quality of American citizens this way. "One of the greatest problems of this decade," the HBAVS wrote in the mid-1960s, "is hapless, unwanted children" whose parents "cannot provide them with the essentials for proper emotional, mental or physical development." Sterilization, the group believed, could help "the poor, the underprivileged, the mentally retarded, and the uneducated adults" to permanently suspend their reproduction, which in turn would help them "become responsible parents."[56]

Most AVS members did not totally abandon their older eugenic allegiances. Instead, they repackaged their ideas to reflect national trends and popular social values in order to attract more supporters to their cause. This continuity of older ideas is evidenced in part by the membership and committee appointments of prominent prewar eugenicists like Dr. Clarence Gamble, Dr. Robert Latou Dickinson, Paul Popenoe, and C. M. Goethe during the early transition years, and the later appointment of population controllers General William Draper and Hugh Moore to the board of directors in the 1960s. Draper led President

Dwight D. Eisenhower's Committee to Study Military Assistance Programs, established in 1959. The committee released the Draper report that same year, which surprised Eisenhower with its recommendations that encouraged the government to become involved in population control and family planning provision abroad in the interest of reducing the threat of Communism and promoting economic progress. Ardent population controller Hugh Moore, seen as an alarmist by many of his peers for his "hysterical" warnings about the risks of overpopulation, served as president of the AVS in the mid-to-late 1960s. So concerned was he about the threats posed by overpopulation that Moore endorsed "coercive measures if voluntary programs failed."[57]

The AVS did make a bold gesture to distance itself from its eugenic past by dismissing founder, spokesperson, executive director, and executive secretary Marion Olden in 1951, who, unlike most of her peers, never renounced her support for the Nazis, even after the regime fell. Olden's strict adherence to traditional eugenics principles of inheritance and fierce anti-Catholicism alienated potential family planning allies and the lay public. Her leadership served as a constant reminder of the organization's eugenic history and stymied the organization's efforts to develop a more nuanced and updated approach to human betterment.[58] As Wood led the transition from the Sterilization League of New Jersey to Birthright, Olden stubbornly refused to accept the changes and clung vehemently to traditional eugenic ideas and the prejudicial attitudes they entailed. In her mission to wrestle "her" organization into submission, Olden squandered her remaining alliances, and the organization ousted her. Her ejection permitted Wood to craft a fresh agenda that simultaneously distanced the AVS from the largely defunct eugenics movement, gained the support of organized medicine, and linked the organization to the nascent family planning and population control movements.

In the 1950s and early 1960s, the AVS drew upon baby boom pronatalism to promote its agenda. As white middle-class Americans struggled to achieve economic stability, settled into suburbs, and endorsed more rigid gender roles, they were troubled by rising illegitimacy rates, persistent poverty, the expansion of public welfare, and, for some, civil rights activism. Many white middle-class Americans believed that these "problems" threatened the security of the American family. In the postwar years, politicians and conservative social critics tied strong family systems to national security by rhetorically positioning the family as a bulwark against Communism. In this context, threats to stable American families could prove devastating and fatal to the nation. Capitalizing on these anxieties, the AVS advocated voluntary sterilization of the poor as a means of preserving the American family in an especially dangerous era. The

AVS reasoned that fewer children in poor families would reduce family expenditures and free parents from excessive child-care duties, allowing them more time to instill "proper" social values in their children and to nurture their marriages. Strengthening these "weaker" families, in turn, would strengthen the nation's ability to repel Communist menaces. Eager to use science to reinforce its message, the group drew upon the research of British sociologist Moya Woodside, who concluded that sterilization improved marriage by stabilizing the family economy and reducing anxiety about unplanned pregnancy.[59]

In 1962, the organization changed its name yet again, adding voluntary and sterilization to its title to become the Human Betterment Association for Voluntary Sterilization (HBAVS). Three years later the organization dropped "Human Betterment" and became simply the Association for Voluntary Sterilization in an effort to emphasize the voluntary nature of its advocacy. Later Wood identified this moment as the point at which the group's "goals, philosophies and emphasis changed." "No longer was our program primarily concerned with those unqualified for parenthood, no longer were we really trying to 'better' humanity," he lectured. Instead, "we focused on selling sterilization to the medical profession and to the public as a sound, effective and rational form of fertility control which, under certain circumstances, might well be the contraceptive method most suitable for many people."[60] The organization formally adopted a neo-eugenic perspective with this final name change. The AVS aimed to make contraceptive sterilization legal and legitimate in the public mind. It hoped to loosen medical and legal restrictions to the procedure and in doing so make it available to the "fit" and "unfit" alike. With some prodding by physicians and family planners, the "unfit" could be directed to permanent contraception in greater numbers than the "fit."

In the 1950s and early 1960s, the organization downplayed the distinction between eugenic and contraceptive surgeries. Members held that it did not matter whether genes or the environment caused defective traits and behavior so long as individuals afflicted with these traits underwent sterilization. Blurring the line between eugenic and contraceptive surgeries, Wood, who spearheaded the transition, focused on outcome rather than motivation for surgery by emphasizing the eugenic effects of voluntary sterilization, effectively straddling the two objectives.[61] In this way, during its transition from a eugenic to a neo-eugenic organization, the group continued to appeal to adherents of traditional eugenic values concerned about the "unchecked" reproduction of the "unfit" and the cost of this reproduction to taxpayers while at the same time rallying support from postwar Americans concerned about domestic stability and security of the American family for the voluntary sterilization of the poor.

The AVS did not abandon its support for the compulsory sterilization of individuals with mental disabilities as it eased into its voluntary sterilization agenda, although it did temper its approach. In its eugenic phase, the AVS argued for the compulsory sterilization of people with mental disabilities on the grounds of racial hygiene. In its neo-eugenic phase, the AVS separated its support for the voluntary sterilization of the poor from its support of nonvoluntary sterilization of people with disabilities in order to legitimize contraceptive sterilization for "healthy" Americans and to persuade public health officials to include the surgery in their programs. The AVS advanced a clear position on the issue of surgery for those with mental "defects" that differed from its earlier eugenic ambitions. Instead of highlighting the benefits to taxpayers that sterilization of "defectives" would have, the AVS promoted the benefits that sterilization would bring to the individual. In a memo to "All Concerned with Helping the Mentally Handicapped," HBAVS president Robert W. Laidlow, M.D., explained that sterilization was "one means of re-establishing these grown children in family and community life."[62]

The group did not discard its eugenic ideas about individuals with mental disabilities; instead, it integrated them into its new agenda. The HBAVS published a pamphlet, *To Protect the Retarded Adolescent*, in which it explained that sterilization could "ease some of the worries and tensions which mount as retarded children grow to physical maturity," and could "help the retarded adolescent and young adult achieve a fuller, happier life."[63] Here, the organization promoted sterilization as a technology with the potential to improve quality of life by freeing those with mental disabilities from institutional care and the restrictions of movement that went along with it. It also argued that as an increasing number of children with mental disabilities lived at home rather than in institutions (where they would have been sterilized), sterilization could relieve some caretaking burdens for parents, especially those fearful that their daughters would be sexually exploited. The HBAVS admitted that "sterilization does not protect the girl against sexual attack," but "it does protect her from illegitimate pregnancy."[64] The privileging of preventing pregnancy over adolescent health exposed the continuity of some eugenic intentions.

Courting Physicians and Family Planners and Creating a Media Campaign

The success of the AVS's efforts to promote sterilization as a solution to social problems rested upon its recruitment of supportive physicians, the only experts trained and licensed to perform surgeries. Like Margaret Sanger and the birth controllers between 1910 and 1930, the AVS envisioned physicians as the central actors in its social experiment and, beginning in the early 1950s, labored to enlist their support. In the Progressive Era, eugenicists and birth controllers competed for doctors' endorsement of their respective movements. In the 1920s, eugenicists successfully persuaded the AMA to sanction sterilization by distinguishing the formal eugenics movement from Sanger's more radical birth control crusade. In the postwar years, physicians focused more on debating their role in family planning than on their use of sterilization. The introduction of the Pill to the market in 1960 "obliged physicians to confront the issue of birth control directly," writes historian Elizabeth Siegel Watkins, because the Pill required a prescription, which many women eagerly requested.[65] The AMA weighed in on the issue in 1964 when it adopted a policy on human reproduction that identified birth control and population control as "matter[s] of responsible medical practice." This policy effectively endorsed physician prescription of contraception.[66] Medical recognition of the legitimacy of birth control was further demonstrated in 1968 when the United Nations declared family planning to be a basic human right.[67] Prescribing contraception in the post-Pill years became normal medical practice, and the AVS exploited this trend in its campaign to secure physicians' support for contraceptive sterilization.

In order to gain organized medicine's endorsement for contraceptive sterilization, the AVS had to reverse eugenicists' earlier distinction between sterilization and contraception and convince doctors that voluntary sterilization constituted a legitimate form of birth control. It did this by presenting sterilization as a medical solution to the contemporary social problems of poverty, illegitimacy, and overpopulation and calling upon doctors to employ their professional authority for the social good by performing sterilizations. Wood articulated this strategy in a 1964 speech to the Kentucky Obstetrical and Gynecological Society in which he asked his colleagues, "Can any rational and intelligent person fail to realize that much of the suffering and misery in the world today stems from medical advances as related to reduction of death rates and that we therefore have a responsibility and even an obligation . . . to ameliorate these economic and social ills?"[68] According to this viewpoint, the population explosion stemmed from medical innovation, and thus physicians bore a particular responsibility to devise solutions to the crisis.

Some physicians articulated similar sentiments in medical journals and emphasized doctors' professional responsibility to intervene in social and population issues. In 1966, physician C. Lee Buxton of New Haven, Connecticut, published an especially adamant article in *Northwest Medicine* entitled "The Doctor's Responsibility in Population Control," in which he reminded his colleagues that "medical responsibility demands more action than just passing resolutions and making recommendations." Buxton urged other physicians to commit to family planning by educating patients, engaging in research, prescribing contraception, and helping family planning organizations to distribute birth control devices and information to the lay public. He advocated sterilization as a solution to the "problem" of unmarried mothers on welfare, whom he described as the "filthy residue of our culture." The "problem" of unwed motherhood "is multiplying itself with dreadful predictability *because the medical profession has controlled the death rate but has done very little about the birth rate*," he proclaimed.[69] Buxton's statement reflects both the continuities and changes in neo-eugenic philosophies of reproductive fitness. Proponents of such ideas continued to view unwed mothers as "unfit" parents whose "irresponsible" behavior taxed valuable government resources, but they also began to tie this "irresponsible" reproduction to the international "problem" of overpopulation. Sterilization, from this perspective, held the potential to attack two important social crises: lack of reproductive fitness and overpopulation.[70]

Identifying sterilization as a solution to the "impending" population problem was perhaps one of the AVS's shrewdest and most effective strategies. In the wake of World War II, a small group of American scientists, reformers, and philanthropists expressed great distress over what they predicted to be an "impending" population explosion on a global scale. Brought together by John D. Rockefeller III in the 1950s, the population control movement sought to bring birth and death rates back into a stable balance. Population controllers predicted that failure to do so would result in an international population crisis of profound social and economic consequences—not least among them, the spread of Communism. Birth rates remained unchecked by death rates because antibiotics and improved nutrition had reduced mortality among infants and children. The nascent population control movement promoted the dissemination of contraception to people in poor nations as a solution to skyrocketing birth rates. The AVS endorsed this idea and presented voluntary sterilization as the best technology in the effort to retard population growth. In a 1966 letter to supporters, President Hugh Moore wrote: "You doubtless have read that the population of the United States is expected to exceed three hundred and fifty million in the next thirty years. The effect on life and living of this doubling of our numbers is beyond calculation. Over-crowded cities, polluted air and water, countless unwanted and suffering children, skyrocketing taxes for welfare! Half of the babies born in some cities are from indigent families on relief. Need we say more?" Moore went on to establish the benefits of permanent contraception and to suggest its utility in combating overpopulation and the "irresponsible" reproduction of poor people.[71]

During the 1960s, population control advocates saturated the American public with newspaper articles, magazine stories, pamphlets, and books warning of the dire threats posed by overpopulation.[72] Stanford biology professor Paul Ehrlich produced the most influential work of this genre, *The Population Bomb*, in 1968. Reprinted thirteen times in only two years, *The Population Bomb* argued that unless Americans took immediate action to combat the problem, overpopulation promised catastrophic effects. The publication of Ehrlich's work also led to the establishment of ZPG in 1969. So concerned about the damages caused by overpopulation, many ZPG members supported coercive abortion and sterilization practices. "Voluntarism is a farce," declared cofounder Richard Bowers. Many ZPG members "entertained notions of licensing parents to conceive, sterilizing welfare dependents," and passing laws to limit population growth. ZPG members were some of the earliest supporters of the movement to legalize abortion, but most supported this goal to combat overpopulation, not empower women.[73] ZPG would align with the AVS and the ACLU in 1971 to challenge hospital guidelines that restricted women's access to sterilization.

Concerns about overpopulation gradually seeped into the mainstream. A 1959 Gallup Poll showed that only 21 percent of respondents worried about the effects of the population explosion. Twelve years later, another Gallup Poll found that 41 percent of respondents viewed population growth as a major problem, and 54 percent believed that the population explosion would seriously affect their families' quality of life.[74] The AVS capitalized on this increasing public awareness to pressure physicians to employ their expert skills in the name of global security. It also used Ehrlich's fame to gain popularity by inviting the biologist to give the keynote address at its 1969 fall conference, which Ehrlich accepted.[75]

The AVS employed several strategies for translating its new ideas into medical practice. First, at the recommendation of Dr. Robert Latou Dickinson, the eugenicist responsible for distinguishing between sterilization and contraception in the 1920s, the AVS established a Medical and Scientific Committee. This committee dedicated itself to promoting research and educating physicians and social workers about the social benefits of voluntary sterilization. Initially chaired by Dickinson, Dr. Alan Guttmacher, leading birth control advocate and chairman of the Department of Obstetrics and Gynecology at Mount Sinai Hospital in New York City, assumed this leadership position in 1952. Second, as "proof" of its neo-eugenic claims, the AVS submitted to medical and popular audiences the research funded by the Medical and Scientific Committee on the uses and benefits of sterilization. In this way, the AVS continued the eugenic tradition of relying upon scientific studies to validate its social engineering goals. Third, in 1951 the AVS hired social worker Frances Dow to survey physicians, community agencies, social workers, and laypersons in New Jersey in order to learn what type of scientific information would convince these individuals to endorse voluntary sterilization. The results of Dow's study augmented Wood's resolve to transform the AVS's eugenic goals into neo-eugenic ones. Dow found that few experts supported eugenic legislation and recommended that the organization cease lobbying for eugenic sterilization bills and focus instead on persuading physicians of the benefits of voluntary surgery. Fourth, the organization invited distinguished physicians and psychologists to join its board and serve on its Medical and Scientific Committee. In addition to electing Guttmacher chair of the Medical and Scientific Committee, the AVS successfully courted several distinguished experts to join its various boards and committees. Finally, AVS representatives attended professional meetings of organizations such as the AMA, ACOG, the American Urological Society, and the American Public Health Association (APHA), where they presented exhibits and papers promoting voluntary sterilization and distributed pamphlets that taught doctors how to identify potential surgical candidates.[76]

In order to persuade physicians that sterilization constituted a legitimate method of birth control, the AVS linked its aims to those of the family planning community. In 1950, the AVS made a formal alliance with Planned Parenthood one of its key goals, but Planned Parenthood proved to be uncooperative. In an ironic reversal of previous positions, Planned Parenthood now feared that the radical taint of sterilization would offend its mainstream supporters at a time when birth control was beginning to gain widespread acceptance among physicians and politicians. Equally as important, Planned Parenthood viewed the AVS as a competitor for funding—and with good reason. In 1945, the AVS field committee led by Clarence Gamble received private funds intended for Planned Parenthood. After this incident, Planned Parenthood ordered its affiliates not to cooperate with the AVS. Relations between the two organizations warmed slowly as a result of their overlapping membership, but Planned Parenthood continued to rebuff the AVS's attempts to establish a formal alliance throughout the 1950s. One critical reason for this continued rejection was that Planned Parenthood's new medical director, Mary Calderone, disapproved of contraceptive sterilization.[77]

Although rebuffed by Planned Parenthood, in 1968 the AVS received endorsements from two prominent birth control advocates: Dr. John R. Rock, who helped develop the Pill, and Dr. Jack Lippes, who invented a popular IUD, the Lippes Loop. The doctors issued a joint statement in support of voluntary sterilization that identified the surgery as a major tool in combating overpopulation. "We believe that in the struggle to control runaway population growth, voluntary sterilization has a vital role to play," they maintained. The *New York Post*, *New York Daily News*, *National Catholic Reporter*, and Associated Press reported this story.[78] In an internal document, probably not released to the public, Rock went further by suggesting that voluntary sterilization could reduce the number of abortion-related deaths. A Catholic opposed to the Church's position on abortion, Rock called for the Church to "give its enlightened support to one of the safest and surest methods of birth control known today—voluntary sterilization."[79] Not only did these leaders in contraceptive research offer their public endorsement of contraceptive sterilization, they also joined the AVS Board of Directors, lending the organization and its goals additional legitimacy and status.[80]

Finally, the AVS published and disseminated pamphlets and brochures designed to sell sterilization to a wide range of populations and undertook an extensive media campaign designed to draw attention to its message. Some of its most popular literature included pamphlets entitled *Now You and Your Wife Can Have Sex without Babies*, *The Physician and Contraceptive Sterilization*, *The Lawyer Speaks on Contraceptive Sterilization*, *The Clergyman Speaks on Voluntary Sterilization*, *Voluntary Sterilization as It Relates to Mental Health*, and *Voluntary Sterilization: Questions and Answers*. The AVS distributed these pamphlets to medical organizations. A 1966 internal report showed that it sent copies of *Voluntary Sterilization: Questions and Answers* and *The Physician and Contraceptive Sterilization* to 2,000 county medical societies. In June of the same year, the organization reported mailing literature to about 20,000 doctors across the country.[81]

An extensive public relations campaign also made both the AVS and contraceptive sterilization featured stories in newspapers, popular periodicals, and professional journals. The *New York Times*, *Medical World News*, *Ob/Gyn Digest*, *American Journal of Public Health*, *Today's Health*, *Redbook*, *Ladies' Home Journal*, *Life*, *Playboy*, *Glamour*, *Sexology*, *Parents' Magazine*, and *Reader's Digest*, among others, ran articles on the AVS or voluntary sterilization during the 1960s. Throughout the 1960s and into the 1970s, AVS president Wood and other prominent AVS members appeared on local and national radio and television programs to raise awareness of voluntary sterilization.[82] Not only did the organization use the media to promote its message, it also attempted to silence opposition. Women's health activist Barbara Seaman wrote an article that questioned the practice of voluntary sterilization in favor of temporary methods of contraception for the *Ladies' Home Journal*. The AVS learned of the article prior to its publication. Deeming it "distorted" and "biased," the organization attempted to have the "article modified or canceled." It failed, and Seaman's article appeared in 1967.[83]

The AVS's public relations campaigns bore tangible results when the organization entered the realm of referrals. For example, in January 1970 the AVS assisted with sixty sterilization operations by providing patients with referrals to doctors in their areas willing to perform the surgery. Of those sixty, thirty-nine listed newspaper, magazine, or television as the means by which they learned of the AVS and its services. The January statistics are representative. Sixty-five percent of people seeking referrals this month learned about the AVS from the popular media. Statistics for the year reveal that 52.5 percent of patients served in 1970 listed their primary source of referral as magazines, newspapers, and books, and 10.8 percent attributed their knowledge of the AVS to television. Sixty-three percent of all surgeries reported that year came from media referrals.[84]

The AVS's Sterilization Services

The AVS's first step to legitimizing voluntary sterilization involved gathering the support of physicians, family planners, and population controllers and creating public awareness of sterilization through educational and promotional campaigns. The second step involved providing the surgery. Beginning in 1956, the AVS ventured into the realm of service provision. It started with a loan and referral program, the French Fund.

In 1956, the AVS received a $10,000 grant (renewable annually) from Philadelphia lawyer and philanthropist Graham French to establish a loan fund for individuals who were "in need" of sterilization but who could not afford the procedure. French's generosity was motivated both by his concern for poor children and, probably more important, by his neo-eugenic politics. In a letter to the editor of Philadelphia's *Evening Bulletin*, French proposed removing the illegitimate children of poor mothers who could not support them and sterilizing fathers who could not or would not support their illegitimate children. He also favored the mandatory sterilization of women on welfare who bore a second illegitimate child. French's donation marked the AVS's first foray into service provision—an enormous step for the organization, which until this point had relied upon other professionals to enact its reforms. The French Fund and the referral service it initiated granted the AVS the opportunity to help provide the sterilization services that it advocated. The AVS did not explicitly endorse French's politics, but it also did not debate the ethics behind accepting his money.[85]

French and the AVS envisioned a loan fund that would support itself: the AVS would pay physician and hospital fees for candidates, who would then reimburse the organization, and these reimbursements would fund subsequent surgeries. This plan never materialized—too few recipients possessed the means to repay the AVS—but the AVS did not mind. In a 1961 letter to a minister who wrote on behalf of a woman unable to repay her loan, Assistant Director Joanna Poletti admitted that "only a very small percentage of this money is ever paid back because those so helped are truly indigent and the money is an outright grant."[86] The organization suggested as much to sterilization candidates when it explained in brochures and personal correspondence that loans could be repaid "without pressure" and at patients' convenience. In personal correspondence to beneficiaries of loans, the AVS stressed that it would accept any payment patients could make, but did not demand immediate repayment. Notably, the organization made no real effort to collect outstanding loans.[87] The French Fund's real goal was to provide sterilization to those individuals who the AVS believed "needed" permanent contraception because of their socioeconomic status.

Initially, the AVS advertised its referral service and loan program to family planners, public health and public welfare departments, hospital social workers, nurses, and physicians—experts who were in direct contact with its target population and whose support the AVS had been lobbying for since the early 1950s. From the mid-1950s through the mid-1960s, about half of the requests that the AVS received were from service professionals seeking "treatment" for their clients. More traditional eugenic concerns like mental retardation and other mental disorders among the poor dominated these letters. A letter written by a social worker from Broward County General Hospital in Florida is fairly representative. In 1964, this social worker wrote to the AVS about a patient who "is so severely retarded that she is unable to give ages of children, cannot even comb their hair or look after any of their needs, according to her mother." The social worker explained that her client "has no idea who the fathers of her various children are, apparently when her mother is at work, men come to the house and she has relations with them indescriminately [sic] with apparently no conception of what may result from these relationships."[88]

In another letter, a Waco, Texas, caseworker described her client having "very low moral character."[89] Other indications for this woman's sterilization included her diabetes and frequent hospitalizations, her unemployed husband, and her conception of a child while her husband was in jail (whether her husband was the father of this child is unclear). The most powerful indication for sterilization, however, came from this woman's "inability" to mother her six children, only four of whom were living. Of the four living children, two resided in state homes, and one lived with an uncle. Similarly, a Kentucky nurse applied for sterilization on behalf of her patients in 1963, a married couple with seven children, ages thirty (husband) and twenty-six (wife). She wrote that "neither parent," but especially the mother, had the "intelligence for following through instructions," and as a result could not use temporary contraception effectively. She later described the father as "not smart" and declared that the mother "is definitely a mentally retarded person" who "does not take care of her children." The nurse pleaded with the AVS to sterilize the husband for the sake of the "pitiful little children."[90] These applications and many others like them were written by social workers guided by more traditional eugenic ideas. The "symptoms" they highlighted were eugenic in nature—mental retardation, disease, poverty, and "deviant" female sexuality—and they spoke of sterilization as a solution to the social costs of caring for "defective" patients. The authors of these letters presumed that unless stopped, the applicant would continue to pass down her or his defects to future generations. For example, a St. Louis social worker applied for sterilization funds on behalf of a female married client and stressed the woman's "poor preparation for motherhood and home-making," which she explained as the result of "having come from a broken home and spending much of her life in institutions." Her emphasis on mothering and her client's own institutionalization and "broken home" suggested that sterilization could stop the reproduction of "defective" social behaviors.[91] Other social workers, nurses, and physicians emphasized the presence of disabled and unemployed spouses, especially husbands (both when they themselves were the applicant for surgery and when their wives were), to indicate the "drain" that future children of these couples would add to precious government resources.[92]

Few social workers wrote on behalf of black clients, but some wrote on behalf of Mexican clients, and frequently pointed to their ethnicity as a "symptom" of their lack of reproductive fitness. Planned Parenthood of Kansas City emphasized one couple's Mexican ethnicity and Catholic religion to the AVS in a July 1958 letter that described a family with nine children in which the thirty-one-year-old mother (pregnant with her tenth child) had cardiac problems and the father was institutionalized for tuberculosis. This family was "completely dependent on relief," the executive director of Planned Parenthood of Kansas City wrote exasperatedly.[93] Implicit in her request for assistance was the idea that these were not the type of people who should be reproducing in large numbers because of their poverty and ethnicity. Similarly, a Polk County Health official applied for sterilization on behalf of a Mexican couple from Des Moines, Iowa, with twelve children who received welfare. In her letter, she reinforced her request for her client's sterilization by admitting her belief that "mexican [sic] people are a bit suspicious anyway."[94]

Although requests for sterilization on eugenic grounds were common in the first decade of the AVS's referral service, the organization also received hundreds of letters from "healthy" couples seeking permanent contraception, many of whom had been referred to the organization by family planning groups like Planned Parenthood (operating on a local level, not national) and state welfare societies. In contrast to the eugenically driven letters described above, the requests sent by patients themselves expressed the desire to limit family size in order to stabilize their families financially and improve the quality of their marriages. Several used the AVS's own rhetoric to explain how sterilization would help them to strengthen their family systems. In 1959, a Los Angeles man referred by Planned Parenthood wrote the AVS: "My wife and I have seven children and are having a hard time trying to support them." He continued, "We have tried several methods of controle [sic] but have all failed. It seems that a sterilization is the only solution to our problem."[95]

Many men and women who wrote to the AVS during this period expressed similar frustration at temporary methods of contraception that had failed them in the past and indicated their desire to limit their family size in order to support the children whom they already had. "Our last child was conceived because of a failure of contraceptives," a New Jersey couple wrote in 1965. "As a result of that experience, we have become increasingly fearful of conventional contraceptives." For this couple, as for others like them, sterilization offered a secure means of preventing future pregnancies that threatened to destabilize their precarious economic situation. The New Jersey couple concluded their letter by saying, "We feel that additional children would deprive the others of our time, affection and material help. We look to sterilization as the most effective means of reducing the strain on our family relationship that stems from the severe economic and emotional crisis that would result from more children."[96] A Fort Lauderdale woman echoed similar sentiments in 1965 when she wrote the AVS to report on her sterilization. "My husband and I have always had good relations, but nothing we did seem [sic] to prevent my getting pregnant. I am so very glad you assisted me for the sterilization because we really can't support any more children."[97]

The French Fund persisted for six years, until French's death in 1962. At this time, with demand for the procedure increasing, the AVS decided to allocate general funds in order to continue the loan program. Generous donations from physicians aided its efforts. In 1965, approximately 135 physicians in thirty-two states donated their services to offer a total of 2,100 sterilizations to the organization. While the AVS arranged far fewer surgeries than the doctors pledged to perform, the volume of the donation indicated the medical establishment's increasing receptivity to the practice of permanent contraception.[98]

From 1956 through 1970, the AVS acted as an intermediary between patients seeking surgery and physicians willing to perform the controversial procedure. In this role, the AVS acted as a true patient advocate.[99] It began all referral proceedings by having an internal review board evaluate patients' requests to determine if medical indications could be identified that might allow patients' to bypass restrictive hospital policies, and to determine the extent to which patients needed financial assistance. It worked directly with patients to locate physicians in their area willing to perform the surgery, often writing to three or four surgeons before finding one willing to help. It arranged logistics for patients who had to travel several hours to meet a surgeon, scheduled surgeries with hospital administrators, and arranged to reimburse hospitals for surgeries covered by its loan fund. The AVS staff also petitioned local hospital boards on behalf of patients whose applications for sterilization had been rejected. By the beginning of the 1970s, however, the demand for referrals exceeded the review committee's ability to process applications. In order to meet the great demand, the AVS discontinued its application process, dismantled the review board, and began to refer patients directly to participating doctors, clinics, and hospitals without conducting intermediary evaluation of applicants. With this new system in place, the AVS provided nearly 17,000 referrals in 1970 alone.[100] Patient demand for referrals demonstrates the increasing popularity of permanent contraception.

The French Fund served several purposes. It brought the AVS into the realm of service provision, which not only increased the number of contraceptive sterilizations performed annually but also led to the development of a vast network of physicians and service providers willing to aid the AVS in its struggle to legitimize permanent contraception. The AVS's referral staff learned how to negotiate hospital policies and insurance claims (some insurance companies would pay for medically indicated surgeries). It also used the referral program to connect to local family planners and public health workers at the grassroots level, an important development given national Planned Parenthood's resistance to the AVS's overtures.

In follow-up questionnaires sent between 1956 and 1965, clients raved that their sterilizations led to dramatic improvements in their marriages and sex lives. In April 1958, Mrs. M.B.P. of Warren, Ohio, wrote on her follow-up questionnaire, "I believe that the operation saved my marriage."[101] Three years later, Mrs. E.S. of Manitowoc, Wisconsin, explained that her surgery improved her husband's relationship with their children. "One thing that I have noticed very much since I have had this operation[,] my husband plays with the children and loves them. Before it was just another child and he would push them away. He helps them with their school work. And it's a wonderful feeling."[102] Similarly, Mr. H.P. of New York City wrote to the AVS in 1958 to report on his successful vasectomy. "Our second child was born in 1952. From that time on, the fear of pregnancy has virtually halted our marital relations," he wrote. "Although the operation seemed like a drastic decision, it has brought us more peace of mind and freedom to enjoy our marriage than at any time since our wedding night."[103] Mrs. O.C. from Syracuse, New York, expressed similar sentiments in December 1962 when she exclaimed, "Since the operation he's [her husband] after me *all* the time" (double underline in original).[104] And Mrs. L.C.G. wrote in March 1965, "Before the operation I was all ways [*sic*] afraid to let go and enjoy intercourse." The operation "has changed my whole life," she continued. "I feel now I can begin to live."[105] Numerous other people expressed great relief that sterilization eliminated their fears of unplanned pregnancy. "My biggest fear is gone," Mrs. H.T. of Hartland, Wisconsin, wrote in May 1961. "I was worn out and tired all the time from being pregnant, and since, I feel just wonderful and can enjoy everything more."[106]

Fauquier Hospital Maternity Clinic

In 1960, the AVS expanded its service activities by contributing funds to a Virginia maternity clinic that provided contraceptive sterilization. This venture constituted the first of several failed efforts to persuade the federal government to provide family planning services, specifically voluntary sterilization, to the poor. The significance of the AVS's investment in Fauquier Hospital Maternity Clinic resides not with its donation, but rather with its public relations efforts. In September 1962, the AVS used the clinic to spark the first national debate about contraceptive sterilization. This debate brought contraceptive sterilization into public discussion and established the terms of many future debates regarding sterilization abuse.

In January 1960, Fauquier Hospital opened its maternity clinic in Warrenton, Virginia, to meet the needs of poor citizens. "Patients kept turning up at delivery. There was no prenatal nor postnatal care," explained Dr. James L. Dellinger, chairman of the hospital's medical staff.[107] Like other local family planning clinics, Fauquier Hospital Maternity Clinic provided prenatal and postnatal care as well as birth control. Unlike other clinics, it included sterilization as part of its contraceptive services. In its first two years, the Fauquier clinic performed only therapeutic sterilizations, or medically indicated surgeries. It expanded its services in March 1962 to include nontherapeutic sterilizations, or those performed primarily for contraceptive purposes. The hospital changed its policy in accordance with a new Virginia law, the first contraceptive sterilization law in the country. The Virginia law explicitly legalized the voluntary sterilization of competent individuals who complied with a thirty-day waiting period and obtained the consent of two physicians. It is significant that Virginia passed the nation's first contraceptive sterilization statute, as the state played a leading role in the eugenics movement, and the landmark eugenic sterilization case, *Buck v. Bell* (1927), upheld Virginia's eugenic code. Virginia sterilized more people than any other state except California.[108]

Fauquier Hospital served Warrington's poor citizens who were referred to the clinic by the Fauquier County Welfare Department. The maternity clinic charged its patients $1.50 per visit, but waived this fee for those unable to pay. Clinic staff offered sterilization to all patients who expressed interest in contraception. It did not, however, offer sterilization on demand. The clinic required the approval of three consulting physicians (the law only required two), and conditioned surgical candidacy upon spousal consent and age/parity restrictions, which required sterilization candidates to be over twenty-one years old and have at least three children. In its first thirty-three months of operation, the Fauquier Hospital Maternity Clinic served 201 patients, delivered 139 women (including twelve mothers who delivered twice), and performed sixty-three sterilizations.[109]

The AVS shined a national spotlight on the clinic on September 1, 1962, when it shuttled approximately twenty international sociologists from Washington, D.C., where they were attending a convention, to Warrenton to tour the facility. That the AVS turned this visit into a media event indicates that it intended to use the clinic's program to provoke a national discussion. The sociologists' responses to the clinic varied. Some expressed their support for the inclusion of sterilization in the clinic's birth control services and wondered why more sterilization programs had not been developed. Others pondered the long-term psychological effects of sterilization on Fauquier's patients, and one questioned the staff's motives. Was the clinic a product of "do-goodism," he asked, or was it a "subtle effort to cut down the welfare rolls"?[110] This second question would become the central issue in the ensuing debate.

On September 9, Archbishop Patrick A. O'Boyle condemned the Fauquier sterilization program in a sermon at St. Matthews's Cathedral in Washington, D.C., and ignited the first national debate over contraceptive sterilization. This particular debate involved religious leaders, but other debates would extend beyond religious communities and involve local grassroots activists as well as national leaders in the civil rights, women's, Chicano/a, Black Power, Puerto Rican independence, and Native American movements. O'Boyle declared sterilization to be "grossly immoral" and a violation of a "natural right which is so profoundly sacred that it may not be taken away from the individual by the State and may not be voluntarily surrendered to the State by the individual."[111] This argument was not new; Catholics had opposed sterilization and contraception on these grounds since the early years of the twentieth century, when Margaret Sanger first called for the legalization of birth control. The archbishop accused the clinic of harboring a eugenic agenda, declaring the true goal of the sterilization program to be to reduce the number of people eligible for welfare in Warrenton in order to lower the tax "burden" of middle-class residents.[112] In September 1962, Catholics, Evangelicals, and Orthodox Jews squared off against Methodists, Unitarians, and Reform Jews in a series of editorials and sermons on the ethics of sterilization. Opponents accused Fauquier physicians of violating natural law and of mutilating their patients, while supporters congratulated these same doctors for validating their patients' reproductive rights.

Like Archbishop O'Boyle, opponents of the sterilization program argued that sterilization constituted an immoral practice. The vice president of the Union of American Hebrew Congregations declared that "voluntary steriliza- tion is 'Playing God,' tampering with the divine economy."[113] Many Christian leaders echoed the rabbi's sentiments. Rev. Walter G. Nesbit S.J., associate editor of the weekly Jesuit magazine *America*, proclaimed, "Such mutilation is against the law of nature and of God. It can never be justified . . . the state should not tolerate it." And when asked by reporters about his position on the Fauquier sterilization program, Baptist Evangelical minister Rev. Billy Graham declared, "I have come out in favor of birth control but sterilization is a crippling of a vital body function."[114]

Methodist and other Protestant leaders supported the program, arguing both that sterilization constituted a compassionate solution to poverty and that Americans held the right to determine the limits of their own reproduction. Rev. Edward H. Redman of the Unitarian Church of Arlington, Virginia, maintained, "I find no virtue in letting the unwed . . . woman go on struggling, all by herself, trying to rear eight to fifteen youngsters, cramped together, ill-fed, ill-clothed, ill- tended. . . . If we have reverence for life . . . our reverence should be a concern that every living person, and every child coming into the world, shall have the means of growth and fulfillment to the highest level of his capacity."[115] In Redman's mind, sterilization offered poor women a means to raise their children with dig- nity and preserved the health and well-being of these children. Methodist bishop John Wesley Lord of Washington, D.C., expressed similar sentiments when he described the hospital's programs as "a beacon of hope and enlightenment."[116]

Despite opponents' allegations, no evidence suggests that Fauquier physi- cians coerced patients into accepting sterilization. In fact, some sources actually provide evidence to counter accusations of abuse, especially abuse directed against blacks. The *New York Times* and *U.S. News and World Report* found that the hospital sterilized blacks and whites at an equal rate, with whites actually demonstrating a slightly greater interest in the procedure. In an article published in September 1962, *New York Times* reporter David Binder declared O'Boyle's accusations unfounded. Examining county welfare records, Binder discovered that the county was not experiencing a "welfare crisis"; in fact, welfare assumed a relatively small portion of the county's total budget. (The total annual relief budget equaled $38,202—less than one-thirteenth of the total budget derived from tax revenue.) Binder also disputed the claim that Fauquier physicians used sterilization to reduce the number of residents eligible for welfare. Of the 298 individuals enrolled in welfare, only 4 sought services at the maternity clinic.[117]

Perhaps most important, patients did not complain of sterilization abuse. In fact, the few patients who contributed to the debate spoke in favor of the clinic. A twenty-eight-year-old mother of seven expressed her deep satisfaction with her surgery. "I've felt better since I've had the operation than any time during the last five years," she declared.[118] In the spring of 1962, Fauquier Hospital conducted a survey of patient satisfaction that found forty of the forty-four patients surveyed to be very satisfied with their surgery. Three of the four outlying respondents reported general satisfaction with their surgery, leaving only one patient dissatisfied with her experience. This woman, the mother of ten children born out of wedlock, reported that her common-law husband and the father of her last four children left her because of her sterility.[119] With forty-three of the forty-four patients who had been sterilized reporting satisfaction, this survey strongly argues against coercion. Moreover, not a single Fauquier patient testified to abuse during the early 1970s, when sterilization abuse became a public concern and victims began to speak out about their experiences.

The apparent lack of coercion in the Fauquier program does not, however, mean that Virginia physicians remained untainted by the politics of reproductive fitness. In fact, the opposite appears to be true. Fauquier physicians positioned themselves at the forefront of the campaign to pass the 1962 voluntary sterilization statute and were the first in the state and the country to establish a freestanding clinic that offered voluntary sterilization. Hospital chairman Dr. James L. Dellinger openly indicated his neo-eugenic sentiments when he described many of his patients as too "ignorant and lazy" to successfully employ temporary methods of birth control. But if the majority of Dellinger's colleagues shared his sentiments, they concealed them from the press. Some Fauquier physicians maintained that reporters and religious leaders exaggerated the role of sterilization at the maternity clinic and argued that patient demand drove the clinic's sterilization provision.[120]

The Fauquier controversy faded by the end of October 1962, but the debates provoked by Archbishop O'Boyle's accusations continued through the late 1970s. This debate set the terms for future contests over the legitimacy of contraceptive sterilization, the practice of forced sterilization, the role of the government in family planning, and the boundaries of Americans' reproductive rights. Opponents were the first to raise questions about coercion, and both opponents and supporters of the maternity clinic were the first activists to publicly weigh the risks and benefits of the controversial surgery. Further, although O'Boyle's accusations seem to have been unfounded in the case of Fauquier Hospital, his predictions had actually already materialized in some southern communities at the time of the debate. Although the archbishop rested his criticisms upon religious doctrine using the language of morality, a decade later feminists, black nationalists, and Native American and Hispanic activists would articulate and expand these same accusations using the language of racial and economic justice.

The Hartman Plan: Bringing Sterilization to Appalachia

The AVS contributed money to the Fauquier program and helped patients obtain surgery through its referral fund, but it finally became directly involved in the administration of sterilization services when it established the Hartman Plan. In the summer of 1964, the AVS inaugurated a pilot sterilization program in Appalachia that launched the organization into actual service provision. A generous donation of $25,000 by Philadelphia businessman and philanthropist Jesse Hartman financed the program, which was designed to persuade federal, state, and local governments to expand their meager roles in family planning. The AVS planned to use private funds to support the establishment of sterilization services within existing family planning programs and then to transfer its financial and administrative duties to local, state, and federal governments. "The Hartman Plan is a pilot program intended to show the way for government to assume full responsibility for similar birth control programs nationwide," it announced in its summer 1964 *Bulletin*.[121] Working in conjunction with state health and welfare agencies, local family planning services such as the Mountain Maternal Health League, and eight local hospitals in twenty-two counties in eastern Kentucky, the AVS funded the sterilization of 195 poor men and women between July 1964 and December 1965.[122] With the Hartman Plan, the AVS finally gained the opportunity to transform its neo-eugenic ideas into practice and to demonstrate to politicians and the public that sterilization constituted a technological solution to the social crises of poverty, illegitimacy, divorce, welfare, and overpopulation. One of its key methods for making these points was to link the Hartman Plan to President Lyndon Johnson's War on Poverty.

From the beginning, the AVS highlighted the connections between its sterilization program and the War on Poverty. When announcing the plan, Hartman claimed, "I'm not a do-gooder, I just want to help in this fight on poverty," and days later the organization's executive director announced that "Mr. Hartman plans to seek 'War on Poverty' funds as soon as we can show results," indicating that the AVS sought to permanently join forces with the administration, which it failed to do.[123] The executive director of the AVS went so far as to send a telegram to Johnson before the president addressed Congress about his Great Society program. In the communication, Ruth Proskauer Smith asked the president to consider sterilization an important weapon in his fight against poverty. "Federal aid to depressed areas such as the Appalachian region, without birth control information is futile," she maintained. "One major cause of poverty is uncontrolled human fertility. There can be no real and enduring prosperity without free access to birth control information." She then asked the president to provide federal funds for birth control and to include sterilization among the services offered.[124] Proskauer Smith was not the only person to petition Johnson's support for birth control. Seventy-six politicians, business leaders, philanthropists, and scholars wrote an open letter to the president in the *New York Times* applauding his attack on poverty and imploring him to recognize "the root cause of poverty—**the present explosive growth of population**" (boldface in original). Citing the financial burden of "unproductive" citizens receiving welfare rather than a wage, these concerned citizens and experts warned that "unless corrective measures are taken 'here and now,' the resulting human misery and social tensions will inevitably lead to chaos and strife at home and abroad," which they concluded "would be grist for the Communist mill."[125]

The AVS repeatedly reminded the public and politicians that the Hartman Plan was in Appalachia, a site of immense poverty and one of Johnson's prime targets. For their part, local and regional public health officials identified large families as one of the primary factors causing Appalachian poverty. Dr. A. S. Holmes, a leading public health officer in the region and one of the program's chief planners, declared that "the problem of too many children in needy families lies at the root of the Appalachian poverty problem."[126] The AVS's Hartman Plan literature promised that by limiting family size and making every child a wanted child, sterilization would break the cycle of deprivation and hardship experienced (and reproduced) by poor Appalachian residents.[127]

The AVS marketed sterilization as a cost-effective alternative to contemporary welfare programs, which were becoming a source of public anxiety as the Great Society expanded federal aid to an unprecedented extent and civil rights victories granted blacks unprecedented access to these services. Harkening

back to older eugenic themes, the AVS suggested that "the poor, the underprivileged, the mentally retarded and the uneducated adults have children in large
numbers, not because they want them but simply because they cannot avoid
having them."[128] The suggestion that these four groups of people could not control their sexual behavior drew upon older eugenic ideas about the "unfit" lacking the morality and responsibility to control their sexuality. Following eugenic
tradition, the Hartman Plan promoted the use of public funds to curb the effects
of this behavior in the interest of reducing government expenditures and
improving the health of society writ large. But its claims held a distinct neo-
eugenic basis, as it tied its efforts to those of the federal government and the liberal domestic programs designed to raise the standard of living of millions of
Americans and quell an "impending" population explosion around the world.
The AVS remained concerned about the economic cost of "unfit" citizens, but
the context in which these concerns existed changed with the times.

One way that the AVS demonstrated its new approach was by employing
the alarmist rhetoric of the population control movement to describe the conditions of rural Kentucky. Suggesting that sterilization constituted the only effective solution to the ticking time bomb of overpopulation, Executive Director
Proskauer Smith wrote in a 1964 press release, "Every family with more children than they can love, nurture, and provide for is a population explosion in
microcosm, with the same damaging impact on the community that an explod-
ing national population has on the world." In the same press release,
the AVS also characterized the Hartman Plan as "a historic attack" on high
birth rates among the poor (which it identified as the primary cause of the
region's economic desperation) and followed this statement with a quote from
Homer N. Calver, chairman of the AVS's Public Health Committee: "I feel
strongly that if the human race is going to protect itself against the invading
horde of the yet unborn, it must look to voluntary sterilization as an important
measure of defense."[129] Drawing upon the popular Cold War themes of national
security and family stability, Calver depicted the Hartman Plan as an offensive
against a marauding force of poor Americans "unfit" to reproduce on the basis
of their poverty and welfare dependency. According to Hartman Plan propaganda,
staving off the "hordes" of poor Appalachians constituted a matter of national
urgency that required immediate and forceful governmental action. "It is
deplorable that many of our people must reproduce in such an irresponsible
manner," the AVS proclaimed, before promising that "sound family planning
leads to an improved total society."[130]

The AVS anticipated great success for the Hartman Plan. A June 1964
memo indicated that the organization hoped that the government would

assume 50 percent of the Kentucky program's cost within one year and the entire cost within three. The organization envisioned replicating this pattern in other states across the country. To this end, the AVS staff wrote to welfare directors in all fifty states offering a matching donation of $25,000 to establish a Hartman Plan in their locales. Only Florida entered into negotiations with the organization, but despite the support of local community leaders, the state ultimately rejected the AVS's offer. Most states simply ignored or flatly rejected the proposal, and as a result the AVS fell far short of its original goal. It received no government aid for its Kentucky program and, after exhausting additional funding from Hartman, terminated the program in December 1965, despite a "sizeable waiting list" of patients.[131] Unwilling to leave these patients "untreated," the Mountain Maternal Health League continued to fund vasectomies through the 1970s, and the E. O. Robinson fund, a private foundation, established a $3,000 account to finance tubal ligations at a local hospital. The AVS's failure to elicit government support from other states for its sterilization program is not surprising, as the federal government was just beginning to subsidize contraception in 1964 and 1965.

The AVS may have failed in its attempt to persuade the federal government to develop a federal family planning policy with sterilization at its core, but it did succeed in convincing many physicians and family planners of the individual and social benefits of contraceptive sterilization. But the AVS cannot assume sole credit for this achievement. Its campaign to legitimize voluntary sterilization was so well received because women, and to a lesser extent men, were searching for highly effective methods of contraception that did not carry health risks. The introduction of the Pill in 1960 and the redesign and redistribution of the IUD in 1964 caused women to expect their birth control to be nearly 100 percent effective. When medicine and the government raised concerns about the safety of these new methods, many couples who had completed their childbearing turned to voluntary sterilization. Their desire for highly effective, safe contraception, set in the context of the sexual revolution and public concern regarding overpopulation, motivated many to begin demanding the surgery from their physicians and hospitals.

Chapter 2

"Fit" Women and Reproductive Choice

Women seeking permanent contraception in the late 1960s confronted several barriers. These included the ambiguous legal status of sterilization, which led some doctors to refuse to perform the surgery for fear of litigation, and age/parity restrictions, which barred young women with small families from obtaining the desired surgery. The high cost of and medical risks associated with tubal ligation also stymied many women. By the early 1970s, advances in surgical technology reduced the costs and the risks of tubal ligation, making the surgery more accessible and attractive to women. Until this time, tubal ligation was open abdominal surgery that required general anesthetic, and several days in the hospital, and included a six-week recuperation period. This changed when physicians revolutionized the technology of female sterilization by introducing laparoscopic methods that significantly reduced the cost and duration of surgery and minimized the medical risks involved, effectively making the procedure safer, more affordable, and less disruptive to women's lives and health. The combination of the AVS's campaign, women's changing expectations of their contraception, and advances in surgical technology intersected to transform sterilization from a procedure associated with eugenics to one of the most popular methods of contraception in the country.

Many couples determined to prevent unplanned pregnancy via surgery found that while tubal ligation was out of reach, vasectomy was not. Most vasectomies were performed in physicians' offices, outside the purview of hospital administrators and policies like the 120 rule, and were far less expensive than tubal ligation. Hundreds of thousands of couples intent on limiting family size turned to vasectomy as a "solution" to their contraceptive problems, and in doing so, granted men a rather unprecedented responsibility for birth control. Likewise, as public concern about overpopulation grew in step with a swelling population control movement, men of all ages concerned about the problem chose to be sterilized as a political act, as a way of "doing their part" in the struggle to limit population size and environmental "dangers" caused by large numbers of people. Of course, men have used condoms for centuries, but condoms do not alter the body's chemistry or physicality like the Pill and IUD do, and as such do not involve the same levels of commitment and risk that women who use these methods assume. The increasing use of vasectomy signaled both a new trend in contraceptive decision making between couples and the medicalization of male contraception. Since the 1930s, physicians dispensed the most effective methods of female contraception (the diaphragm, the Pill, and the IUD), while the most popular method of male birth control, the condom, remained available in drugstores and without a prescription. As vasectomy gained popular and medical support, men found themselves following women and turning to physicians for help controlling their reproduction. Men who had a vasectomy also assumed a historically female responsibility for birth control. Having adopted a method that was nearly foolproof, these men released their partners from the duty of employing contraception and the worry that it might fail.

Sterilization as an Alternative Contraceptive

The introduction of the Pill in 1960 and the redesign of the IUD in 1964 caused women to revise their expectations regarding contraception. These technologies offered women reliable birth control that did not interfere with the sex act, existing as attractive alternatives to less-effective, messy diaphragms, jellies, and condoms. The Food and Drug Administration (FDA) approved the first birth control pill, Enovid, in 1960, and within five years of its arrival on the market, the Pill became the most popular form of contraception in the country. The introduction of the Pill to the United States market ushered in new contraceptive behaviors and created a cultural phenomenon. Eager to try the revolutionary technology, millions of women (largely white and middle class) began to demand that their physicians prescribe the Pill for them. Their demands shifted the balance of power in the doctor-patient relationship to grant more authority to women, who assumed the role of health care consumer. In the 1960s, women entered doctors' offices with their own diagnoses and treatment plans; they wanted to avoid pregnancy and to take the Pill. Generally, patients approach physicians for medical advice and assistance, assuming a submissive position, which was magnified for women on account of their sex. But women seeking the Pill rejected this model in favor of a more consumer-based one in which they approached a physician for a prescription, and if he refused their requests, they took their business elsewhere. In the pre-HMO era, not all physicians could risk such financial loss, which led some physicians who were ambivalent about prescribing the Pill to comply with women's requests for it.[1]

Women across race and class demanded the Pill, but doctors preferred to prescribe it to white women, especially middle-class women, those deemed reproductively "fit" on the basis of their race and class status and, as such, sufficiently "responsible" to take this female-controlled method of birth control. Physicians advocated the use of the IUD—a device controlled by physicians that women could not remove—as an appropriate contraceptive for "unfit" women both in the United States and abroad.[2] That the IUD was not as effective as the Pill was less important to family planners and population controllers than the device's reliance on physicians to insert. Physician and president of Planned Parenthood Alan Guttmacher viewed the IUD as a tool to reduce the reproduction of poor women to the benefit of society. "No contraceptive could be cheaper," he explained to the president of pharmaceutical manufacturer G. D. Searle, "and also, once the damn thing is in, the patient cannot change her mind. In fact, we hope she will forget that it is there and perhaps in several months wonder why she has not conceived."[3] This approach to contraception at once continued and diverged from Planned Parenthood's founder Margaret Sanger's politics of birth control. In the 1920s and 1930s, Sanger appropriated eugenic rationales in order to gain physicians' support for her cause. But eugenics undermined the feminist ideas that originally drove the birth control movement. Many physicians endorsed contraception to control the reproduction of "fit" and "unfit" women according to their own politics rather than to guarantee women reproductive self-determination. Sanger succeeded in gaining medical advocates, but in doing so she compromised the feminist impulse of her movement and undermined some women's ability to control their reproduction. Guttmatcher's statement reflects one of the consequences of her actions.[4]

Ideas of reproductive fitness were still at the center of American family planning in the 1960s. Physicians preferred to prescribe the Pill to white middle-class women and the IUD to poor women, especially poor women of color, because the IUD granted them greater control over "unfit" women's behavior. Guttmacher viewed the IUD as an effective method of contraception for individuals in "underdeveloped areas where two things are lacking: one, money and the other sustained motivation."[5] Although Guttmacher never explicitly identified poor women of color as appropriate recipients of the IUD, he insinuated such through statements like the following: "For most private patients and more highly motivated clinic patients, the pill may give the best protection. Where there is less motivation, the IUD is superior."[6] "Private patients" and "highly motivated patients" referenced white middle-class women. Less-motivated clinic patients referred to poor women with several children, and likely meant women of color, whose fertility in the postwar and post–baby boom years had become a source of public anxiety and discussion.

Medical concern about the Pill's safety for all women began one year after its release. This apprehension peaked in 1969 following announcement of an FDA study that found Pill users to be four-and-a-half times more likely to develop blood clots than nonusers. The Pill controversy culminated in early 1970, when Senator Gaylord Nelson conducted a series of Senate hearings regarding the safety of the new technology that led the FDA to order pharmaceutical companies to include an educational insert in each package of birth control pills.[7]

The majority of Pill users were white and middle class. In part this reflects ambivalence in the black community about this technology; in part it reflects doctors' preference in prescribing the Pill for this population; and in part it reflects the cost of the drug. Until the late 1960s, the Pill was prohibitively expensive for working-class and poor women.[8] White middle-class women articulated the greatest interest in sterilization during the Pill scare because they constituted the majority of Pill users.

Concerned about their health and/or dissatisfied with side effects from the Pill, which included nausea and weight gain, thousands of women threw away their Pill dispensers and adopted an alternate form of contraception. Many chose sterilization, the only other contraceptive method that could match the 99 percent effectiveness rate of the Pill. Demographers' statistics capture this decision. Between 1961 and 1970, the percentage of Americans undergoing sterilization rose steadily (with the exception of a sharp but quick decline followed by a rebound in 1966). Significantly, the percentage of Americans undergoing sterilization spiked between 1969 and 1970, during the height of the Pill scare. As figure 2.1 shows, the total percentage of Americans undergoing sterilization rested at about 10 percent in 1969. By 1970, this figure had risen to about 33 percent.[9] Like the Pill, sterilization required physician compliance, and women who had already positioned themselves as active health care consumers when they sought the Pill now applied this experience to their requests for tubal ligation. In addition, increasingly open discussions of sex and sexuality ushered in by the sexual revolution likely led many women to be more forthright with their physicians about their contraceptive needs.[10] By the late 1960s, many Pill users had become accustomed to the medicalization of contraception and were thus comfortable with requesting permanent birth control from their doctors.

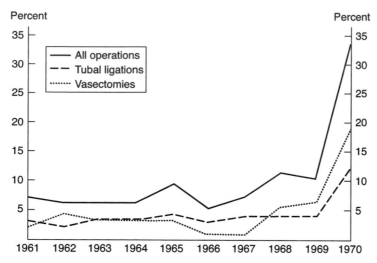

Figure 2.1 Larry L. Bumpass and Harriet B. Presser, "Contraceptive Sterilization in the U.S.: 1965 and 1970," *Demography* 9, no. 4 (November 1972): 534. Courtesy of the Population Association of America.

Notably, the sharpest increase in sterilization came from male surgeries and white men. Vasectomies and tubal ligations occurred in roughly equal numbers between 1963 and 1965, but the relationship between the two surgeries shifted in 1967, and by 1968 the percentage of vasectomies had overtaken that of tubal ligations. Not all men rushed to be sterilized. White men's interest in permanent contraception caused the sharp rise in surgery; very few black men chose vasectomy. In 1970, only 1 percent of the black male population had undergone vasectomy, as compared to 9 percent of the white male population. (The reverse was true for tubal ligation; 12 percent of black women had undergone sterilization in the same year, while only 6 percent of white women had.) Region also shaped sterilization trends. Demographers found that contraceptive sterilization was most prevalent in the West, although other regions witnessed increases between 1965 and 1970. "In the West, vasectomies were about five times as numerous as tubal ligations," one study found, while "in the Northeast, tubal ligations outnumbered vasectomies two to one."[11]

Urologists noticed this demand for vasectomies, linked it to the Pill scare, and alerted the mainstream press. In November 1970, the *Wall Street Journal* reported that "doctors across the country say requests for vasectomies have risen 100 percent to 200 percent since Senate hearings earlier this year gave wide publicity to some adverse effects of the pill."[12] Earlier the same year, the *New York Times* told of a Rhode Island urologist who experienced a "tripling in requests for male sterilization procedures (vasectomies) since the Senate hearings." One month later, the doctor reported continued demand for surgery. To meet this demand, he operated during his lunch hour and agreed to work on Easter Sunday in order to accommodate a couple "dismayed" by his overbooked schedule.[13]

The surge in vasectomies during the height of the Pill scare was not coincidental. Many couples that decided to seek sterilization as an alternative to the Pill chose vasectomy over tubal ligation because it was the more accessible of the two procedures. Hospital restrictions on tubal ligations made it difficult for many women to obtain their desired method of contraception, but because most vasectomies were performed in urologists' offices rather than hospitals, these women's partners did not face the same barriers, which one doctor described as the "dictatorial policies of hospital administers."[14]

Free from hospital oversight, urologists established their own rules to govern which patients they would sterilize. Their policies proved to be less rigid than the 120 rule. Although each doctor could create his own policy, many shared two general practices: they refused to sterilize young men, especially childless patients, and insisted upon spousal consent to surgery. Office standards were discussed openly at medical conferences and in medical journals in the late 1960s and early 1970s. In a 1969 speech to the section on urology at the Southern Medical Association annual meeting, Dr. Hjalmar E. Carlson explained his policy. "Personally," he said, "I think all couples capable of having children should have the experience and to do vasectomies on these immature adults would be morally wrong." For Carlson, the main factor in determining a patient's eligibility was his status as a parent. "If a husband is 25 years old and the couple has 4 children, I will do a vasectomy," he explained.[15] In a 1973 article published in the *Journal of Obstetrics and Gynecology*, urologists Robert E. Hackett and Keith Waterhouse reported that most of their colleagues operated according to a 50 rule, which classified any individual over twenty-five years old with at least two children a qualified candidate for vasectomy. But they also admitted that "few patients are rejected."[16] The Margaret Sanger Vasectomy Clinic in New York, established in 1969, allowed an individual who did not fulfill its eligibility requirements (patients had to be twenty-five years old and married or in a stable relationship) to meet with a team of experts (including a psychiatrist, urologist, endocrinologist, and geneticist). If the individual could obtain the approval of two consultants, he could be declared eligible for surgery.[17]

Vasectomy was not only more available than tubal ligation; it was also a much cheaper and simpler surgery and involved far fewer medical risks. As such, it was a logical choice for many couples seeking to limit their family size, especially those individuals whose motivations included achieving financial stability. Before the development of endoscopic methods in the early 1970s (which will be discussed later), tubal ligation was open abdominal surgery that required general anesthesia and a hospital stay of several days. Costs ranged from $500 to $1,400. Vasectomy, on the other hand, could be performed in a physician's office on an outpatient basis under local anesthesia in fifteen minutes, involved a recovery time of only two weeks, and cost between $50 and $200. Even before the Pill scare, the AVS recognized the cost-effectiveness of vasectomy in relation to tubal ligation. It pushed the male surgery in its referral and loan programs and in its Hartman Plan in Appalachia, with the goal of sterilizing the maximum number of people with its limited budget.[18]

Couples across the country told journalists that concerns about the safety of the Pill motivated them to seek permanent contraception. "I don't want to continue to disrupt the chemical balance of my body," a forty-two-year-old mother of two explained as she described her decision to undergo sterilization to the *New York Times Magazine* in a 1974 article that made the front cover. "I've known since my last child was born that I didn't want any more children," she added.[19] Committed to preventing additional pregnancies but also concerned about the side effects and long-term risks associated with the most effective methods of temporary contraception, this woman chose permanent sterilization. In 1976, *Good Housekeeping* ran an article titled "Sterilization: The Growing Alternative to the Pill," based upon a questionnaire administered to women and men between the ages of twenty-five and forty. Results of the survey found that women deemed the Pill "too chemical, too dangerous," and they complained that it caused them to gain weight. Many found the IUD to be unreliable, often because they had become pregnant while using it. One respondent, Susan Herner, claimed the Pill caused her to develop "crippling arthritis" in her arm. This mother of four swapped the Pill for an IUD, but became pregnant with her fourth child within months of having the device inserted. After giving birth, she returned to the Pill, but soon her arthritis returned as well. Feeling that she "had to be *sure*" that she would not become pregnant again, Herner and her husband chose vasectomy.[20] Other respondents shared similar stories of health difficulties with the Pill and pregnancies conceived with the IUD, some of which ended in abortions. But having once experienced "worry-free" contraception, few women were willing to return to older, less reliable methods; they wanted sterilization.

Individuals who wrote to the AVS during the Pill scare described similar experiences. As vasectomy was more accessible than tubal ligation at the time, many husbands vocalized the contraceptive dilemmas they shared with their wives in these letters. For example, in 1969 a thirty-year-old husband explained how disappointment with temporary methods of contraception led him and his wife to sterilization: "We have been using condoms for the ten years of our marriage and now feel this means of birth control leaves something to be desired. . . . My wife has tried the pill and found it makes her sick."[21] In another application written in February 1970, a couple described their difficulty locating an effective, safe method of contraception. Distrustful of the diaphragm and condoms, the wife tried birth control pills. "This relieved the anxiety over becoming pregnant and lead [sic] to a renewed sexual life for the both of us," her husband wrote in 1970. "However with all the latest controversy over the pill and with the possible side effects of blood clots etc. we decided that we would discontinue the use of the pill," he concluded.[22] Another couple worried about the long-term side effects of the Pill. In 1968, a husband wrote that his wife experienced "breakthrough bleeding and other difficulties" while on the Pill. "She has used several brands," he continued, but "is afraid of the effects they might have on her by taking them for 20 or 30 years more." Another man seeking a vasectomy the same year explained, "The side effects caused by the pill have forced her [his wife] to discontinue taking them." As a result, "we are back where we started with the fear of pregnancy always in our minds."[23] Accustomed to highly effective contraception, these couples sought to avoid both pregnancy and the anxiety caused by the constant fear of pregnancy. Sterilization was the only form of contraception that could meet their qualifications, and often vasectomy was the only surgery they could access.

A few husbands touted the health and marital benefits of sterilization. Dick Manning, a New England minister and father of four, offered a fairly feminist explanation for his decision to undergo vasectomy to *Good Housekeeping*. "I just felt it was my turn. This is one way a man can sort of balance out what the woman has done in bearing the children. It's a husband's gift to his wife," he declared.[24] The AVS sent follow-up surveys to its patients, and patients' responses offer insight into the ways concerns about the safety of the Pill led couples to choose permanent contraception. In his 1965 follow-up evaluation, a husband from Rockville Centre, New York, suggested that more Americans follow his lead and adopt vasectomy as an alternative to the Pill. "If more men knew how easy [the] operation is more would have it. Recently announced side effects of pills . . . could be avoided," he maintained.[25] One year later, a man from Long Beach, New York, reported that if he had the opportunity to make the decision to undergo sterilization again he would because now "my wife doesn't have to worry about taking the pill or any effects from it."[26] A husband from Pittsburgh expressed the same sentiments in 1970 when he wrote that as a result of his vasectomy, his "wife no longer fears long range effects of [the] pill."[27] Choosing vasectomy constituted a strategy adopted by couples seeking effective contraception but concerned about long-term side effects and dangers associated with the Pill. Notably, men functioned as the contraceptive agent in these situations, assuming a role in their marriage usually reserved for women. Some, like Dick Manning, viewed surgery as their responsibility; others viewed it as their only option given administrative and financial constraints.

Women's magazines brought the option of vasectomy to their readers' attention with stories like "At 22, My Husband Chose Sterilization," written by a young woman with three children and married to her high school sweetheart. Difficulties with the Pill, dislike of condoms and diaphragms, and an unplanned pregnancy conceived while using withdrawal created considerable strain, financial and emotional, on her marriage. This couple chose vasectomy and described the results as "truly liberating."[28] *Ladies' Home Journal* published similar stories, as did magazines seeking both male and female readership like *Reader's Digest*, the *New York Times Magazine*, and *Life*.[29] Print media played a critical role in educating Americans about vasectomy, and most of these stories presented sterilization as a safer, easier option than the Pill, and certainly a more effective option than condoms, diaphragms, and other, older methods of contraception.

The disastrous effects of the Dalkon Shield IUD also contributed to American women's desire for permanent contraception. The steadily climbing rates of female sterilization spiked again between 1973 and 1975, when women fitted with the Dalkon Shield began to report grisly stories of infection, uterine perforation, septic abortion, and infertility. Altogether, the Dalkon Shield caused eighteen deaths; over 200,000 infections, miscarriages, hysterectomies, and other gynecological complications; and an untold number of septic abortions.[30] Unwilling to risk their health with temporary contraception, yet also unwilling to trust less effective barrier methods, an increasing number of women gravitated toward sterilization. Concern about the safety of the IUD led Gladys Meyers, who lived in a suburb of New York City, to have the device removed. But this left the question of what form of contraception to use. "I hated the thought of starting over with something else. I was thirty-five," she explained, "and I felt I'd been through all of that." Her gynecologist suggested tubal ligation, and four months after quitting the IUD, Meyers was sterilized.[31] Meyers was part of a national trend. In 1973, 37 percent of couples married between ten and twenty-four years relied upon sterilization. By 1975, this figure had increased to 55.7 percent.[32]

Contraceptive Sterilization for Population Control

Both women and the AVS recognized that surgeons were the gatekeepers of sterilization. Like the AVS, women concerned about the health risks of the Pill played upon their physicians' concerns about overpopulation in their efforts to persuade doctors of the surgery's benefits. Some did so solely out of self-interest, hoping to use physicians' politics to gain access to surgery, while other women and their partners were genuinely attracted to sterilization because they believed it to be a solution to the "problem" of overpopulation and wanted to do their part to help the cause. The AVS referral applications and follow-up questionnaires reflect this trend, which strengthened over time. For example, in 1962 a twenty-six-year-old man and his twenty-four-year-old wife applied to the AVS for a vasectomy. When asked to list the couple's reasons for considering sterilization, he wrote, "We both feel that it is basically immoral to contribute to the overpopulation of the world, and wish to limit our family accordingly. This is a sincerely held belief and in fact the most important reason [for surgery]."[33] In 1970, another man echoed this sentiment when he wrote on his follow-up questionnaire, "My wife and I did not want to share in the overpopulation of the world."[34] A third vasectomy patient told the *New York Times* that he underwent sterilization for entirely political reasons. "It's all linked directly to the population explosion," he asserted. "I felt that if I was going around talking about population problems, then I'd better set a good example."[35] In March 1970, *Life* ran a story about this trend titled "One Man's Answer to Overpopulation," which chronicled a New Jersey man's decision to undergo vasectomy.[36] The presence of this story in such a mainstream, conservative magazine testifies to the popularity and acceptability of this man's decision.

Concern about overpopulation intersected with couples' decisions to bear smaller families than those created during the baby boom. By the mid-1960s, birth rates had declined from their baby boom highs, and at the beginning of 1968 birth rates fell below the "replacement rate."[37] Steadily climbing rates of female employment, coupled with feminists' emphasis on women's autonomy and independence from men, contributed to this trend. Women seeking to balance motherhood and paid employment in the post–baby boom years regulated their fertility differently than women who remained primarily in the home a generation earlier. One way that women navigated this difficult balance was by having two children in fairly rapid succession, effectively condensing their years of intense child care. While this allowed women to negotiate paid work easier than if they entered and exited the workforce repeatedly, it also left couples vulnerable to unwanted pregnancies for several decades after achieving their ideal family size. Demographers publishing in the 1970s found that couples seeking to limit their family size faced between twenty to thirty years of continued fertility after the birth of their last planned child. An estimated 30 percent of IUD and Pill users experienced an unintended pregnancy in the interim between the birth of their last child and menopause, making unplanned pregnancy a real risk. Many couples that completed their families while still quite young viewed sterilization as a promising means of eliminating the risk of unplanned pregnancy, especially after concerns about the Pill and IUD surfaced.[38]

Unwilling to risk an unintended pregnancy but worried about the risks associated with the new temporary technologies, in the late 1960s and early 1970s an increasing number of younger women leaned toward sterilization. A 1972 study of the acceptability of contraceptive sterilization between 1965 and 1970 published in *Family Planning Perspectives* found that 40 percent of couples studied "adopted sterilization before the wife turned 30."[39] (The study followed married couples, not singles.) The study also measured popular interest in sterilization among women and men of different age groups. While sterilization was least prevalent in women and men under twenty-five years of age, individuals in this demographic demonstrated considerable interest in the procedure. The authors of the study, Harriet B. Presser and Larry L. Bumpass, read this "serious interest" coupled with rising rates of surgery to be "indicators of *current acceptability* of sterilization." They found that in 1970, 64 percent of couples surveyed with a wife under twenty-five years old said that they would seriously consider either a male or female operation.[40] Men and women under twenty-five often had not completed their childbearing, but this study showed that many were looking ahead to the point at which they sought to permanently limit family size, and they looked to sterilization as a solution to the problem of unexpected pregnancy. "At 28, I had too many fertile years ahead," said a mother of three, explaining her attraction to sterilization.[41]

Other women saw sterilization as a way to free themselves from repeated childbearing and long-term child care. Another mother of three who underwent tubal ligation at age twenty-seven explained, "I used to be exhausted by the kids. I was saturated. I felt trapped." Sterilization allowed her to see an end to time spent caring for young children. Another woman said that "it takes a special kind of person to have a large family, and I'm not that kind. When there's a lot of chaos, I'm not happy." Another couple chose to be sterilized after having one child. The wife, Virginia, was sterilized after undergoing two abortions and the insertion of an IUD that failed, causing one of the two unplanned pregnancies. She credited sterilization with providing time for her to explore new passions. In addition to working part-time for a cancer researcher, Virginia took up sculpting, started to study Italian, played tennis three times a week, and hoped to learn to play the piano. "There's so much I want to do," she exclaimed. Freedom from additional pregnancies allowed her to begin doing some of these things.[42]

Alice Lake wrote the 1976 *Good Housekeeping* article about women's preference for sterilization over the Pill. She collected stories like Virginia's and concluded that feminist ideas had trickled down into the mainstream to cause this change in women's attitudes toward contraception and motherhood. Women "unaware of any influence from the feminist movement" seemed to be "touched" by feminist ideas, Lake found. The women she interviewed, she wrote, "are learning to value themselves as persons, not just baby-making machines. The concept that if a woman can't bear children she is damaged goods is being diffused." Lake viewed sterilization as a tool of women's liberation, as a means through which women disinterested in feminist politics could break down traditional gender roles. Sali Horowitz's understanding of her poststerilization transformation reinforced this point. "I used to be a homebody" who "did my own cooking and baking, and that's all I did," she maintained. But "now [postsurgery] that I have no more babies, I play tennis. I work in a dentist's office twice a week. I've lost 40 pounds. People notice that I'm different. 'Now you're standing on your own two feet,' they say."[43]

Not only did Americans show a preference for smaller families in the 1970s, but an increasing number of Americans actively chose to remain childless and saw sterilization as a method of realizing this goal. Some even created an antinatalist movement in the early 1970s committed to reducing population growth and/or to lifestyles that did not involve children. Members of the National Association for NonParents (NON), established in 1972, and similar groups advocated the environmental, population control, and personal benefits of childlessness. For many antinatalist Americans, these three issues were deeply intertwined. For example, a Berkeley, California, couple, Michael and Pamela Shandrick, were featured in a *U.S. News and World Report* article in 1976. Both cited an "unfettered lifestyle" as factoring in to their decision not to have children. "We're just too selfish to have children at this point," Michael explained. "We would rather buy the things we want than sacrifice for children." He continued, "We like the independence of getting up and taking off whenever we want." Pamela endorsed her husband's views and offered two more to support their nonparent lifestyle: commitment to zero population growth and feminism. A member of Zero Population Growth (ZPG), she declared, "I am doing my part from [sic] keeping the world from trampling itself to death with human beings in another 100 years." Pamela's language reflected the values of ZPG, a population control organization that advocated the use of coercive measures to limit population. Feminist ideas also shaped her commitment to childlessness. She cited high divorce rates and the very real possibility of single motherhood that many women faced, a situation she sought to prevent by not bearing children. In addition, Pamela endorsed the feminist effort to separate womanhood from motherhood when she stated, "I'm sure raising a family is a career for some women and a rewarding experience, yet it is not for everybody."[44]

Other couples, like Mary and Nat Freedland, profiled in a 1970 *Newsweek* article, stressed similar concerns. "Everything is such a mess," Mary complained, "the water and air are slowly being polluted. We're getting more and more crowded. . . . It's silly to have a child if you can't insure him a decent future." For her, responsible citizenship and environmental awareness led her to decide that her initial desire to have children when she married was an "ego thing," and that the condition of the planet and her desire to improve it trumped her maternal ambitions. Her husband placed his decision not to reproduce in a more personal perspective. "I have other things to live for," he insisted.[45] Other women and men chose to remain childless to focus on their careers. A thirty-one-year-old woman married eight years decided to undergo sterilization for this reason. "I feel very strongly that I'm a person defined by my work," she explained. "I'm ambitious and I'm a perfectionist. I'm just not cut out for having children."[46] Sterilization allowed her to dedicate herself to her work and to eliminate the risk of an unplanned pregnancy that could disrupt her focus.

NON, founded by Ellen Peck, author of *The Baby Trap*, and her husband, William, undertook a campaign to legitimize "childfree" lifestyles. NON achieved considerable media popularity, and its message resonated with the hundreds of childless people who wrote to the AVS in the mid-1970s requesting help locating a surgeon willing to operate on them. For example, a woman from Scottsdale, Arizona, wrote the AVS in May 1974. "I have just completed reading the book entitled 'The Baby Trap' by Ellen Peck," she began, adding that Peck listed the AVS in her book as an "agency for people needing help with voluntary sterilization." She explained, "I am 20 years old, single, and have no children. Of course, I am aware that my age and marital status will probably prove to be a hindrance, however, I am deeply devoted to my beliefs and have been for several years. . . . Please send me the names of any doctors, hospitals, or agencies who would consider such a procedure under the given circumstances."[47]

Peck articulated neo-eugenic ideas and praised the AVS in *The Baby Trap*. She attacked welfare and housing policies for encouraging poor women to reproduce and accused women on welfare of having children in order to draw a larger check from the government. "Children allowance seems the poorest of reasons for producing children, it is reason enough for many women," she wrote. Peck saved her most vehement attack for Housing and Urban Development (HUD). "The larger the family, the larger the subsidy . . . basically that's the way it works. That plan not only forces taxpayers to contribute money to bail irresponsible baby-breeders out of their partially self-created financial difficulties; it also encourages those who receive money from H.U.D. to remain poor." She also included sterilization in her chapter about abortion and birth control. Peck explained both tubal ligation and vasectomy and credited both with the ability to liberate recipients by freeing them from fear of unplanned pregnancy. (She credited the Pill with this success, too, and downplayed the medical risks highlighted in the Nelson hearings.) Not surprisingly, she challenged the necessity of the 120 rule and snidely quipped that if the rule remained, "when I'm 120, I can have mine [sterilization]." Peck concluded the chapter by championing the AVS and its executive director, John R. Rague, whose efforts to liberalize sterilization policy she believed would move the childless movement forward by increasing adherents' access to surgery. To encourage readers to contact the AVS, Peck included the AVS's mailing address in the first sentence that referenced the organization.[48]

Although NON's membership peaked at 2,000 people in 1976, its presence and popularity in the national media symbolized a larger cultural shift away from the child-centered families of the 1950s and 1960s. Sterilization offered Americans seeking to avoid parenthood a secure means of achieving this goal. The AVS's referral service and vast network of supportive providers proved to be a critical resource for individuals committed to "childfree" lifestyles. After the mid-1970s, when male and female sterilization had become accessible to the majority of Americans, nonparents' requests became the majority of those the AVS received.[49] Increasingly, they came from younger women and men, like a woman from Spokane, Washington, who wrote to the AVS in 1974. She had read about the organization in *Family Circle* magazine and contacted the organization for help. "I have tried every method [of birth control] from pills to IUD's and they have all proved inadequate. As a result I have had two abortions," she wrote.[50] She did not want to undergo another abortion and thought she could not rely on temporary methods of contraception. But she could not find a doctor willing to sterilize her, even though her husband supported her decision. The AVS suggested she contact Planned Parenthood in Spokane for a referral. It also gave her the name of an outpatient clinic in San Francisco that did not employ age restrictions and could provide financial assistance.[51]

"Vasectomania"

In the late 1960s, independent vasectomy clinics sprang up to meet the growing demand for the surgery. To a large extent, these independent entities represented the culmination of the AVS's and women's attempts to legitimize contraceptive sterilization. A 1966 Gallup Poll reported that 64 percent of Americans approved of permanent birth control for women who bore more children than they could support, and 78 percent approved of voluntary sterilization when additional pregnancies endangered a woman's health. By 1972, a study sponsored by the Commission on Population Growth and the American Future indicated that 80 percent of Americans approved of voluntary sterilization. As public support for the surgery grew, the AVS launched its first successful sterilization clinic, rather ironically, at the Margaret Sanger Research Bureau in New York City. After witnessing its success, dozens of other providers followed the AVS's lead and established outpatient clinics of their own. Sterilization rates rose accordingly.[52]

In 1969, the AVS pledged $30,000 to the Margaret Sanger Research Bureau to establish the country's first freestanding vasectomy clinic in New York City. Built in the bureau's basement, the Margaret Sanger Vasectomy Clinic opened on October 2, 1969, with a backlog of patients. In the first year alone, the clinic responded to 5,147 requests for information, conducted 379 interviews of surgical candidates and their wives, and performed 262 surgeries. By its second anniversary, the clinic had performed over 1,000 vasectomies. The AVS and the Sanger Research Bureau intended for the clinic to "act as a catalyst in the stimulation of more public and medical interest in the method [sterilization] and in the establishment of other similar facilities in the country."[53] They succeeded magnificently. By June 1971, 124 outpatient sterilization clinics had been opened in thirty-three states, including at least five facilities dedicated to female sterilization.[54] The majority of clinics were for vasectomies at this time because of the medical risks involved with tubal ligation. The laparoscopic methods that would reduce the medical risks and ease the cost of tubal ligation were just entering medical practice. With the 120 rule in effect in the majority of institutions, investors likely saw outpatient clinics for the controversial female surgery as risky.

Across the country, vasectomy clinics opened to high patient demand, which led to the creation of long waiting lists. In its first week of business, a Cincinnati clinic cultivated a waiting list holding the names of 160 men. At the same time, the Milwaukee Planned Parenthood Vasectomy Clinic boasted a waiting list of 200 names, while the Ann Arbor (Michigan) Vasectomy Clinic had 400 men waiting for surgery. Over a year after opening, in February 1971, the Sanger clinic in New York reported being "booked solid until July."[55] Planned Parenthood Rhode Island opened the first vasectomy clinic in New England at the end of September 1970. By November, the clinic "had received over 175 applications, and 122 men were waiting for appointments."[56] And in

March 1971, a Houston vasectomy clinic that performed thirty-six surgeries a week had a six-week "backlog" of patients waiting for surgery.[57] Even with the explosion of new clinics, vasectomy providers could not keep up with demand for their services.

In 1971, the AVS assisted with the development of another vasectomy clinic, the Midwest Population Center in Chicago, when it loaned the center $5,000 interest free. The AVS was a secondary financial supporter of this clinic. The facility received the majority of its funding (in the form of a grant and loan) from the Playboy Foundation. The Midwest Population Center viewed the vasectomy clinic as part of a larger initiative to educate the public about over-population and sterilization. In addition to creating the clinic, the center provided office space to ZPG and the Congress on Population and the Environment Inc., planned to organize programs to educate experts and graduate students on sexuality and population issues, and intended to develop a speakers bureau.[58]

Although the Midwest Population Center distributed pamphlets intended to appeal to working-class men, Director Rev. Don C. Shaw claimed that the center's target audience was middle-class men because "it is the middle and upper classes who are contributing the most to the population explosion."[59] The majority of men who underwent vasectomy in the late 1960s and 1970s were white, middle class, and married. They were not the AVS's original target population. As sterilization gained popularity in the late 1960s and early 1970s, an increasing number of working-class and poor men gravitated toward the procedure. Dr. Aquiles Sobrero, director of the Sanger clinic, noticed a diversification in the socioeconomic status of his patients. "At the beginning, we got mostly white-collar workers, doctors, professors, and so forth. Now, the picture is mixed. We are serving almost anyone," he told *Look* magazine in 1971. John R. Rague, executive director of the AVS, confirmed Sobrero's observation: "The people we refer to physicians cut across all classes, from Ph.D.'s to illiterates."[60] A 1973 *Journal of Obstetrics and Gynecology* article on recent vasectomy trends reported that "applications for vasectomy come from individuals of all walks of life."[61] But despite these observations, demographers identified the overwhelming majority of vasectomy patients as white middle-class educated men.[62]

In 1970, just 1 percent of black men had been sterilized as compared to 9 percent of white men.[63] Black men tended to reject sterilization for one of two reasons (or sometimes for both reasons): they equated sterilization with genocide and/or racial oppression, or they mistakenly conflated sterilization with castration. A long history of abuse contributed to these sentiments. From the eighteenth to the early twentieth centuries, white Americans wielded the scalpel as a tool of racial supremacy. In eighteenth-century Virginia, slaves who were found engaging in sexual relations with white women faced castration, and in 1855 the territory of Kansas passed a law that punished black and mixed-race men accused of rape with castration. (Kansas later erased the mention of race from this law, making it applicable to all men convicted of rape.) Other states attempted to pass similar laws, and although they failed, the act of introducing such legislation shows that policy makers attempted to formalize the myth of the black rapist into law. Later in the nineteenth and early twentieth centuries, lynch mobs brutally castrated their victims in order to emasculate black men and terrorize black communities. By the 1930s, the majority of the black community supported birth control, although a few prominent leaders accused white birth control activists of distributing contraception in order to reduce the numbers of blacks in the United States. These concerns increased in the 1960s as family planners began to distribute the Pill and the IUD through newly established family planning clinics that received state funding. The Black Panther Party and the Nation of Islam were especially vocal in their accusations that state-supported family planning was a form of genocide. Most black women, however, did not agree with this position. In Pittsburgh, for example, local black women successfully protested the efforts of militant William Haden to close Planned Parenthood clinics in the Homewood-Brushton neighborhood and other black communities in the city. "We cannot help but notice that most of the anti–birth control pressure is coming from men, men who do not have to bear children," the Welfare Rights Organization of Allegheny County proclaimed. It continued, "We're speaking for the women and we want the Planned Parenthood Centers in our neighborhood."[64]

While black nationalists criticized the politics of permanent contraception, insurance companies debated the economics of sterilization. As the cost of sterilization decreased and the procedure gained medical and public acceptance, private insurance companies began to fund vasectomies and tubal ligations, although many continued to refuse to cover temporary methods of contraception like the Pill. Insurance companies most likely changed their policies to include contraceptive sterilization in an effort to increase the cost-effectiveness of their policies.

Insurance companies' increasing willingness to pay for contraceptive sterilization both shaped and reflected the growing legitimization of the surgery as well as the profitability of the outpatient clinics. As it expanded its referral service in the 1960s, the AVS learned that some insurance companies covered sterilizations performed for medical reasons, which led the organization to search patients' records for a possible medical indication to use in an insurance claim. The AVS's referral service pushed insurance companies and prodded state Medicaid agencies to cover sterilization in order to reduce the financial burden of the procedure on patients and itself. If a patient's insurance company paid, the AVS did not have to administer a loan to this individual and could use its funding to sterilize another "needy" person. This motivated the organization to investigate private insurance coverage of male and female sterilization. In 1969, the AVS released results of a survey measuring third-party coverage of contraceptive sterilization. It found that Blue Cross paid for hospital expenses related to sterilizations performed for medical and socioeconomic reasons in thirty-two of the thirty-nine states it served and paid for medically indicated surgeries (but not socioeconomic ones) in four additional states. For its part, Blue Shield funded surgeries performed for both medical and socioeconomic reasons in thirty of the forty-two states it served. It funded medically indicated surgeries only in six more states.[65] Apparently, these insurance companies had adopted the AVS's rationale that socioeconomic factors were valid indications for sterilization.

Because the AVS worked with many poor people who did not have access to private insurance, the organization also tracked state Medicaid coverage of sterilization and involved itself in public policy debates regarding coverage. In particular, the AVS aimed to persuade states to cover contraceptive sterilization through Medicaid. Under President Lyndon Johnson, the federal government involved itself directly in the provision of family planning services. In 1964, the government awarded Corpus Christi, Texas, a $9,000 grant to provide contraception to poor adults. The Office of Economic Opportunity (OEO) funded similar programs in St. Louis; Austin, Texas; Buffalo, New York; Nashville, Tennessee; and Oakland, California. The OEO expanded its funding of contraception in 1964, and Congress, invigorated by the Supreme Court's ruling in *Griswold v. Connecticut* legalizing contraception for married adults, began to debate bills that authorized federal funding of contraceptive services with the goal of reducing the cost of welfare. During Johnson's tenure, Congress authorized the federal government to fund contraceptive services through existing agencies like the OEO; the Department of Health, Education, and Welfare; the Public Health Service; and the Children's Bureau. The goal of these programs was to reduce the birth rate among the poor and, in doing so, reduce welfare expenses.[66] In 1964 and 1965, the AVS had failed in its attempt to use the Hartman Plan to convince states to include sterilization in their welfare and family planning programs, but a few years later government-supported family planning lost its political taint. The AVS hoped to capitalize on this change and persuade states to expand their Medicaid programs to include contraceptive sterilization.

The AVS was especially engaged in New York State policy debates, in part because it was based in New York City. As the federal government increased funding of family planning services at the state level, states across the nation began to redefine their contraceptive policies. The AVS inserted itself into some of these debates in an effort to broaden states' definitions of contraception to include sterilization and thereby achieve its goal of promoting sterilization as a "solution" to poverty, welfare, overpopulation, and the reproduction of "unfit" Americans. In 1967, the state commissioner of social services in New York contacted the state attorney general to clarify state policy on Medicaid coverage of sterilization for medical and contraceptive purposes. At issue was a 1934 attorney general opinion that determined the state should not assume payment of sterilization "in the absence of legislative authority." Without a law specifically legalizing contraceptive sterilization in New York, the current attorney general refused to allow state funds to cover such surgeries, although he allowed medically indicated surgeries to be covered.[67] The AVS wrote multiple letters to New York state officials urging them to change the policy, but none would without legislative mandate. In 1971, such a bill was introduced. The AVS threw its support behind the legislation, which drew opposition from the commissioner of social services, who continued to favor state funding of medically indicated surgeries only.[68]

Other state legislatures soon followed New York's lead, debating and sometimes passing bills specifically legalizing contraceptive sterilization. The AVS began to assume a watchdog role in the enforcement of these new statutes. When it received letters from men and women and their advocates describing denial of coverage by state officials, the AVS wrote letters to these individuals and their institutions informing them of current policy and asking them to comply with these new rules.[69] Intent on making sterilization accessible to all who wanted and/or "needed" it, the AVS viewed Medicaid as integral to its plans.

The AVS tracked coverage of sterilization in federal/state Medicaid programs (the federal government contributed funds to state services). Its insurance survey found that forty states had Medicaid programs, thirty-four of which covered voluntary sterilization, as did the Virgin Islands and the District of Columbia. Additional surveys reported that coverage for voluntary sterilization grew over the next few years, as family planning expanded with the addition of federal funds. In 1971, the AVS reported that forty-eight states paid for voluntary sterilization under Medicaid programs. Thirty-three of these covered procedures performed for socioeconomic and medical reasons; the remaining programs covered only medically indicated surgeries. By 1973, forty of forty-eight federal/state Medicaid programs covered voluntary sterilization for socioeconomic reasons. Private and public insurance adhered to similar policies. In 1971, Blue Cross covered surgeries performed for medical and socioeconomic reasons in forty-two states. A much larger study of insurance coverage published in 1978 in *Family Planning Perspectives* found female sterilization to be covered by thirty-four of thirty-seven commercial carriers surveyed and vasectomy to be covered by twenty-seven of the thirty-seven carriers.[70]

Insurance coverage coupled with the rapid explosion of vasectomy clinics made sterilization accessible and affordable for American men. The AVS surveys showed that 750,000 vasectomies were performed in 1970, and about 800,000 surgeries were performed the following year. In 1973, the *American Journal of Obstetrics and Gynecology* reported that "the number of vasectomies being done is rapidly approaching one million each year."[71] Women could not say the same about tubal ligation.

Revolutionizing the Technology of Female Sterilization

Two barriers to women's easy access to tubal ligation remained in the early 1970s. First, the technology of female sterilization was stagnant. Before about 1970, tubal ligation required open abdominal surgery, general anesthesia, and a hospital stay of several days.[72] The development of endoscopic methods of surgery radically changed this reality and made sterilization affordable and attractive to many women. Second, age/parity policies continued to obstruct women's access to surgery. Until these barriers were removed, women seeking sterilization continued to be stymied by restrictive hospital policies.

Motivated by the desire to combat overpopulation in poor nations, American physicians began to experiment with endoscopic sterilization techniques in the 1960s.[73] This is not surprising given both population controllers' increasing presence in American politics and federal funding of family planning and population control measures abroad in this decade. In 1965, the Agency for International Development (AID) allocated $2.7 million to combat overpopulation abroad, and two years later Congress passed the Foreign Assistance Act, which allocated $35 million for family planning under Title X. The AID funding supported "assistance" such as the development of clinics and population surveys, but did not include direct provision of contraception to people in nations struggling with population problems. Title X, however, authorized the president to fund private and government programs involved in the distribution of contraception. The same year that Congress passed Title X, it also granted AID the ability to fund birth control as part of its population control efforts. As a result of this legislation, "population control was an integral goal of U.S. economic programs abroad."[74]

Supported by federal grants, American physicians concerned about over-population abroad strove to develop an operative technique that could hasten the spread of permanent contraception in poor countries by reducing the cost and duration of the surgery, as well as by minimizing the invasiveness of the procedure. The laparoscopy, a technique based on the use of an instrument called a laparoscope—a long, narrow "light pipe" with electrified forceps attached—accomplished all of these goals. With the laparoscope, physicians operated through one or two tiny incisions in a woman's navel; the technology eliminated the need for open abdominal surgery entirely. The small incisions, in turn, allowed physicians to replace general anesthetic with a combination of local anesthetic and light sedation and reduced or eliminated the need for a long hospital stay. Female sterilization could now be performed on an outpatient basis. Surgeons nicknamed the laparoscopy "Band-Aid" or "belly-button" surgery because patients left the hospital or clinic with only Band-Aids covering their navel wounds. The laparoscopy left no visible scars after the incision healed. These innovations lowered the cost of surgery by hundreds of dollars, reduced the risks of surgery and postoperative complications, and cut the time it took to perform the procedure from one hour to fifteen minutes.[75]

Having attained success with this technology abroad, some surgeons sought to import the technology back to the United States. Johns Hopkins University gynecologist Clifford Wheeless placed himself at the forefront of this trend. Wheeless trained physicians in Nepal and El Salvador to perform laparoscopic female sterilizations. In 1969, he and Dr. Bruce Thompson (also of Johns Hopkins University School of Medicine) undertook a pilot study of the laparoscopic methods in Baltimore to determine the "feasibility of outpatient sterilization" in American medical practice. The pilot study produced promising results, leading the surgeons to begin a twenty-eight-month study of female outpatient sterilization at Johns Hopkins University that involved 666 laparoscopic surgeries, 72 percent of which were performed outpatient. More than half of the patients (61.5 percent) in the study received subsidized health care. The remaining 38.5 percent were private patients. Patients' income determined who would perform their operation. Residents operated on public patients, while attending physicians sterilized private-pay patients. Put another way, the more experienced surgeons treated private-pay patients while the less experienced surgeons operated on patients who received subsidized health care. Thompson and Wheeless described the "racial distribution of patients" to be "approximately equal," which likely means about half of the patients were black women and half were white women. When they published their findings in *Obstetrics and Gynecology* in 1971, the physicians did not discuss the consent process.[76] Without any mention of informed consent, it is difficult determine if coercion occurred or if the physicians involved in the study respected patients' rights.

In the 1971 article, Thompson and Wheeless concluded that laparoscopic surgery had "significant advantages over former sterilization techniques. It is less expensive, offers better utilization of hospital facilities, and patients return to full function in a shorter period of time." They also maintained that laparoscopy held lower rates of complication than older methods.[77] By 1973, Wheeless had performed over 4,000 laparoscopies in Baltimore. He became so adept at the surgery that he could complete a procedure in eight minutes. The doctor did not underestimate the impact of his work. In 1976, he bragged to *New York Times* journalist Jane Brody that although he was "no women's libber," he had "liberated more women than Gloria Steinem ever thought of."[78]

Wheeless was one of a few surgeons practicing noninvasive methods of tubal ligation in the United States in the early 1970s. Other colleagues, like Dr. Martin Clyman of Mount Sinai Hospital in New York City, performed slightly different versions of the same surgery. Clyman used a tool called the culdoscope, an instrument similar to the laparoscope but used slightly differently; instead of being inserted through the abdomen, the culdoscope was inserted through the vagina.[79] Other surgeons preferred the mini-laparotomy method of tubal ligation. The mini-lap, as physicians called it, was distinct from the other two procedures because it did not involve the use of any rodlike tools, and for this reason was not considered to be an endoscopic method. The mini-lap did not require any additional technologies because the incision in this procedure occurred at the pubic hairline, which allowed for direct visualization of the fallopian tubes. With this method, a surgeon made a small incision at the pubic hairline, retracted the abdomen walls, then used a uterine elevator to bring each fallopian tube through the incision and stitched the tubes together. All three methods of female sterilization achieved popularity in the 1970s. The laparoscopy, however, was physicians' preferred method because it held a low rate of complication and infection and because it allowed physicians to most accurately visualize the pelvic organs, a critical factor when treating patients with suspected abnormalities. General acceptance of the laparoscopy within the profession came in 1973 when the American College of Obstetricians and Gynecologists (ACOG) promulgated formal "Guidelines for Gynecologic Laparoscopy," which included specific qualifications for surgeons using the technology.[80]

Many women learned about these new technologies from the popular media. Women's magazines like *Good Housekeeping*, *Redbook*, and *Mademoiselle* ran articles announcing the availability of these new surgical methods, and many offered testimony from satisfied patients who had been "liberated" from additional pregnancies and financial worries by them.[81] In 1976, *Mademoiselle* ran an article titled "On Being 29 and Having a Tubal Ligation," in which the author, the mother of a two-year-old son, celebrated the certainty she felt regarding her decision to undergo laparoscopy. "Having had a baby, having loved having that baby in every way, I felt I didn't need to do it again. I often look back, but I never go back. Once bottles and diapers were over, I want them over for good."[82] Such sentiments were common among more conservative women's magazines. Women who had been sterilized celebrated their decision to terminate their fertility while at the same time affirmed their mothering capabilities and the joys that motherhood brought them. They also lauded what *Mademoiselle* described as "the simplicity" of laparoscopy. *Good Housekeeping* even titled a 1975 article "A Simple New Kind of Sterilization for Women," which began by describing laparoscopic surgery as "the safest, quickest, most efficient means of sterilizing women."[83] But these magazines did not just celebrate sterilization; they also reminded readers about the permanence of the surgery and cautioned readers not to decide to undergo sterilization quickly, and some offered a series of questions readers should ask themselves before deciding to be sterilized.[84]

The number of female sterilizations performed in the United States doubled between 1970 and 1975, demonstrating the popularity of endoscopic surgery. In 1970, 201,000 tubal ligations were performed in hospitals; by 1975 the number had increased to 550,000. (These numbers do not include independent clinics.) By 1975, tubal ligation had become the third most common surgical procedure on women between the ages of fifteen and forty-four (behind elective abortion and diagnostic dilation and curettage [D&C]).[85] But women's attraction to endoscopic methods only partially explains these numbers. Even with these technological advances, many hospitals refused to rescind their age/parity guidelines. Not until women filed suit against the institutions and individuals who refused their requests for surgery did most hospitals begin to change their policies.

Chapter 3

Sterilizing "Unfit" Women

The practice of involuntary sterilization existed throughout the twentieth century, but it changed over time, with a critical transition occurring in the late 1950s and early 1960s, during the shift from eugenics to neo-eugenics, and another occurring in the late 1960s concurrent with the development of federal family planning. In both moments of transition, region and race intersected to create distinct trends. First, physicians, social workers, and members of state eugenics boards exploited existing eugenic statutes to sterilize poor black women with the specific intention of reducing the number of blacks eligible to receive public assistance. Some southern physicians performed what black women colloquially referred to as "Mississippi appendectomies," or the secret sterilization via hysterectomy of poor black women who entered hospitals for abdominal surgeries—like cesarean sections and appendectomies—and left, unknowingly, without their uteruses. Women of color in other regions came under scrutiny during the second transition. The establishment of federal family planning functioned as a catalyst for this change but was not the only factor responsible for it. Neo-eugenic attitudes and policies also contributed. Physicians who treated patients receiving government aid benefited from the legitimization of contraceptive sterilization and the absence of hospital policies governing informed consent. Physicians recorded forced sterilizations as voluntary, and rising rates of female sterilization in the 1960s and 1970s "hid" their coercion. As contraceptive sterilization gained legitimacy and as federal family planning brought together poor women, especially women of color, and physicians who sought to control their reproduction and funded these interactions, forced sterilization increasingly occurred during childbirth.

The exact number of women involuntarily sterilized between roughly 1950 and 1980 remains unknown. Neither medical institutions nor federal agencies collected the necessary statistics—perhaps an impossible task, as physicians recorded most coercive sterilizations as voluntary, and many women chose not to file formal complaints. Few sterilizations appear suspect when read through the official medical record. Consequently, the burden of verifying abuse fell to victims, an especially difficult task during a decade of rapidly evolving definitions of informed consent and consent policy. Many victims believed their coercive sterilizations to be isolated incidents, and cultural stigmas attached to infertility shamed other victims—especially Native American and Hispanic women—into secrecy.[1] The threat of racial violence prevented still more victims from demanding recourse. "Me? Getting a white lawyer to go against a white doctor?" civil rights leader and sterilization abuse victim Fannie Lou Hamer exclaimed. "I would have been taking my hands and screwing tacks into my own casket."[2] Although exact statistics are not available, experts and contemporary activists have estimated that the total number of forced sterilizations ranged between a few thousand to several hundred thousand.[3]

Images of and Policies to Control the "Welfare Queen"

In the first half of the century, racial segregation created a semiprotective barrier between many poor black women and eugenicists.[4] Largely excluded from state and federal aid and institutions because of their race, many black women escaped eugenicists' grasp. But once civil rights activists threatened to integrate state facilities and the law mandated the inclusion of minorities in the welfare state, some opponents of integration seized sterilization as a weapon to combat racial equality and drew upon neo-eugenic ideas to do so. Integration proved to be bittersweet for victims of sterilization abuse. The Civil Rights Act of 1964 granted people of color full access to federal programs and services such as welfare, public housing, and occupational training, but it also brought them into intimate contact with social workers, physicians, lawyers, welfare workers, and judges who provided family planning services, some of whom who took it upon themselves to sterilize "defective" women in order to reduce their dependence on welfare.

As ideas about reproductive fitness changed, so, too, did images of the "unfit." Women continued to receive the majority of attention because of their ability to bear children, but the ethnicity and race of those targeted changed as Cold War society struggled to accept civil rights, Mexican immigration, an expanding welfare system, and a rise in illegitimacy. Two new stereotypes directly linked ideas about reproductive fitness to poor women of color: the "welfare queen" and the "pregnant pilgrim." Together, these images solidified links between women of color, dependency, lack of reproductive fitness, and single motherhood in the public mind. These stereotypes promoted and reinforced postwar standards of reproductive fitness designed to privilege the reproductive capabilities of white middle-class women. They also affected welfare policy.

The image of welfare recipients changed in the 1950s from that of a sympathetic white widow who had lost a male breadwinner through no fault of her own to a licentious, single black woman who chose welfare over work and bore additional children out of wedlock in order to collect more money from the state. Female recipients of welfare have historically been seen as less deserving of public assistance than men who lost their ability to work because of injury, illness, or old age, but the stereotypes of women on welfare did not become profane until welfare expanded and black women gained access to the rolls.[5] Between 1940 and 1960, Aid to Dependent Children (ADC, renamed Aid to Families with Dependent Children [AFDC] in 1962) expanded from 372,000 to 803,000 families (although the numbers dropped briefly during World War II), and its budget escalated from $133 million to $994 million. By the mid-1950s, unwed mothers and minority women had displaced white widows as the primary recipients of federal aid, and blacks had become overrepresented on the case rolls. Normal population growth and high fertility rates coupled with increasing rates of divorce and desertion among all Americans had caused the number of single women across race seeking aid to rise. On top of these national trends, black families faced high rates of unemployment that stressed household resources, especially among families in the South, where mechanized agriculture displaced workers and segregation pushed blacks into the lowest-paying jobs or out of the market altogether. The intersection of these factors caused black women to become overrepresented in the ADC caseload, although whites remained the largest group receiving aid.[6]

These trends accelerated in the 1960s. Between 1961 and 1967, the total number of recipients jumped from roughly 3.5 million to 5.0 million, and by 1967 single women constituted three-quarters of all AFDC cases. The cost of AFDC grew as well, from $994 million in 1960 to $2.2 billion in 1967.[7] Three factors caused this expansion. First, Congress inaugurated President Lyndon B. Johnson's Great Society, and the Johnson administration actively recruited eligible citizens to enroll in these new programs. Second, civil rights victories, most notably the Civil Rights Act of 1964, granted blacks access to federal aid, which automatically increased the number of black women eligible for AFDC. Third, the Supreme Court dismantled discriminatory state welfare practices such as midnight raids, residency requirements, home checks, and man-in-the-house policies in 1966 and 1967. As a result, by 1970 the number of welfare recipients had increased by 35 percent.[8]

Conservative white Americans, especially those upset by integration, ignored these factors and instead blamed recipients' "immorality" and "irresponsible" reproduction for the increased enrollment. Many worried that their tax dollars were being used to support an underclass of dependent women who rejected the values they endorsed as central to maintaining a strong nation during the Cold War. A Gallup Poll conducted in 1964 reflected these concerns. Pollsters asked, "What proportion of persons do you think are on relief for dishonest reasons—most, some, hardly any, or none?" Sixty-one percent of respondents believed "at least 'some' dishonesty" existed among welfare recipients.[9] This suspicion is connected to the development of the "welfare queen" image that portrayed welfare recipients as conniving and deceitful.

The media chronicled this suspicion. A 1966 *Wall Street Journal* article depicted white animosity against welfare recipients. "I know of young Negro girls who get themselves deliberately pregnant so they can go on welfare," a Philadelphia secretary reported. A Fall River, Massachusetts, garage owner proclaimed, "The only ones benefiting from the way they're running things now are bums, deadbeats, and people who just don't give a darn about earning a living." The Catholic magazine *America* ran an article on "welfare backlash" the same year. This piece defended welfare programs as "one of the most humane features of American society," but conceded that "there are, of course, malingers on the relief rolls. There are pitiable people who make a vocation of welfare— men and women congenitally allergic to honest toil." Even this article, written in defense of welfare and of the "honest and helpless poor," expressed the neo-eugenic notion that some people were "inherently" "unfit," dishonest, and unworthy of government support.[10]

Public ideas about the purpose of welfare changed during the baby boom years. Once a program of child aid used by respectable mothers caught in difficult circumstances, in the 1950s welfare became characterized in popular discourse as a program of mothers' aid exploited by "welfare queens." The city of Newburgh, New York, sparked the first national debate about welfare, which solidified the association between black illegitimacy, welfare, and immorality in the public mind. In 1961, the city enacted a thirteen-point plan to overhaul its welfare system with the intention of expelling the "undeserving" from its rolls. Other northern cities followed. The plan's author, City Manager Joseph Mitchell, infused his welfare policy with the politics of race by accusing blacks, especially migrants, of enrolling in public assistance programs in order to avoid paid labor. Linking dependency to illegitimacy and accusing poor black women of deliberately becoming pregnant in order to extort government subsidies, Mitchell held that the city's welfare system encouraged a "culture of welfare" that bred violence and criminality.[11] The term "culture of welfare" referenced common neo-eugenic ideas about reproductive fitness that cited culture as the way in which "unfit" women reproduced their immorality and defects. Mitchell and his supporters did not want their government to support the reproduction of "defective," "lazy" citizens who they assumed would raise their children with the same values of shiftlessness and immorality.

Mitchell's policy drew upon existing strategies used by Congress and the states to reduce the welfare rolls, shame recipients, and force single women into nuclear family households. In 1951, Congress passed the Jenner Amendment, authorizing states to publicize the names of welfare recipients under the guise of curbing welfare fraud. States took even more drastic action during the next decade. They removed thousands of women and children from the rolls by reducing their welfare expenditures and shrinking public services. Nearly half of all the states also employed man-in-the-house, suitable home, or substitute father policies, which assumed that recipients' boyfriends provided for their children and hence such families no longer required public aid. In theory, "suitable home" policies sought to ensure that poor children resided in nurturing, safe environments. In practice, they punished illegitimacy by withholding aid from unwed mothers, especially women of color. Most states employed a single criterion to define an "unsuitable home": illegitimacy. These policies targeted black women, who constituted a disproportionate number of unwed mothers enrolled in federal programs. For example, in Louisiana in 1960, 66 percent of children receiving ADC were black, and 98 percent of these children were born out of wedlock.[12]

These policies reflected the belief that women who received state aid should relinquish reproductive self-determination as a condition of receiving assistance. In legislators' and supporters' minds, the "privilege" of reproductive decision making resided with the government and the taxpayers who financed the welfare system: poor women had no right to bear children whom they could not support. The welfare system itself institutionalized this assumption. Between 1910 and 1920, mothers' pensions provided poor single women with stipends on the condition that they submit to government regulation of their private relationships and family life.[13] Their successors, ADC and AFDC, advanced similar stipulations, such as requiring recipients to submit to unscheduled home visits. The Supreme Court struck down especially intrusive practices like midnight raids in 1967 and man-in-the-house policies in 1968, but the neo-eugenic notion that middle-class taxpayers held a direct investment in, and thus the right to determine, the reproductive choices of welfare recipients continued to gain favor as the decade progressed and America entered the 1970s.

The welfare queen stereotype chastised poor black women for "choosing" to engage in "deviant" sexual behavior while simultaneously suggesting that their "inherent" promiscuity and hypersexuality drove this behavior. In this way, the myth integrated biological, moral, and economic determinism. This synthesis of eugenic and neo-eugenic logic reflected contemporary scientific trends; by the 1940s social and biological scientists had resolved the nature-nurture controversy by declaring genetics and the environment to be interdependent variables.[14] By naturalizing black women's "deviant" sexuality, neo-eugenicists ensured that this behavior could only be attributed to black women. White women could never be accused of possessing the same "vulgar" sexual appetites and "inherent" licentiousness as black women because they would never be black. With the number of illegitimate births rising (the illegitimacy rate tripled between 1940 and 1957), neo-eugenicists used the fixed variable of race to distinguish between white and black unwed mothers and to reinforce a social hierarchy that preserved white supremacy during a period when white women's illegitimacy rates rose faster than those of black women.[15]

In the post–baby boom era, poor black women, especially unwed mothers, were considered "unfit" by definition. Neo-eugenicists placed poor black women in a double bind: they criticized them for their lack of reproductive fitness while simultaneously upholding standards of fitness based upon race and class that prevented these women from ever achieving an "acceptable" level of fitness. The myth of the welfare queen ensured that poor black mothers could never be "fit" so long as they remained poor and black—and because women could not change their race and punitive welfare policies and a lack of economic opportunities prevented many recipients from rising out of poverty, this population became "destined" to exemplify the "pathological" behavior ascribed to their race and poverty. In the 1960s, unwed black mothers came to represent the "pathologies" of the black family and community. The myth of the welfare queen nurtured this association, as did Senator Daniel Patrick Moynihan's infamous 1965 report on the black family, which blamed black crime, unemployment, single motherhood, and other social "pathologies" upon black "matriarchs."[16] Both stereotypes naturalized race and class differences by grounding these differences in a language of cultural deficiency that could be reproduced across generations.

In the late 1950s, lawmakers began to introduce bills designed to control the reproduction of "welfare queens," to use public policy to regulate "unfit" women's behavior and punish them for bearing children out of wedlock. State legislators proposed bills that criminalized illegitimacy among welfare recipients and sentenced "unfit" women (and occasionally men) to sterilization. Across the nation, but especially in southern states, legislators drafted bills to punish welfare recipients who bore two or more illegitimate children with incarceration, sterilization, a fine, or a combination of all three. In 1960, the Maryland Senate debated a bill that would subject any woman convicted of bearing two or more children out of wedlock to a fine of up to $1,000 or a prison term of under three years, or both. Under this bill, a woman convicted of the crime of illegitimacy would be declared unfit to parent and would lose custody of her children. The Maryland bill passed the senate by a vote of twenty-three to three, but suffered defeat in the House of Delegates.[17] Two years earlier, the Mississippi legislature debated "An Act to Discourage Immorality of Unmarried Females by Providing for Sterilization of the Unwed Mothers." The act read, "The birth of a second illegitimate child to any unmarried female shall subject her to the provisions of this act and a proceeding to have the unmarried female temporarily or permanently sterilized."[18] The bill died in the house, but in 1964 another Mississippi legislator took up the cause and introduced a similar bill, but with a few crucial differences. Under the second bill, parents convicted of being involved in the birth of an illegitimate child could be subjected to incarceration for one to three years. This bill was distinctive because, unlike the others, it aimed to punish both women and men for illegitimacy. Parents convicted of illegitimacy a second time would face between three and five years of jail time, but they could "submit to sterilization in lieu of imprisonment." The house approved the bill by a vote of seventy-two to thirty-seven, but public backlash caused Mississippi lawmakers to modify the bill significantly. They dropped sterilization altogether, reduced the jail time to between thirty and ninety days, and decreased the fine to less then $250.[19]

Numerous states proposed similar bills, but only two states succeeded in criminalizing out-of-wedlock births—although neither law included sterilization penalties. Several bills intended to punish illegitimacy with sterilization passed both houses only to be killed by a governor. Others passed only a single house, and still others died in committee. All, however, generated public debate about "proper" standards of reproductive fitness and whether the government held the right to legislate the reproduction of citizens receiving welfare. Politicians on both sides of the debate campaigned on the issue, local and national newspapers reported on the progress of proposed illegitimacy bills, and activist groups like the American Civil Liberties Union (ACLU) and Student Nonviolent Coordinating Committee (SNCC) vocalized their dissent through press releases and publications like SNCC's *Genocide in Mississippi* (1966) that brought the debate to a national level. The ACLU's criticism of the proposed bills is consistent with its commitment to civil rights, begun in the 1950s.[20] Although the ACLU would later commit to defending American women's reproductive freedom when it formed the Reproductive Freedom Project in March 1972, in the early-to-mid-1960s the organization had not yet established a clear position on women's reproductive rights, and thus its opposition centered on racial discrimination rather than women's rights. This is not surprising, as *Griswold v. Connecticut* (1965), legalizing contraception for married couples, had just been decided, and both the second-wave feminism and abortion rights movements were in their infancy.[21]

Debates about legislators' ability to regulate the reproduction of welfare recipients extended beyond the introduction of bills aiming to punish poor Americans who bore children out of wedlock. In 1965, *U.S. News and World Report* published an interview with Stanford physicist and Nobel Laureate William Shockley titled, "Is the Quality of U.S. Population Declining?" Basing his claim on his statistical analyses, Shockley suggested that whites were inherently more intelligent than blacks and urged his fellow scientists to take up the study of race and intelligence in an effort to evaluate the effectiveness of President Johnson's antipoverty programs.[22] Shockley's interview and subsequent scholarship on the topic set off national debates about genetic differences between whites and blacks that reinforced the prejudices inherent in the welfare queen stereotype and lent "scientific" authority to this bigotry. The physicist spent the next decade actively promoting his theory of dysgenics, or "retrogressive evolution," which held that the unrestrained reproduction of the poorest and least intelligent citizens would eventually lead to the "unfit" out-"breeding" the "fit."[23] Shockley was not alone in his musings about the role of genetics in shaping social dynamics. One year earlier, Dwight J. Ingle, a University of Chicago physicist, published an article in *Science* in which he declared that "the very high birth rate among indolent Negroes is a threat to the future success of this race."[24] Both scholars continued the eugenic tradition of employing scientific evidence to support their claims of inherited differences between the races. Richard J. Herrnstein and Charles Murray used a similar framework in *The Bell Curve: Intelligence and Class Structure in American Life*, published in 1994.[25]

A few years after President Johnson inaugurated his Great Society, some scholars began to assess the program's impact, and a minority began to use claims of genetic difference to support their rejection of antipoverty initiatives, especially when used to bolster the socioeconomic status of blacks. These scholars questioned Johnson's efforts to link civil rights and antipoverty initiatives by suggesting that blacks were inherently less intelligent than whites and therefore unable to effectively participate in federal programs designed to raise their socioeconomic status. In 1969, Arthur Jensen, a professor of educational psychology at the University of California, Berkeley (who met Shockley in 1968 when he accepted a fellowship at Stanford's Center for Advanced Study of Behavior Sciences), published a controversial article in the *Harvard Educational Review* titled "How Much Can We Boost IQ and Scholastic Achievement?" in which he intended to explain why the War on Poverty was not more successful. Jensen suggested that the inferior intelligence of black Americans could account for the relative failure of many programs. "But such a hypothesis," he maintained, "is anathema to many social scientists. The idea that the lower average intelligence and scholastic performance of Negroes could involve not only environmental, but also genetic, factors has been strongly denounced. But it has been neither contradicted nor discredited by evidence."[26] Shockley proved to be one of the few scholars who supported Jensen's thesis.[27] If in fact blacks were not as intelligent as whites, he repeatedly postulated, then Head Start and other Great Society programs designed to improve the socioeconomic status of black Americans must be rethought since environmental changes could not alter genetic "deficiencies."

As noted scientists working at premier universities and publishing in respected journals, Shockley and Jensen possessed the status necessary to have their work taken seriously by their colleagues and the media. Shockley's ideas grew increasingly radical as the 1960s gave way to the 1970s. "We fear that 'fatuous beliefs' in the power of welfare money unaided by eugenic foresight may contribute to the decline of human quality," he insisted in March 1970, the same year he established the Foundation for Research and Education on Eugenics and Dysgenics (FREED).[28] FREED boasted several prominent scientists as members as well as connections to the few individuals and organizations that remained committed to traditional eugenic ideas and practices. R. Travis Osborn, a member of the Executive Committee of the International Association for the Advancement of Ethnology and Eugenics, who served as an expert witness for segregationists attempting to overturn *Brown v. Board of Education* (1954), assumed the role of adviser to the organization.[29] One of FREED's major sources of financial support was the Pioneer Fund, created in 1937 by Wycliffe P. Draper to fund eugenic-related research. In 1977, the *New York Times* found that the Pioneer Fund contributed over $179,000 to Shockley. Remaining traditional eugenicists felt invigorated by Shockley and attached themselves to his organization, as did segregationists and members of the Ku Klux Klan (KKK) and the Citizens' Council, who appropriated "scientific" ideas that validated their racial prejudices.[30]

All three scientists—Ingle, Jensen, and Shockley—challenged the effectiveness of welfare and other government programs to improve the socioeconomic status of the poor, especially of poor blacks. If intelligence is largely determined by genetics, they maintained, then alternative solutions to poverty, illegitimacy, criminality, and joblessness must be identified. Two of the three—Ingle and Shockley—recommended sterilization as a plausible alternative, and in doing so followed the lead of state legislators working to criminalize illegitimacy in order to shrink the welfare rolls. Ingle believed sterilization to be appropriate for "all who, either because of genetic limitations or poor cultural heritage, are unable to endow children with a reasonable chance to achieve happiness, self-sufficiency, and good citizenship." He proposed the quarantine of "defectives" in what psychologist William Tucker calls "low IQ housing."[31] Shockley advanced several sterilization proposals, which he called "thinking exercises," that drew upon fears of overpopulation. His first plan called for government regulation of reproduction. In this system, citizens would be issued "deci-child" certificates that could be used for a pregnancy, or bought or sold on the market or through members of the New York Stock Exchange. The consequence of this plan (which he outlined in detail) would be that "only people who want and can afford children will have them."[32] This plan clearly intended to reduce the welfare "burden" and to appeal to those offended by "welfare queens." In a second plan, Shockley proposed to pay "a bonus rate of $1,000 for each point below 100 I.Q.," and again linked his proposal to anxiety about overpopulation. "We have to deal with [the] population explosion," he implored. To ensure that those not "bright enough to learn of the bonuses on their own" would be reached, Shockley actually suggested using bounty hunters to track down the "unfit."[33]

Scientists who linked race to intelligence and who argued that blacks were inherently less intelligent than whites and therefore needed to have their reproduction controlled for them represented a minority opinion in this era of civil rights and black nationalism. Jensen faced considerable backlash from his colleagues, the public, and students who picketed his office and demand that he be fired. Shockley's talks met with frequent protests from university students.[34]

Although Shockley's radical theories constituted a minority perspective, they continued to draw audiences and controversy for over a decade because Shockley tapped into neo-eugenic sentiments within the general population. Letters written to Shockley by nonacademics, by people who had seen him on television or read about his ideas in the papers, indicate that his concerns resonated with many whites at the grassroots levels, especially those attracted to the conservative politics of the era. Many conservative working- and middle-class whites viewed integration as a direct assault on their social and economic status; Shockley's theories provided them with a "legitimate" defense of the privileges of whiteness they sought to protect. Several writers used Shockley's ideas to reinforce their own prejudicial ideas about differences between the races. "As a white female employee of one of America's leading airlines I have daily encounters with the black race at Detroit Metropolitan airport," one woman wrote in 1973. She continued, "perhaps knowing 'why' would help me better understand the stupidity, ignorance, and harassment which I must contend with each day."[35] A man from Inglewood, California, wrote in 1973, "I am by no stretch . . . a racist, but I have been a student of history throughout most of my life. . . . I have been at a loss to explain the lack of progress in history by the Black populace throughout the world. My professors could not, or/nor would not, explain the Blacks' apparent lack of development compared to other racial groupings."[36] This man believed that Shockley had provided such an explanation. Similarly, a white substitute teacher of biology and science in Wichita, Kansas, wrote that Shockley's findings confirmed her own experiences in public schools. She claimed to have witnessed "the inability of almost all black students to grasp complicated concepts."[37] An Oklahoma City woman wrote to Shockley in 1974 to inform the professor that his theories reinforced her own ideas about inherent intellectual and cultural differences between blacks and whites. "I have lived around two generations of Negroes & while I am very fond of the man who has worked for me for years, & his college-educated children," she wrote, "I can't help but believe they just have a different culture or something inherently different from that of the white man."[38] This woman's use of Shockley's theories to explain her own prejudices reflects a powerful and popular trend in neo-eugenic thought: it did not really matter whether differences between the races were ascribed to genetics or environment, what mattered was that a difference could be "scientifically" identified and used to legitimize ideas of racial difference.

Shockley and his likeminded colleagues and supporters focused most of their attention on antipoverty initiatives related to education, but their sterilization theories extended into the realm of welfare. Shockley, in particular, explicitly used the language of overpopulation and eugenics to urge Americans to take action to reduce an "inevitable" drag on the nation's genes by large poor families, especially black ones. In this way, Shockley's ideas intersected with popular stereotypes like the welfare queen that suggested that poor black women could not manage their reproduction "responsibly" and that their failure to do so would have profound consequences on American society. "Our society is being profoundly irresponsible," he declared. Linking this "irresponsibility" to welfare, he warned that "our nobly-intended welfare programs may be encouraging dysgenics."[39]

The stereotype of the welfare queen caused so much resentment among white middle-class conservative Americans for the same reason: because it was the antithesis of the values they sought to embody. Postwar prosperity brought an unprecedented number of white Americans into the middle class. Roughly ten years after the conclusion of World War II, nearly 60 percent of Americans had achieved middle-class status (as opposed to only 31 percent of Americans before the Depression).[40] Many of these newcomers to the middle class had advanced economically because of government subsidies in the form of the GI Bill, which financed education and supplied homeowner and business loans for veterans. But the new middle class distinguished itself from other classes that received government aid. Most of its members believed themselves to be "worthy" and "deserving" of these benefits, which they viewed as very different from welfare and other "handouts."[41]

Politicians who employed the image of the welfare queen pitted the interests of white middle-class families against those of poor black women and declared the latter to be undeserving of federal support while simultaneously reinforcing the deserving nature of the former. In addition, Cold War conservatives had already linked the preservation of the white nuclear family to national security by declaring the family to be a bulwark against Communism.[42] The welfare queen stereotype took this one step further by suggesting that preventing the "undeserving" from "leaching" onto the welfare system for support was an act of patriotism, a reaffirmation of the postwar democratic values of thrift, hard work, and the nuclear family. In this context, sterilization, as suggested by Shockley and conservative politicians, appeared to be an effective means of protecting white middle-class values and their attendant privileges.

Racializing Reproductive Fitness: "Pregnant Pilgrims"

The "welfare queen" became a popular stereotype in the 1960s that paved the way for other racially constructed negative images of poor women of color to emerge in the 1970s. Although it never became a national image to the extent that the "welfare queen" did, the "pregnant pilgrim" became a popular image in California in the 1970s, especially in southern cities like Los Angeles that witnessed a rise in Mexican immigration. Conservative Californians, concerned about overpopulation, the expansion of welfare, and changing ethnic demographics, began to accuse new immigrants of deliberately fleecing the state welfare system. A 1973 study found 8 to 9 percent of welfare recipients to be undocumented immigrants who received $100 million a year in social services. Los Angeles County commissioned a special report to investigate the "fleecing" of local services by these "undeserving" immigrants. The results conflicted with popular sentiment: the study reported that a "negligible" number of "aliens" received welfare. This disconnect characterized the public debates surrounding the issue of whether illegal immigrants could receive state aid. In general, public anger far exceeded the actual "problem."

One specific stereotype emerged from these discussions: the "pregnant pilgrim," which described a pregnant Mexican woman who crossed the border in order to give birth in an American hospital to an American citizen eligible for welfare. Newspapers like the *San Antonio Express*, *El Paso Times*, and *Arizona Republic* published a host of articles about this "problem" in the mid-1970s. One such article claimed that 45 percent of women who delivered in a Los Angeles County hospital "involve illegal alien women giving birth to brand new U.S. citizens."[43] Letters written by "concerned citizens" to the Sierra Club and Zero Population Growth (ZPG) echoed similar sentiments. In personal correspondence to the leader of ZPG, one man linked issues of immigration to those of population control and environmental preservation when he complained that Mexican immigrants "cancel the benefits of conservation." "The foreigners raise large families and defeat the birth control program," he proclaimed, adding, "Besides, there are many in our jails, mental institutions, and on welfare which cost us millions."[44] In 1973, California's Social Welfare Board weighed in on the debate when it reported that "aliens in California are getting at least $100 million in services to which they are not entitled."[45]

At the core of these editorials, news stories, and the debates they ignited was the issue of who should be able to legitimately access public services. Like criticisms of "welfare queens," debates about "pregnant pilgrims" featured the voices of white middle-class Americans who believed that the payment of taxes granted them the authority to determine how their contributions would be spent. These critics insisted that "if you worked hard you would be a success." Many social conservatives in Southern California and the Sun Belt, where the conservative movement developed in the postwar years, felt strongly that citizens should bear responsibility for their own welfare and believed that if recent immigrants and the poor would only adopt a Protestant work ethic, they, too, would succeed. They challenged the government's efforts to redistribute wealth and expressed anger that local and state governments expanded welfare programs without consulting middle-class taxpayers, whose money funded public assistance programs.[46]

In California and other border states experiencing a wave of Mexican immigration during the 1970s, issues of ethnicity and class also shaped the discussion, as did fears of overpopulation. The "pregnant pilgrim" constituted a threat not only because critics believed her to be "unethical" in her pursuit of American welfare (that is, getting paid for not working) but also because they believed her to be hyperfertile as well (her "contributions" to society were negative and detrimental). The two issues were linked in the public mind: hyperfertility contributed to the dependence of a "pregnant pilgrim" on welfare because she chose to have more children than she could support on her own. Like eugenicists decades earlier, social scientists of the era produced research, especially population-related studies, that reinforced the popular notion that Mexican women were dangerously hyperfertile, and this scholarship lent a scientific legitimacy to immigrant opponents' calls to close the border and deny Mexican immigrants access to public services. Despite claims of objectivity, some of this scholarship reflected researchers' own racial assumptions about Mexican women and their fertility.[47]

Social scientists and politicians were not alone in their evaluations of Mexican women's fertility and the demographics of Mexican families. Population controllers and environmental groups also expressed concern about the negative consequences of Mexican immigration. The Sierra Club wanted to restrict Mexican immigration as a means of preventing overpopulation, but chose not to lobby for federal legislation for fear of appearing racist. ZPG had the same fears, but approved a platform seeking an end to illegal immigration and a huge reduction in legal immigration in 1974. The following year, the organization made immigration a central issue and drew upon the expertise of population control expert and activist Paul Ehrlich to elicit public support for the cause. Ehrlich cautioned that Mexicans were immigrating in families, sometimes with pregnant members, with the intention of settling permanently. He warned about the economic consequences of this trend, estimating that illegal Mexican immigrants were "costing American taxpayers an estimated $10 to $13 billion a year in lost earnings and taxes, in welfare benefits and public service."[48] Ehrlich's message was clear: those who allowed illegal immigration to continue did so at their own financial risk. The threat of pregnant immigrants added another dimension to the issue, as those women who bore children in the United States produced citizens legally eligible for welfare. The president of the Los Angeles chapter of ZPG reiterated this concern when she maintained that California was overflowing with "Mexican immigrants with a baby-producing culture that won't quit."[49]

ZPG's derogatory attitude toward Mexican immigrants sheds light on its contraceptive sterilization-related activism in the early 1970s. In 1971, the

Association for Voluntary Sterilization (AVS), ZPG, and the ACLU joined together to launch a series of lawsuits designed to overturn restrictive hospital policies and make contraceptive sterilization available on demand (which will be discussed later). A few years after opposing punitive sterilization legislation, the ACLU had begun to develop a position on reproductive freedom, and it undertook these suits in the interest of defending women's right to contraception without arbitrary interference. The AVS and ZPG, however, sought to open access to sterilization in order to increase its prescription for poverty, dependence on welfare, and illegitimacy. For California-based ZPG and its founder, biologist Paul Ehrlich, Mexican women constituted the population most in need of permanent contraception, and ZPG members believed they had the academic evidence to prove it. They fought for sterilization on demand not to expand women's reproductive freedom, but instead to promote the surgery among the poor in the interest of reducing the threat of a population explosion and the cost of welfare.

As they had with the "welfare queen," critics viewed sterilization as a potential solution to overpopulation, a way to ensure that "hyperfertile" women could not "fleece" the welfare system and receive benefits that they did not deserve and that taxpayers did not want them to receive. Ten years passed between the appearance of these two images. In the late 1950s and early 1960s, critics of the "welfare queen" put forth formal legislative proposals for sterilization. In the late 1960s and early 1970s, physicians at public hospitals undertook their own sterilization plans, using the opportunities provided by the development of federal family planning and the legitimization of permanent contraception. Lawmakers in the early 1960s attempted to establish a system that would bring women into contact with public health providers and fund their sterilization. By the 1970s, such institutions were already in existence, and forced sterilization flourished.

When Legislation Fails, Try the Courts

In the late 1950s and early 1960s, state legislators failed to pass laws that punished illegitimacy with sterilization, but judges proved more successful in forcing the "unfit" to accept permanent contraception. In 1959, three grand juries in Georgia considered recommending sterilization for mothers of illegitimate children. In the early 1960s, California judges actually implemented similar plans.[50] Two California cases merit closer inspection because they expose the social engineering imperatives that drove these judges to overextend their prescribed authority and sentence "unfit" men and women to sterilization.

The first case involved Miguel Vega Andrade, a father of four who in 1960 injured his back, lost his job, and separated from his wife. For the first two years after his injury, he received $200 a month in medical compensation and paid $120 of that to his wife in child support. When these payments ceased, in the fall of 1963, his wife charged him with nonsupport. Andrade pleaded guilty in December, and the county prosecutor recommended probation. Pasadena Municipal Court Judge Joseph A. Sprankle ignored this recommendation and instead offered Andrade the choice of sterilization and marriage to his current girlfriend or jail. Andrade chose the first option, got married, had a vasectomy, found a job washing dishes, and resumed child support payments. In February 1964, Sprankle granted him probation. Later that year, Andrade decided to have children with his new wife. His lawyer petitioned the California Supreme Court for a writ of habeas corpus and asked the U.S. Supreme Court to hear the case, but both courts denied the appeal. Judge Sprankle expressed surprise at Andrade's regret, telling *Time* magazine that, until he met Andrade, he had "counseled" vasectomy in several hundred nonsupport cases without complaint.[51] Apparently, this judge believed that men who were unable to pay child support should lose the ability to bear children and that he held the authority to compel those who came before him to "choose" surgery. Sprankle's logic reflects neo-eugenic attitudes of the era, but his policy is distinctive because it targeted men, not women. Most other judges and physicians involved in punitive sterilization directed their actions at women because of their ability to become pregnant.

Andrade's case received brief national attention, but failed to spark considerable public debate about the ethics of sterilization sentences and the boundaries of citizens' reproductive rights. Nancy Hernandez's case did. Her story remained national news for days, and immediately after newspapers announced her sentence, more than 300 people offered to sign a petition in protest.[52] In May 1966, Santa Barbara Municipal Court Judge Frank P. Kearney found Hernandez guilty of a misdemeanor for occupying a room that contained marijuana. Estranged from her first husband with whom she had a daughter, Hernandez, age twenty-one, had been living with her boyfriend, Joseph Sanchez, and their daughter. When police raided the drug dealer's apartment, they found Hernandez in the same room as Sanchez's marijuana stash and charged her with the misdemeanor.[53]

Judge Kearney offered Hernandez a choice between probation with permanent sterilization or a six-month jail term. At her probation hearing, before her attorney arrived, Hernandez accepted sterilization and probation. "I was shocked and didn't want to go to jail and leave my children," she later explained.[54] A local priest, a physician, and several family members intervened and convinced Hernandez to reverse her decision. Judge Kearney, in turn, revoked her probation and sentenced Hernandez to three months in jail effective immediately.

Hernandez's lawyer quickly submitted a writ of habeas corpus and petitioned for her client's release from the court order she described as "unreasonable, capricious, illegal, and unconstitutional," and designed "to shock the moral sense of the community."[55] Describing Judge Kearney's decision as "arbitrary and outside the law," Superior Court Judge C. Douglas Smith granted both petitions and reprimanded Kearney. "Judges may not ignore a law simply because they do not like it or believe in it."[56]

Municipal Court Judge Kearney based his decision on neo-eugenic principles. He assumed that because Hernandez lived with a drug user, committed adultery, and bore an illegitimate child, she would inevitably descend into the criminal world of drugs and illicit behavior. "It seemed to me she should not have more children because of her propensity to live an immoral life," Kearney maintained.[57] Similarly, like physicians who coercively sterilized their patients, the judge extended his professional authority to advance his own social welfare agenda. Rather than enforcing established policy through his legal interpretations as the law required, Kearney designed and implemented his own public policy in the courtroom. He sentenced Hernandez to sterilization in the interest of reducing the state's welfare expenditures and preventing the reproduction of subsequent generations of "unfit" citizens, something he considered "inevitable" given Hernandez's lifestyle. He also never questioned his authority to dictate Hernandez's reproductive decisions, a trait he shared with physicians who performed forced sterilizations. Evaluation of Hernandez's maternal fitness lay far beyond the bounds of the case—which involved the defendant's proximity to marijuana, not her parenting skills—yet Kearney located it at the center. Superior Court Judge Smith acknowledged this when he overturned Hernandez's sentence. He reminded Kearney that while "law-abiding taxpayers" may resent supporting the poor with "their hard-earned tax dollars," the issue of Hernandez's reproductive fitness was entirely unrelated to the drug-related misdemeanor she faced.[58]

Yet even after Kearney's ruling was overturned, the judge insisted that he had acted within his jurisdiction. Kearney claimed Hernandez's sentence represented "nothing novel, legally, medically, or sociologically," and noted that he did not order Hernandez to be sterilized; instead, he had offered sterilization as an alternative to incarceration.[59] The logic underlying his offer remains fuzzy. Even conservative social critic William F. Buckley Jr. criticized the incongruity between the crime and punishment in Hernandez's case. Writing for the *National Review*, Buckley editorialized, "the act of sterilization is no more symmetrical to the charge of drug-taking, than, say, a frontal lobotomy is to drunken driving." Further ridiculing Kearney's ruling, Buckley snidely predicted that "it would only be a matter of time before he [Kearney] started offering, in lieu of stiff jail sentences, the rack, or the whipping post."[60] Judge Kearney defended his order by arguing that California law gave courts "the right to place a defendant on probation on terms aimed at the reasonable rehabilitation of the defendant."[61] Exactly how sterilization would have rehabilitated Hernandez for occupying a room with marijuana remains a mystery. But for Kearney, as well as other neo-eugenic judges and lawmakers, establishing congruity between the crime and the punishment was not the critical issue; preventing "unfit" women like Hernandez from bearing children was of primary importance.

Andrande's and Hernandez's cases serve as a bridge between eugenics and neo-eugenics in American judicial practice. They involve judges developing their own punishments for "deviant" social behavior that raise questions about citizens' private rights. Eugenic statutes were premised on the idea that the state's interest in the health of its citizens and the reproduction of a healthy society granted it the right to revoke certain citizens' ability to reproduce, specifically citizens "shown" to have been physically "defective" in some way. But neither case followed established eugenic law; instead, they involved judges operating outside of established legal boundaries to inscribe their personal politics on the bodies of "unfit" individuals who appeared before them for unrelated matters. The concept of reproductive rights did not enter public discussion until the late 1960s, after the Supreme Court identified a constitutional right to reproductive privacy in *Griswold v. Connecticut* and after feminists began to demand the legalization of abortion. Yet the extent to which the state could legally interfere in its citizens' reproductive decisions and to which citizens could protect themselves from such interference was contested in these early cases. In subsequent years, doctors would replace judges as the experts who sentenced the "unfit" to sterilization.

Early Sterilization Abuse

Changing images of "unfit" mothers coupled with changing welfare and family planning policies contributed to changing sterilization practices. The number of sterilizations performed under eugenic statutes fell dramatically during World War II and never returned to the prewar levels. But although the number of eugenic sterilizations decreased after the war, the practice of forced sterilization did not end; rather, it transformed to reflect new social and cultural anxieties and respond to new technologies like the laparoscopy. The surgeries performed in the 1950s and early 1960s represent a transition from the eugenic surgeries of the first half of the century to the neo-eugenic surgeries of the late 1960s and 1970s. In the 1950s and early 1960s, forced sterilization was confined largely to the South and assumed two forms: use of existing eugenics laws to sterilize poor unwed black mothers, and "Mississippi appendectomies." By the 1970s, new trends in forced sterilization had spread from the South to the rest of the country through federal family planning, and forced sterilization was increasingly performed under the guise of voluntary contraceptive surgery.

In the late 1950s, southern neo-eugenicists opposed to integration and resistant to the civil rights movement began to employ existing state eugenic statutes to force poor black women to undergo unwanted and unnecessary tubal ligations. North Carolina was one of a few states to continue its eugenic sterilization program in the postwar years. Designed to reduce welfare rolls and prevent the reproduction of "feebleminded" citizens "destined" to dependency on the state, North Carolina's eugenic laws remained active and in use in the 1950s. But in the 1960s, the target demographic changed from poor white women to poor women of color, who were increasingly labeled "unfit," as welfare expanded and the previous barriers to public aid for people of color were lifted. Blacks constituted 23 percent of those sterilized by the state in the 1930s and 1940s. By 1966, blacks made up 64 percent of those sterilized under North Carolina's eugenic code.[62]

Determining the boundary between consent and coercion can be very tricky as historically it has been murky and flexible. Indeed, women have not always been victims of eugenic sterilization; some have been active agents in a complex process of negotiation involving themselves, welfare workers, and medical authorities in which women used public health services for their own purposes. From the 1930s through the early 1970s, some women "willingly accepted—and in some cases, even sought out—eugenic sterilization as a form of contraceptive control."[63] They manipulated their state eugenics boards to gain access to the one form of effective contraception they could obtain: sterilization. This was true even after the Pill emerged on the market in 1960 and before the creation of federal family planning later in the decade, especially for poor rural women who lacked access to reproductive health services for both financial and geographic reasons.[64] White middle-class women were not the first American women to conceive of sterilization as a legitimate method of contraception. Unlike their poor sisters, however, middle-class women could not have themselves sterilized under eugenic statutes because they could not point to poverty as a "symptom" of lack of reproductive fitness. When they bumped up against restrictive hospital policies prohibiting contraceptive sterilization in the late 1960s and early 1970s, middle-class women turned to the courts, not the state eugenics boards. Some poor women took their cases to the courts at this time, but increasingly they did not need to because although sterilization might not have been available, contraception now was, thanks to the creation of federal family planning. Fewer poor women needed to manipulate the system to obtain the sterilization once highly effective methods of temporary contraception became available.

While North Carolina appears to have been the only state to employ its eugenics statute so forcefully against healthy, noninstitutionalized women, it was not entirely alone. Other southern states also employed their existing eugenics codes to achieve neo-eugenic goals, albeit less frequently. Although the vast majority of forced sterilizations occurred in the South, neo-eugenicist policy makers, social workers, and physicians in other states also exploited existing eugenics laws. Washington State so heartily embraced the association between illegitimacy, mental incompetence, and poverty among black women that it sterilized one woman twice. The state ordered a tubal ligation for her at age fifteen after her first pregnancy. The surgery failed. When she became pregnant again at nineteen, the state mandated the pregnancy be aborted and forced her to undergo a hysterectomy.[65]

Social workers, physicians, and members of state eugenics boards identified poverty and unwed pregnancy as "symptoms" of "feeblemindedness" and used these "symptoms" to justify the sterilization of poor unwed black mothers under eugenics laws. Sometimes their patients welcomed this advocacy; other times, as the instance of Nial Ruth Cox indicates, they did not. In these latter instances, sterilization abuse occurred. On November 24, 1964, Cox, barely eighteen, gave birth to a child out of wedlock. Shortly thereafter, a North Carolina welfare worker threatened to discontinue her family's welfare payments unless she consented to sterilization. Cox later insisted that the social worker described the surgery as reversible.[66] Living with her mother and eight siblings (her father died when she was six) in a home without running water, electricity, or a stove, the teenager could not risk noncompliance and submitted to the surgery—although she never provided her consent. As a minor, under twenty-one years old, Cox could not legally consent to her own surgery. Instead, a social worker obtained the mother's consent, which Cox's mother provided because she was also under the impression that the surgery was temporary. Years later, Cox recalled her experience: "I got pregnant when I was 17. I didn't know anything about birth control or abortion. When the welfare caseworker found out I was pregnant, she told my mother that if we wanted to keep getting welfare, I'd have to have my tubes tied—temporarily. Nobody explained anything to me before the operation. Later on, after the operation, I saw the doctor and I asked him if I could have another baby. He said that I had nothing to worry about, that, of course, I could have more kids. I know now that I was sterilized because I was from a welfare family."[67]

As in many of these cases, the county director of welfare who petitioned the state eugenics board failed to produce concrete evidence of Cox's purported mental deficiency, relying instead on her poverty, race, unwed pregnancy, and family's welfare status to indicate her supposed mental incompetence. This information proved definitive enough for the state eugenics board to accept as valid. As was common practice, the eugenics board approved the petition for surgery without convening a formal hearing and without supplying a court-appointed representative to protect the patient's interests. The board also failed to offer Cox a forum in which to contest its January 25, 1965, decision. Consequently, Dr. A. M. Stanton sterilized Cox on February 10. It was another five years before Cox learned that her sterilization was permanent.[68]

Elaine Riddick Trent had a similar experience with the North Carolina Eugenics Board. On March 1, 1968, the fourteen-year-old entered a hospital in Edenton, North Carolina, to deliver her first child. During her confinement, hospital staff sterilized her without her knowledge or consent at the order of the North Carolina Eugenics Board. The board did not request that Trent undergo psychological evaluation to determine her mental status, but instead interpreted Trent's out-of-wedlock pregnancy and dark skin as evidence of her "mental incompetence" and authorized her surgery on this basis, without convening a formal hearing.[69] Hospital staff did obtain the "consent" of Trent's illiterate grandmother, who marked an "A" on a form presented to her, although it appears that the grandmother did not understand the significance of her mark. Had the grandmother understood the content of the document she signed, it is more than likely that she would have communicated this knowledge to Trent, who did not learn of her sterility until 1973.[70]

In the late 1950s and early 1960s, some southern physicians with neo-eugenic politics also began to practice "Mississippi appendectomies." Civil rights activist Fannie Lou Hamer was victimized this way in 1961 when she entered Sunflower City Hospital in Alabama to have a uterine tumor removed. Having lost the battle to preserve Jim Crow segregation, some southern whites looked for other ways to demonstrate their racial power. Performing an unwanted and unknown surgery on a black patient who had no recourse or evidence (in the form of a medical chart) to support her claims was one method that some southern physicians used to exert their influence over a black community demanding equality. Physicians frequently failed to document the sterilizations they performed, leaving women no direct evidence to link the violations of their bodies to their physicians, and sometimes leaving patients without the knowledge of their violation. A physician who performed an unauthorized surgery that terminated the fertility of an unknowing patient who lay unconscious and vulnerable on the operating table exercised considerable power over her. At a time when civil rights victories granted black women and men access to health care and other government programs that refused to serve them for so long, forced sterilization functioned as one way that the whites in charge of public health could continue to assert racial supremacy without directly challenging new policies of integration. It also functioned as a reminder of black patients' dependence upon white doctors' goodwill. Aware of these covert sterilization practices, women in need of abdominal surgery who chose to be treated by undergoing cesarean sections, having tumors removed, or undergoing appendectomies had to accept the risk of forced sterilization when seeking medical care.

Physicians performed "Mississippi appendectomies" primarily in rural communities overwhelmed by racial struggle. In the years preceding the establishment of federal family planning, sterilization abuse remained generally confined to southern states, where most surgeons operated without their patients' knowledge or informed consent. However, by offering contraceptive services through the Office of Economic Opportunity (OEO), the Department of Health, Education, and Welfare (HEW), and the Public Health Service (PHS), legislators in the Johnson and Nixon administrations unintentionally created an institutional network that encouraged new practices of forced sterilization.

Federal Family Planning: Creating the System That Fostered Abuse

The end of legal segregation, the development of federal family planning services, and the legitimization of sterilization as a method of birth control intersected to create an environment conducive to a new pattern of forced sterilization. Instead of exploiting eugenics statutes and removing women's uteruses without their knowledge or consent, in the late 1960s some physicians began to force women to consent to unwanted surgeries. Instead of secretly performing a "Mississippi appendectomy," physicians began to require their patients to sign consent forms to surgeries they did not want or did not understand. The existence of signed consent forms allowed abusive physicians to avoid administrative suspicion and protected them against litigation. When victims began to file lawsuits against their abusers, physicians submitted the signed medical consent forms as evidence of their patients' desire to undergo sterilization. In this way, they shielded themselves from liability and blamed victims for their own sterility.[71] This new pattern of forced sterilization developed and spread from the South to the rest of the country as a result of federal family planning and the absence of hospital policies governing informed consent.

President Johnson announced his commitment to controlling overpopulation abroad in his 1965 State of the Union address, but he proved more hesitant to develop family planning initiatives at home. Over the course of his term, Johnson's administration gradually expanded existing public assistance programs to include family planning services. It was not until 1967 that Congress formally entered the realm of domestic family planning on a national level, when it amended Title V of the Social Security acts. The amendment stipulated that at least 6 percent of the monies allotted to the AFDC maternal and infant care fund be directed toward family planning services. It also required that states develop family planning programs and make family planning services available to adults on welfare. Congress also offered federal grants to private nonprofit family planning organizations like Planned Parenthood for the first time. Surprisingly, the amendment passed quietly. In part, this is because legislators considered family planning policy while debating welfare reform, and the controversy generated by the latter issue overshadowed the former. But it is also because politicians on both sides of the aisle believed that family planning offered a "solution" to the "problems" of illegitimacy and welfare.[72]

The federal government delved further into the provision of family planning services with the election of Richard Nixon in 1968. Under President Nixon, Congress not only increased funding for existing programs but also developed a host of new services.[73] Nixon based his support for family planning on cost-benefit analyses that showed that it was cheaper to fund contraception for poor women than to support their children. Congress passed the Family Planning Services and Population Research Act on December 24, 1970. This legislation provided $382 million for family planning services, research, and training, and authorized Title X of the Public Health Services Act, the second largest single source of federal funding for family planning next to Medicaid.[74] The 1970 law signaled a clear and firm federal commitment to family planning services.

Congress placed two restrictions on the use of these funds. First, attempting to guard against coercion, legislators stipulated that participation in federal programs "shall be voluntary and shall not be a prerequisite to eligibility for or receipt of any other service."[75] But legislators neglected to develop actual safeguards to protect patients against coercion; they naively assumed this proclamation sufficient to deter abuse. Second, the 1970 act mandated that no federal monies be used for abortion. Earlier legislation prohibited the use of federal funds for both abortion and sterilization. In 1970, legislators lifted the restriction on sterilization for HEW and PHS programs. Operating under different legislation, however, the OEO continued to ban the procedure. Nevertheless, the ban failed to prevent some OEO providers from performing sterilizations—some voluntary, some coercive.[76]

The OEO's ban on sterilization reflected both the agency's ambivalence about providing family planning and its concern for patients' rights. A few federal agencies administered their own family planning programs prior to passage of the 1967 Social Security amendments. The OEO was one such agency. In November 1966, Sargent Shriver, the director of the OEO, published regulations for his agency's family planning project grants. Shriver's list of regulations reflected the Johnson administration's reluctance to enter the realm of family planning. Conservative in its application, the policy entitled only married women residing in two-person households to utilize OEO-sponsored programs and prohibited the use of agency funds for abortion or sterilization. The AVS and the ACLU opposed this policy, but aside from letter writing, did not take action to change the rules. Despite its cautious nature, Shriver's proposal privileged patients' rights by mandating that participation in all OEO-funded programs be voluntary and by forbidding providers from conditioning federal aid upon receipt of contraception. Shriver's attention to patients' rights suggests that at least one federal agency recognized the potential for coercion within federal family planning programs from the outset. Despite frequent and fervent objections to OEO policy by the ACLU and the AVS, the ban on sterilization and abortion remained in effect until May 18, 1971, when the OEO lifted the restriction on sterilization, but not abortion.[77]

The OEO reversed its ban on voluntary sterilization in 1971 in response to increasing pressure from state providers, who reported heavy demand for the service from their female clients.[78] A 1970 OEO survey of family planning programs found that 80 percent of respondents supported including sterilization among their services.[79] Unlike HEW, which simply expanded its programs to include contraceptive sterilization under the Family Planning Services and Population Research Act, the OEO delayed implementing sterilization services until it could develop protective guidelines. Although Shriver was no longer at the OEO, his fear of coercion continued to shape the antipoverty agency's policy. Protecting patients from coercion also proved to be a central concern of Dr. George Contis, director of the Family Planning Program, Office of Health Affairs at the OEO. In a memorandum addressed to all agencies receiving OEO family planning funds dated June 28, 1971, Contis wrote: "We are more concerned that the patients be protected and provided with high quality medical care. Therefore, we are developing a set of guidelines and clinical standards for the provision of sterilization services. . . . We plan to have these available for use by the family planning projects and comprehensive health centers by

September 1, 1971." He then instructed his affiliates, *"Please do not begin providing sterilizations until you receive these guidelines."*[80]

Despite Contis's promise, OEO affiliates did not receive the guidelines in September. Instead, they received another letter from the director of Family Planning dated November 5, 1971, stating that regional health specialists and national health professionals had reviewed the guidelines on September 7, and determined that they required further revision. Thanking providers for their patience, Contis predicted that the formal guidelines would be released within a few weeks.[81]

Finally, on January 11, 1972, the OEO printed the long-awaited guidelines, *OEO Instruction 6130–2, Voluntary Sterilization Services*. This eighteen-page document carefully outlined conditions for voluntary sterilization under OEO programs. Most important, the document reiterated Shriver's 1965 edict that all OEO sterilizations be voluntary. Specifically, sterilization was to be provided "only to those persons who request it," who "must be well informed enough to make a meaningful choice," and who held "the legal capacity" to consent to surgery. Equally as important, the guidelines mandated that "no sterilization procedure shall be conducted unless the individual patient has given his informed written consent to the procedure."[82] The guidelines included sample consent forms and standards and rules for record keeping.

Although the OEO printed the new guidelines, the agency did not distribute them due to political pressure from the White House. In late 1971, Dr. E. Leon Cooper became the new director of Health Affairs at the OEO. A physician opposed to contraceptive sterilization, Cooper objected to the now extremely delayed guidelines because of his own personal skepticism about permanent contraception and because he feared that the cost of sterilization would strain his agency's budget.[83] On January 31, 1972, one day before a press conference scheduled to announce the guidelines, Cooper suspended release of the new policy, a move sanctioned by the White House. In meetings between the OEO and the Office of Management and Budget, White House officials expressed President Nixon's concern about the political implications of an explicit federal policy condoning voluntary sterilization in an election year. Specifically, Nixon feared a Catholic backlash. The president "definitely didn't want us to go ahead" with the publication of the guidelines, OEO Deputy Director Wesley Hjornevik recalled.[84] At the combined request of the White House and Cooper, the OEO transferred 25,000 copies of the guidelines to a warehouse in northeast Washington, D.C., where they remained until news of the forced sterilization of fourteen-year-old Minnie Lee Relf and her twelve-year-old sister, Mary Alice, in the summer of 1973 prompted a federal investigation into their whereabouts.[85]

Because it never authorized the performance of sterilizations, the OEO never tabulated the number of sterilizations performed by its family planning affiliates between May 1971, when the sterilization ban was lifted, and July 1973, when it transferred its family planning responsibilities to HEW. An unpublished OEO study estimated that the department funded 2,000 sterilizations in 1972, at least 15 of which involved minors.[86] Likewise, although HEW affiliates began to provide sterilizations after Congress passed the Family Planning Services and Population Research Act in December 1970, the agency also failed to collect and maintain accurate records of its activities until 1974, when evidence of sterilization abuse forced it to implement strict record-keeping protocol. At the time, HEW could only estimate the number of sterilizations performed with its funds in the early years of its family planning activities. For example, it claimed to have funded approximately 16,000 female and 8,677 male sterilizations in 1972.[87]

It remains unclear how many OEO officials knew that their providers performed unauthorized sterilizations between 1971 and 1973. The acting director of the OEO from January through June 1973 testified at Senator Edward Kennedy's hearings on human experimentation that he had no knowledge of these practices during his tenure. However, *Medical World News* reported that Cooper, director of Health Affairs, had received two memoranda (one dated March 30 and the other April 4, 1972) that openly discussed sterilization in OEO programs, which indicates that Cooper and other administrators in OEO's Family Planning Division knew about the unauthorized surgeries. "Programs are being besieged by requests for voluntary sterilization services and some programs, we understand, are providing these services in response to popular demand," read one memorandum.[88] This memo suggests a disconnect between OEO policy and practice that was tacitly acknowledged at the highest levels of the agency but never addressed explicitly until victims publicized their abuse.

Minnie Lee and Mary Alice Relf

Sterilization abuse finally became a national issue in the summer of 1973 when Minnie Lee and Mary Alice Relf filed suit against the government agencies and individuals responsible for their involuntary sterilizations. The black girls, ages fourteen and twelve, respectively, had been sterilized without their knowledge or informed consent on June 14, 1973. Minnie Lee's and Mary Alice's abuse epitomizes the neo-eugenic values underlying this new practice. Family planning workers funded by the OEO identified the girls as appropriate surgical candidates on the basis of their race and class and tricked their illiterate mother into "consenting" to her daughters' sterilizations. No evidence suggested that the girls were at risk for an unintended pregnancy, and neither the girls nor their parents solicited family planning services. The Relfs' experience is not representative of sterilization abuse incidents during this era because of the extremity of their case and the publicity it generated. It is instructive, however, because it magnifies the prejudicial attitudes and assumptions about reproductive fitness inherent in forced sterilization and because it was the case that brought forced sterilization to national attention.

Minnie Lee and Mary Alice Relf lived with their parents and older sister, Katie, in public housing in Montgomery, Alabama. Local family planning agents at the Montgomery Community Action Agency, an OEO-sponsored program, approached the girls about contraception as soon as the family moved into the housing project in 1971. They predicted that because Minnie Lee and Mary Alice were poor and black, they would engage in unprotected sexual activity and bear illegitimate children, whom they would ask the state to support. No evidence suggested that the Relfs were sexually active when family planning workers solicited their consent to contraception. Community Action Agency workers had merely observed that "boys were hanging around" the girls.[89]

In 1971, the family planning agency began to administer the contraceptive injection Depo-Provera to Katie, then fourteen years old. Community Action Agency staff did not obtain parental consent for these routine injections of the controversial drug, which was in clinical trials at the time. In March 1973, again without consulting her parents, nurses took Katie to a family planning clinic and forced her to accept an IUD. Katie protested, but clinic staff dismissed her objections and inserted the device, telling the teenager that she needed it.[90]

Sometime after Katie began receiving Depo-Provera at the clinic, family planning workers began to administer the three-month injections to Minnie Lee, who was then twelve, and Mary Alice, who was then ten. Again, the staff did not obtain parental permission to perform these injections, nor did they adequately explain the injections to the girls. Most medical professionals today consider Depo-Provera to be a safe, effective, and popular method of contraception. However, in the early 1970s Depo-Provera was an experimental contraceptive in its early clinical trial phase, and clinicians administered the injections to welfare recipients like the Relfs at federally funded clinics. The Food and Drug Administration (FDA) terminated this round of clinical trials of Depo-Provera in the spring of 1973 after a preliminary study linked the drug to cancer in beagles. Rather than substitute another form of temporary contraception or simply stop administering contraception to the sexually inactive girls, family planning workers decided to sterilize them.[91]

On June 13, 1973, a family planning worker from the Montgomery Community Action Committee escorted Minnie Lee, Mary Alice, and their mother from their home to a doctor's office and then to a hospital, where the Relfs were told that the girls would receive more shots. Hospital staff obtained Mrs. Relf's consent to what she believed to be Depo-Provera injections and helped her home. Mrs. Relf, who was illiterate, had no way of knowing that the form she signed had authorized her daughters' sterilizations. "I put an X on a piece of paper, and she told me that they were going to give them some shots. That is what she told me," Mrs. Relf testified at a Senate subcommittee hearing convened by Senator Edward Kennedy in July 1973. "They didn't say anything about giving them no operation," she contended. "They told me they were going to give shots."[92] Her husband corroborated this account, testifying at the same hearing that "the girls had been getting some birth control shots for some time, and the clinic nurses come here and said they wanted to give them some more. But they just took 'em away instead and then taken the life right out of them."[93] When asked by Kennedy if she would have willingly consented to her daughters' sterilization, Mrs. Relf replied, "I would not have let them do that." Her husband reiterated his objection to the offense, "I didn't want it done and I'm still upset."[94]

Concerned about his daughters, Lonnie Relf, a fifty-six-year-old unemployed contractor crippled by a back injury, traveled to the hospital around nine or ten o'clock on the evening of June 13 to check on them. Hospital staff refused to allow Mr. Relf to see the girls, informing him that visiting hours were over and that he would have to wait until the following day to see his children. Lonnie Relf returned home puzzled about the cause of his daughters' hospitalization.

The next morning Mrs. Relf returned to the hospital where her daughters "told me they had been operated on." "That was the first I knew about it," she testified.[95] Although a nurse claimed to have explained the procedure to the girls, her competence is questionable. If she did in fact explain the surgery to the girls, she did an extremely poor job of communicating its permanence. Joseph Levin, general counsel of the Southern Poverty Law Center and attorney to the Relfs, maintained that Mary Alice did not understand that she could not bear children, and while Minnie Lee appeared to understand the consequences of her surgery, she continued to speak of reversing the procedure and having children in the future.[96]

Orelia Dixon, director of the Montgomery Community Action Agency's Family Planning Project, insisted that Mrs. Relf understood the nature of the surgery to which nurses asked her to consent. "There is no doubt in my mind that they knew what that meant," she maintained. "We explain everything and don't use words that people can't understand."[97] Unable to continue injecting the girls with Depo-Provera after the FDA terminated clinical trials, but unwilling to trust the girls to take birth control pills consistently, Dixon contended that family planning nurses determined sterilization to be an appropriate method of contraception for the young girls. When accused of racism in the press, clinic staff pointed out that "the nurses who took the girls from their home were also black."[98] This defense intended to suggest the nurses' clinical objectivity by implying that black women would not victimize other black women.

Perhaps the girls' sterilization constituted a genuine, albeit terrible, misunderstanding between the clinic staff and the Relfs. Regardless, the neoeugenic intent of the clinic workers' actions remains clear, as evidenced by the clinic staff's insistence that sterilization constituted an appropriate alternative to Depo-Provera for two sexually inactive preteen girls. Clinic personnel identified Minnie Lee and Mary Alice Relf as "unfit" to reproduce on the basis of their race and class and sought to render them infertile before they could bear illegitimate children who would become dependent upon the state. Clinic records suggest that the staff did not confine this practice to the Relfs; they targeted other poor black girls whom they also predicted would bear children out of wedlock. In 1973, the Montgomery Community Action Agency sterilized eleven females. Ten of the eleven patients were black, and five, including the Relfs, were between the ages of twelve and seventeen.[99] These records show that in the early 1970s, forced sterilization had evolved beyond the targeting of those who had born children out of wedlock; some family planning clinics had begun to sterilize "unfit" girls who, they predicted, would become unwed mothers.

Exposing Sterilization Abuse

Although a physician sterilized Minnie Lee and Mary Alice Relf without their knowledge or consent, the majority of forced sterilization incidents in the late 1960s and early 1970s (the peak years of abuse) involved physicians coercing patients to consent to unwanted surgeries when they entered the hospital for labor and delivery. Most often, physicians, nurses, and social workers forced patients to consent to surgery by threatening to revoke their public aid if they refused, leading them to believe that tubal ligations could be reversed, or pressuring them to agree to surgery while under duress or on medication, especially during labor and delivery. In the years following the Relfs' disclosure, victims' testimonies and lawsuits, federal investigations, private studies, and congressional hearings revealed the existence of widespread sterilization abuse across the nation. New York, California, North Carolina, Mississippi, and Alabama stood out as particularly egregious offenders.

Sterilization abuse assumed multiple forms and ranged from subtle persua-
sion to oppressive harassment. It also bore a distinct regional and racial/ethnic
pattern. In the South where blacks and whites continued to struggle with integration, black women remained targets for those who performed forced sterilizations. In California and the Sun Belt, where issues of Mexican immigration
dominated, physicians and medical staff targeted Mexican and Mexican
American women for sterilization as a method of reducing the population and
shrinking the welfare rolls. Puerto Rican and black women in New York City
became targets for physicians who endorsed the myth of the welfare queen and
who believed that Puerto Rican women's "hyperfertility" and poverty made
them appropriate candidates for surgery. Finally, Native American women living on reservations experienced very high rates of forced sterilization as the
medical staff serving this population sought to reduce dependency by preventing their patients from bearing children.

As sterilization gained acceptance as a legitimate method of contraception
and as federal family planning funded the procedure, surgeons and social
workers stopped secretly sterilizing women or using eugenic statutes to sterilize poor women who bore children out of wedlock, and instead started to
demand that patients consent to permanent contraception. Most physicians
approached potential surgical candidates during labor and delivery, and many
deceptively marketed sterilization in order to secure patients' consent to the
procedure. One physician explained, "Women seem to accept the procedure
more readily if the word 'operation' is not used." He routinely described tubal
ligations to patients as "a stitch in the vagina" that protected against pregnancy.[100] Another physician established a policy of informing patients of the
permanence of tubal ligation only if they asked.[101] Still other doctors "neglected"
to inform their patients that sterilization was permanent. A San Francisco intern
reported, "If the patient asked, yes she'd be told it was permanent. If there was a
big rush, the staff wouldn't bother."[102] And an Ohio physician bluntly admitted, "The alternatives were rarely gone into with a black welfare patient who
had two or more kids."[103]

Many Mexican, Puerto Rican, and Native American women found that
physicians exploited the language barrier between them when patients did not
speak English fluently. A pediatric intern at New York's Bellevue Hospital
explained: "There was a large Puerto Rican population and I think a lot of
women didn't know the full consequences of what was happening to them.
There was a language problem. Many of them thought their tubes could be
untied."[104] By referring to sterilization as the "tying of tubes," physicians suggested that surgery could be easily reversed. Elena Orozco became a victim of

this type of abuse. "What I was signing, I understood it to tie my tubes, not to sterilize. If they would have put the word 'sterilization' there, I would not have signed the papers," the Los Angeles woman revealed.[105] Another woman sterilized without her informed consent at the University of Southern California, Los Angeles County Medical Center (USC L.A. County Medical Center) explained in a deposition, "We [her husband and herself] both believed that my tubes could later be untied if I desired to have more children. . . . At no time did any member of the medical center's staff inform me that my tubes were going to be cut and that I would be permanently sterilized."[106] As both women learned too late, doctors generally cauterized or cut the fallopian tubes entirely, making reversal difficult, if not impossible.

Pressuring non-English-speaking women to consent to surgery using English forms was another way in which physicians exploited the language barrier in order to force patients to accept sterilization. Physicians and other hospital staff made few efforts to find translators for these patients. When Dr. Bernard Rosenfeld, a resident at the USC L.A. County Medical Center, opposed the sterilization of a twenty-six-year-old Spanish-speaking woman who "spoke no English," but whose "operation consent form [was] signed in English," the physician responsible for the patient told Rosenfeld, "We're doing her a favor."[107] Sterilizing the patient was far more important to this physician than making sure she understood and consented to the procedure.

Physicians aggressively "sold" tubal ligation by repeatedly approaching women during labor and delivery and, if this proved unsuccessful, during the subsequent hospital stay. Patient records from the USC L.A. County Medical Center indicate that physicians approached women during active labor, when they were distressed and often under the influence of anesthesia or pain medication. Consent forms were frequently signed just before surgery began.[108] For example, a thirty-year-old Los Angeles woman was in labor for nineteen hours and thirty minutes before consenting to sterilization. During this time, she received the drugs Demerol and Visteril. Her last dose of Demerol was administered forty-five minutes before she signed the consent form.[109] Another woman treated at the same hospital recalled submitting to sterilization after being worn down by labor, pain medication, and her doctor's insistence. "I told the doctor that I did not want to be sterilized since my husband and I planned to have another child," she explained. "I was groggy from the drugs, exhausted from the labor, as well as from the doctor's constant pressuring. Finally, I told the doctor, 'Okay, if it's a boy, go ahead and do it.'"[110] Although she delivered a girl, this woman awoke from anesthesia to learn that she had been sterilized. She was not alone in learning of her surgery after the fact. Admitted to the hospital on

June 5, 1972, thirty-three-year-old Maria Gomez remembered that the doctor who was to perform her emergency cesarean section asked her about sterilization just before surgery began. "I don't remember very much after this," she explained in an affidavit, because "I was very drowsy and drugged. They gave me some funny anesthesia." A postpartum check-up confirmed that she had been sterilized. Sterilization proved especially devastating for Gomez; her baby died twenty-four hours after birth.[111]

Some women who successfully resisted surgery during delivery were pursued by resentful physicians for the remainder of their hospital stay. Dr. Juan Nieto recalled that in the Colorado hospital where he trained, physicians harassed poor Mexican women from the moment they entered the hospital to deliver until they consented to surgery. Nieto explained, "They would get a young woman, maybe 19 or 20, who was having a baby and start right in on her in the delivery room. . . . If she said no, they would all stand around her bed every morning while on rounds and repeatedly suggest that she have the operation."[112] Ralph Nader's Health Research Group's (HRG) 1973 *Study on Surgical Sterilization* confirmed this practice. Its primary author, Dr. Bernard Rosenfeld, remembered his chief resident's instructions upon learning that a woman scheduled for a tubal ligation after delivery refused the surgery. The chief resident told him, "Go in there [the postpartum room where women stay for a few hours after delivery] and see if you can talk her into it."[113]

Ricardo Cruz, a Los Angeles lawyer involved in litigation on behalf of Chicanas sterilized without their knowledge or informed consent, compiled a list of 190 women sterilized during labor at the USC L.A. County Medical Center between 1970 and 1974. The list also included copies of portions of these women's medical record, most likely copied and interpreted by Dr. Rosenfeld. None of the women had any medical indication for sterilization, and few had large families. Seven of the 190 women listed had no living children at the time of surgery. Fifty-three had only one living child at the time of sterilization, and the same number of women had two living children when sterilized. Only 21 of the 190 patients had more than five children.[114]

The Cruz documents reveal several specific patterns of coercion at the USC L.A. County Medical Center, which became notorious for its forced sterilization of Chicana patients who arrived at the hospital for delivery. On several occasions, patients' refusal to consent to surgery is charted, then followed by a second note listing the day of sterilization.[115] For example, the chart of a twenty-five-year-old reads, "No history of desiring sterilization in clinic. Admitted 6/1/71[.] Pre Op Note states, 'Doesn't want tubal at time of surgery.' Cesarean section and tubal ligation done 6/2/71."[116] Another chart of a thirty-nine-year-old woman

includes a note that states, "Doesn't desire bilateral tubal ligation." This is followed by a description of a subsequent blood transfusion, indication for cesarean
section, and confirmation of "cesarean section and sterilization done."[117] Notes
on another patient's medical record indicate that the twenty-eight-year-old
mother of four was "in hospital 3 days before labor began; not asked until labor
was in progress if she desired tubal ligation even though cesarean section was
known to be needed before labor began."[118] Clearly, the physicians treating her
made an effort to approach her about surgery when she was most vulnerable.

Sometimes the phrase "no consents signed" was followed by a second one
stating: "physician's certificate of emergency: 'This is to certify that the delay
necessary to obtain complete consent for treatment would endanger this
patient's life or chance of recovery. We believe emergency operation is necessary.' "[119] On the one hand, an emergency situation would warrant the bypass
of consent under common standards of informed consent, which were just
being developed (but not yet formalized) in the early 1970s as abuse occurred.
On the other hand, sterilization is not an emergency procedure, although a
cesarean section is. If a pregnant patient's health depended on immediate delivery, an emergency bypass of consent for the cesarean section would make
medical and ethical sense, but not so for elective tubal ligation. Physicians preferred to perform cesarean sections and tubal ligations in tandem to minimize
risks associated with infection and anesthesia, as well as to reduce medical
costs. It appears that at this hospital, physicians who performed emergency
cesarean sections sometimes used the opportunity to persuade a woman to
accept permanent contraception.

Coercion caused by the failure of hospital staff to adequately explain the
consequences of tubal ligation is evident in records in which patients questioned their fertility status after surgery. For example, notes from a patient's follow-up check-up revealed that she did not know whether she had been
sterilized while undergoing a cesarean section. "Patient states she's nervous
because she doesn't know if her tubes were ligated with c/s 1970," the chart
read.[120] Frequently patients' lack of knowledge about their fertility status
appeared in requests for contraception. One patient, described as "Spanish-
American, Mexican" with one living child, was sterilized in June 1972. She
returned to her family planning clinic about six weeks after delivery and
requested birth control pills, but was given an IUD because her varicose veins
constituted a counterindication to Pill use. A pathology report in her chart dated
July 20, 1972, indicated that both of her fallopian tubes had been removed during
her cesarean section. As of August 1973, however, the IUD remained inside the
patient, suggesting that she did not understand the consequences of her surgery

and that medical staff had failed to explain them to her. Her chart offers a possible explanation for the confusion. The patient had "signed [her consent] in markedly distressed handwriting 6/20 for cesarean section and sterilization" after she experienced a full twenty-four hours of labor, numerous doses of Demerol and Visteril, and an unsuccessful attempt at a forceps delivery.[121] Similarly, postpartum clinic notes on the chart of a twenty-nine-year-old black woman sterilized after a cesarean section on March 16, 1972, read, "Birth control method wanted—diaphragm."[122] The chart indicates that the patient consented to sterilization, but one must wonder about how well the procedure was explained to this patient given that she requested temporary contraception at a postpartum check-up.

Physicians who failed to elicit consent before surgery sometimes required their patients to sign consent forms *after* surgery to ensure that they had a signature to protect themselves against potential litigation. In one instance, a patient signed her consent forms at 9 A.M. for a cesarean and tubal ligation that occurred three and a half hours earlier. When she returned for her postpartum visit, she requested a diaphragm, indicating that she, like so many others, did not fully understand the consequences of her sterilization.[123]

The absence of official hospital protocol for obtaining patients' informed consent to surgery allowed these patterns of abuse to develop and grow. The practice of forced sterilization at delivery began in the interim period between the start of medical and public discussion of patient protections in the late 1960s and the actual implementation of these policies in the early-to-mid-1970s. In the late 1960s, consumer groups and health activists started to demand increased oversight over medical practice, the establishment of strict standards of informed consent, and the strengthening of the patient's position within the inherently unequal doctor-patient relationship. Their demands led to the creation of clear standards of informed consent and the adoption of these standards by hospitals across the country, which slowed forced sterilization upon delivery by prohibiting physicians from obtaining consent from patients under duress and the influence of anesthesia and pain medication, requiring that they explain all the risks and side effects of surgery, and mandating that non-English speakers have surgeries explained to them in their native language. In 1970, the Joint Commission on the Accreditation of Hospitals (JCAH) adopted a Patient Bill of Rights, which the American Hospital Association (AHA) endorsed in 1973.[124]

In the interim between demands for standards of informed consent and the actual adoption of these protective mechanisms, physicians devised their own sterilization policies, some more explicit than others. Rosenfeld believed that "it's mainly a question of the doctor's prejudice. Or their feeling that they have a social right to determine how many children a woman should have."[125] Physicians across the country affirmed Rosenfeld's contention. A doctor trained in North Carolina reported that his colleagues "pushed them [sterilizations] on anyone delivering their second or more child."[126] In the experience of a resident who studied at Wayne State Medical School in Detroit, the number of children a woman bore played a greater role than age in doctors' choices of sterilization candidates. "We had a lot of young girls come in . . . thirteen and sixteen and they'd have two or three children. . . . There were so many young girls and most of them had a real low mentality. We'd tell them about birth control and they wouldn't take it. It would get some of the residents real mad."[127] An intern from Milwaukee reported that she witnessed physicians sterilizing minors "if they had two kids."[128]

Another common form of sterilization abuse involved physicians persuading poor patients to accept hysterectomies instead of tubal ligation solely for the purpose of practicing a more complicated surgery. A 1973 HRG study on sterilization confirmed this practice, as did patients' own reports. Physicians who acted in this manner placed their own education over their patients' well-being, as hysterectomy involved a greater medical risk and recovery period. A 1972 *American Journal of Obstetrics and Gynecology* study found that the complication rate for hysterectomy was ten to twenty times higher than for tubal ligation. As sociologist Adele Clark maintains, "this is a classic example of professionals exercising their autonomy over and against that of patients."[129]

Residents' comments to HRG investigators revealed institutional acceptance of the practice of using poor patients to develop young surgeons' skills. One resident at Boston City Hospital reported, "We like to do a hysterectomy, its [sic] more of a challenge . . . you know, a well-trained chimpanzee can do a tubal ligation . . . and it's good experience for a junior resident." Another medical student at the same hospital recalled that "on many occasions, patients requesting sterilization . . . usually by tubal ligation, were talked to for several days until they agreed to hysterectomies." A staff doctor admitted to HRG investigators, "Let's face it, we've all talked women into hysterectomies who didn't need them, during residency training." Likewise, when one student questioned whether the size of a supposed fibroid tumor (a benign growth in the uterus that is sometimes an indication for hysterectomy) necessitated a hysterectomy, the presiding resident replied, "We don't know. The guy that sent her in thought there might be." Besides, he added, "She's 42 and doesn't need a uterus."[130] Likewise, a physician trained at a southwestern hospital recalled that one of his colleagues would lie to women whom he believed had too many children and tell them that they needed hysterectomies when no medical indications for surgery existed. He remembered one instance in which this colleague actively covered up his misdiagnosis, saying, "'We're going to have to make sure the pathology report does not get back to the woman and make up a reason why she needed to have it taken out.'"[131]

Native American women who lived on reservations and received health care through the Indian Health Service (IHS) also experienced an extremely high rate of sterilization abuse. Between 1970 and 1976, IHS hospitals and affiliates sterilized between 25 and 42 percent of all Native American women of child-bearing age.[132] The IHS provided poor health care in run-down, underfunded, understaffed, and underequipped hospitals and clinics that could not meet the needs of Native Americans. Understaffing prevented many Native Americans from receiving health care quickly. To compensate, the IHS contracted out its services, which encouraged forced sterilization, as the IHS made no effort to regulate contract facilities. Set in the context of poor health care, which contributed to short life spans, and the decades-old practice of removing children from Native American homes and sending them to white schools to be assimilated, forced sterilization exacerbated an existing population problem that threatened the health and well-being of Native American tribes and cultures.[133]

The introduction of forced sterilization to an already dwindling population imperiled the reproduction of many tribes and tribal cultures and led some tribal advocates to accuse the federal government of using sterilization to reduce population size in order to claim more Native American land.[134] These claims bore a similarity to cries of genocide leveled against the government by black nationalists in the same era. "There are only 5,000 of us," Tribal Judge Marie Sanchez of the Northern Cheyenne exclaimed. "This is another attempt to limit our population—but this time, they're doing it in the noble name of medicine."[135] Dr. Constance Uri, an outspoken advocate of patients who had been sterilized, approached the issue from another perspective. "Zero population growth may be all right for the white man, because he's crowding this continent. But for the Indian, it's genocidal," she declared.[136]

In the early 1970s, Dr. Uri witnessed a significant rise in the number of young, sterile Native American women. She first confronted the issue in 1970 when a twenty-year-old woman asked her for a "womb transplant." "I've heard of kidney transplants," the patient said, "and I want to know if you can give me a new womb." Uri had to explain to her young patient—who was engaged and planning a family—that her uterus had been removed and could not be replaced. An IHS physician had performed a hysterectomy on her six years earlier when she struggled with alcoholism and told her that the surgery was reversible.

Although this woman sought assistance from Uri, fear of forced sterilization led many women to avoid the IHS providers: Uri and two colleagues held clinics in a tepee in order to provide services for patients in a "safe" environment.[137]

Concerned that an epidemic of abuse was under way, Uri contacted Senator James G. Abourezk of South Dakota, who requested a Government Accounting Office (GAO) investigation of sterilizations performed through the IHS and its contract facilities. The GAO studied the incidence of sterilization in four regions (Oklahoma City, Oklahoma; Aberdeen, South Dakota; Albuquerque, New Mexico; and Phoenix, Arizona). But it asked only one question: Did the sterilizations comply with the 1974 HEW guidelines? These guidelines (which will be discussed in detail later) prohibited the sterilization of individuals under the age of twenty-one, required that patients be informed of all risks and benefits of the surgery before consenting to it, and standardized the process of informed consent. The GAO study found that between 1973 and 1976, the IHS funded 3,406 female sterilizations and 142 vasectomies. Of the 3,406 female surgeries, 3,001 involved women of childbearing age. The GAO identified several violations of the waiting period and informed consent process, but ultimately concluded that most sterilizations performed through the IHS did not constitute abuse.[138] This conclusion contradicts the evidence provided by tribal leaders, some of who conducted their own studies. Had investigators broadened their study to examine the conditions under which these surgeries occurred, rather than measuring compliance with the 1974 guidelines, they would likely have uncovered the blatant evidence of abuse already documented by Native American activists and victims of sterilization abuse. Various violations of the 1974 guidelines, such as the thirty-six sterilizations of women under twenty-one years of age and the GAO's conclusion that most physicians caring for Native Americans were unaware of the new federal guidelines, suggests that abuse was common on reservations.[139]

Tribal leader Lee Brightman collected his own evidence of abuse. In 1979, he reported that during a weeklong visit to the Rosebud Reservation in South Dakota, he encountered seven women sterilized without their informed consent. Two women had entered an IHS hospital to have their appendixes removed and left without their ovaries. One sixteen-year-old awoke from anesthesia administered during delivery to learn she had been "fixed so that she wouldn't have more kids until she was eighteen."[140] Another young woman had gone to the hospital to have an ovarian cyst removed and left without her uterus. Finally, IHS surgeons sterilized a young postpartum patient by falsely informing her mother that without surgery, her daughter would die. IHS physicians later convinced the same mother that she, too, would die unless she accepted sterilization.[141]

Chief Tribal Judge Marie Sanchez also investigated sterilization abuse among Native Americans. Sanchez interviewed women in Lame Deer, Montana, and found that thirty women had been sterilized between 1973 and 1976. She found two girls under fifteen who were victims of "Mississippi appendectomies." They entered the hospital to have their appendixes removed but later learned they had been sterilized. Sanchez met another woman with severe migraine headaches. Doctors attributed her headaches to hormones and suggested a hysterectomy. Surgery did not eradicate her headaches; she was later found to have a brain tumor.[142] Sanchez found the practice of physicians pushing hysterectomies on otherwise healthy patients to be common on reservations, as it was in other public hospitals. "The doctors that come to us are young, often fresh out of medical school and they want to practice on someone," Sanchez stated.[143] Dr. Uri's investigation also uncovered unnecessary hysterectomies in patients as young as eighteen who had undergone the surgery without comprehending its permanence.[144]

The most well known case of Native American women and forced sterilization occurred off the reservation, in western Pennsylvania. In 1970, Norma Jean Serena received a visit from a welfare worker from Armstrong County Welfare Services in Pennsylvania who responded to a complaint that Serena and her two children were living in squalid conditions with a black man who was not her husband. Social workers insisted on taking the two children, a boy and a girl, both under four years old, to Children's Hospital in Pittsburgh for medical examination. After the exam, they told Serena that her children were too sick to leave the hospital, although the physician's report indicated that the children were "healthy and alert."[145] Subsequently, caseworkers placed the children in foster care, telling Serena that the arrangement was temporary, but informing the foster parents that it could be made permanent.[146]

Serena was pregnant with her fifth child at the time (the oldest two children did not live with her). The Child Welfare and Board of Assistance in Pittsburgh removed the baby from her care after birth and placed him in the foster system in August 1970, claiming that Serena was too ill to care for him. Serena was sterilized after delivery. Sources offer two conflicting stories about how and when Serena discovered her sterilization. One says that she learned about her surgery the following day when physicians approached her to sign a consent form. Another, that she found out days after the surgery when she "overheard a conversation in her hospital room."[147] Doctors recorded their motivation to sterilize this patient on her chart. "We find from observation and examination of Norma Jean Serena," they wrote, "that she is suffering from the following ailment or conditions . . . socioeconomic reasons . . . and that another pregnancy would, in our opinion, be unadvisable. Therefore, we are of the opinion that it is medically necessary to perform the sterilization."[148] The note on Serena's chart makes clear the association between poverty, illegitimacy, and women of color and highlights the authority that white physicians assumed in making the most intimate decisions on behalf of their patients without consulting the patients themselves. Her lawyer, Richard Levine, agreed, stating, "These people [the defendants—welfare officials, doctors, and so forth] wield enormous power in the name of benevolence. If this case does nothing else it will put a bridle on that power."[149]

Serena filed suit against the institutions and individuals complicit in removing her children and sterilizing her without her informed consent. She was only partially successful. In 1973, a jury ruled in her favor, determining that her children had been removed under false pretenses. It awarded her $17,000 and ordered her children released back to her. In 1979, Serena lost her case against the physicians and social worker involved in her sterilization after the doctor who sterilized her testified that he had explained the procedure carefully to her and that she demonstrated an understanding of it.[150]

Understanding Physicians on Forced Sterilization

How does one explain why physicians who practiced forced sterilization acted as they did? Were they all malicious? Did some act out of benevolence, however misguided such logic may have been? How did changing trends in the practice of medicine and the doctor-patient relationship influence physicians involved in abuse?

Most physicians appear to have operated with relatively benevolent intentions, genuinely believing that sterilization would raise their patients' standard of living and improve their quality of life. They functioned according to an outdated, paternal model of professional conduct, which granted doctors the authority to make life-and-death decisions on behalf of their patients. Medical paternalism functioned relatively effectively in the first half of the twentieth century when doctors practiced within their local communities and community members trusted their physician to act on their behalf. But by the mid-1960s, these once familiar public figures had become strangers. Postwar changes in medical practice—specifically, the consolidation of services within the hospital movement toward specialization, advances in diagnostic technology, and the migration of hospitals out of rural communities—disrupted the close relationships doctors once shared with their patients. With these changes, the doctor ceased to be a general practitioner residing within his local community and instead became a specialist operating in a large, impersonal institution.

Without a shared community, patients became estranged from their doctors and began to question these experts' ability to act on their behalf.[151] Despite patient skepticism, many physicians retained their right to make medical decisions on behalf of patients. While doctors held tight to paternalism, patients increasingly invoked their right to make their own medical decisions. Even after the courts and legislatures established formal protocols for medical decision making, many doctors stubbornly refused to concede their professional authority to patients, bioethicists, lawmakers, and judges. Many involved in forced sterilization acted according to outdated precepts, genuinely believing sterilization to be in the best interest of a particular patient, but failing to understand that they no longer controlled reproductive decision making.

A minority of doctors operated with more neo-eugenic intentions. Blaming poor minority women for the expansion of welfare, which they believed to directly threaten their own economic security, these doctors deliberately sterilized their patients in order to reduce the number of "defective" citizens and "undeserving" poor. As a North Carolina physician explained, "A doctor who had just got his income tax back and realized it all went to welfare and unemployment was more likely to push it [sterilization] harder."[152] Exploiting their professional authority, these physicians literally inscribed their politics upon their patients' bodies.

Both groups of doctors exploited the economic, gender, and racial disparities between themselves and their patients to intimidate patients and pressure them to consent to unwanted sterilization. As one physician commented, poor women "were uneducated and trained to do what the doctor told them."[153] Victims of sterilization abuse often reported being overwhelmed by physicians who embodied social power and prestige far above their own. In an extreme example, Guadalupe Acosta recounted the delivery that resulted in a forced sterilization. "There were two doctors just pushing down on my stomach and ... I couldn't stand it. I pushed one doctor because I couldn't stand the pain. When he came back, he hit me in the stomach and said, 'Now lady, let us do what we have to.' "[154]

Having relinquished bodily control to their doctors, victims of sterilization abuse possessed few tools of resistance. Isolated from friends and relatives, without the economic resources to change providers (and for women in labor, the time to insist upon an alternate provider), many victims of sterilization abuse lacked the means to resist their abusers effectively. Those in labor could not leave the delivery room, and those who did not speak English fluently could not fully understand the surgery being pushed on them. Those under the influence of pain medication often lacked the ability to consent to permanent contraception. Those whose doctors threatened to revoke their welfare benefits if they refused the procedure conceded rather than consented, fearful that continued resistance would cause them to lose support they desperately needed. Every woman who experienced forced sterilization witnessed the incredible imbalance of power between doctor and patient. The majority understood the racial and socioeconomic politics that created the situation. A few women forcibly sterilized continued to fight their victimization after surgery by filing lawsuits in defense of their violated reproductive rights and seeking compensation for the loss of their fertility, but even the few who succeed could not retrieve their lost fertility.

Chapter 4

"Fit" Women Fight Back

In 1971, with the aid of several Newark, New Jersey, attorneys working together with the American Civil Liberties Union (ACLU) and the Center for Constitutional Rights in New York, Anne and Barton Yohn sued Riverview and St. Barnabas hospitals for refusing Anne's request for tubal ligation after the birth of their second child. According to their lawsuit, the Yohns "had decided to limit their family to two children, feeling that this was the best and most economical [*sic*] feasible family unit for them."[1] Although her doctor was willing to perform the surgery, he was prevented from doing so by the 120 rule governing sterilization at the hospital. After giving birth, Anne resumed the use of oral contraceptives, but side effects forced her to seek an alternative form of birth control. Unable to receive the permanent contraception she desired, Anne chose an IUD. Five months after its insertion, the device failed, and Anne became pregnant with the couple's third child. In April 1969, while pregnant, Anne again requested a postpartum tubal ligation from St. Barnabas. The hospital told her it would grant her request if "she would submit to having a psychiatrist certify that she was mentally unfit to deal with the burdens of a fourth child."[2] It appears that Anne refused this option because when the family moved from Essex to Monmouth County in New Jersey in June 1969, she contacted a local physician on staff at Riverview Hospital about her request for sterilization. Unfortunately, she learned that this hospital also refused to provide healthy women who failed to meet the standards set by the age/parity formula (used by hospitals to determine eligibility for sterilization) with contraceptive surgeries unless their lack of mental fitness was "certified" by three doctors—two gynecologists and a psychiatrist. Unwilling to give up, Anne telephoned the administrator of Riverview Hospital, who not only affirmed his institution's sterilization policy but also informed Anne that vasectomies did not require the same type of regulation as tubal ligations because "it's nobody's business what a man does."[3]

The Yohns filed a class action lawsuit against both hospitals in 1971 after making a final request for surgery at St. Barnabas that was, not surprisingly, denied. In their complaint, the coupled alleged that the hospitals' sterilization policies violated several of Anne's constitutional rights, including the right to due process and equal protection under the law. Attacking the sexism expressed by the Riverview administrator, the couple alleged that women were not receiving equal treatment as men at these institutions because female sterilization was subject to regulations to which male sterilization was not. Perhaps the most controversial aspect of their claim, however, lay with the damages they sought to collect. The Yohns asked for $500,000 to compensate them for the pain and suffering of an unwanted pregnancy and childbirth, medical expenses related to that pregnancy, the financial costs of raising a third child, the loss of Anne's "earning capacity" for the last two years, and the disruption of the couple's "life plan and life style."[4] The complaint was feminist in its allegations. It sought equal treatment for men and women seeking sterilization. The plaintiffs wanted the hospitals and the courts to recognize the costs—physical, mental, and financial—associated with unplanned pregnancy in the years before abortion was legal. Their demand for compensation related to Anne's loss of wages indicates the importance of these wages for their family and highlights the value of Anne's productive and reproductive labor. It also reflects the shifting of American gender roles in the 1970s as feminists challenged rigid baby boom norms and as women, especially middle-class white women like Anne Yohn, became more visible in the workforce beginning in the late 1960s.[5]

In the end, the Yohns settled out of court in September 1972. The details of the settlement remain private, but the settlement appears to have been reached after the hospitals agreed to overturn their sterilization policies.[6] The Yohns' case is representative of a series of lawsuits filed by white women who wanted voluntary sterilization but who failed to meet the criteria established by hospital policies like the 120 rule. Committed to preventing future pregnancies and unwilling and/or unable to use temporary methods of contraception, these women used the courts to demand that their local hospitals change their outdated pronatalist policies and replace them with more contemporary rules that recognized women's expanding reproductive rights.

The Yohns were assisted by the Association for Voluntary Sterilization (AVS), Zero Population Growth (ZPG), and the ACLU, which united in 1971 to form Operation Lawsuit, a legal campaign designed to overturn restrictive hospital policies. The three groups maintained unique and sometimes conflicting motivations for participating in this action. Concerned with overpopulation, ZPG viewed access to sterilization as a necessary component of its efforts to curb an "impending" population explosion. The AVS viewed Operation Lawsuit as the next step in its campaign to legitimize permanent contraception. The ACLU's involvement had nothing to do with population control or neo-eugenics. Instead, the ACLU's participation reflected its commitment to a woman's right to make her own reproductive decisions without the interference of medicine or the law. Operation Lawsuit was only one part of the ACLU's reproductive rights activism. Other ACLU activities included defending women's access to legal abortion and representing victims of forced sterilization. Notably, only the ACLU worked on behalf of both women denied access to permanent contraception and women forced to accept the surgery. The AVS spoke out against sterilization abuse when women began to tell their stories in 1973, but neither it nor ZPG involved itself directly in the defense of the reproductive rights of poor women of color. Given these groups' concerns about the reproductive fitness of poor women of color, it is not surprising that they did not actively defend victims' right to reproductive self-determination, although they did not condone the practice of forced sterilizations either.

Operation Lawsuit recruited plaintiffs who had been denied permanent contraception and sought to overturn the policy that obstructed their access to surgery. With the help of the three groups, plaintiffs petitioned the courts to issue injunctions against age/parity restrictions like the 120 rule and to compel offending institutions to grant their requests for surgery. They also asked the courts to strike down spousal consent requirements and to force private denominational hospitals (primarily Catholic) to rescind their moral bans on sterilization. The AVS, the ACLU, and ZPG hoped that Operation Lawsuit victories would force hospitals to abandon restrictions on voluntary sterilization and usher in an era where women who wanted to be sterilized could receive the surgery on demand.

Operation Lawsuit never generated the controversy that *Roe v. Wade* or other abortion-related lawsuits did in part because sterilization has been less controversial than abortion in American culture. Abortion involves both a woman and her fetus and raises the unresolved question of when life begins, a question that pits scientists, theologians, and women (on both sides of the debate) against each other. Sterilization, on the other hand, had become an accepted method of contraception by the majority of Americans by the early 1970s, when Operation Lawsuit began, and did not entail the same ethical concerns that abortion did. As a result, plaintiffs did not need to convince judges or the general public of the legitimacy of their demands, as plaintiffs involved in abortion cases did. Operation Lawsuit plaintiffs also benefited from recent precedents in birth control and abortion policy that legalized contraception and abortion in the first two trimesters. Instead of advancing novel legal arguments, plaintiffs simply asked the courts to expand existing precedent just enough to include voluntary sterilization. The courts generally complied.[7]

Operation Lawsuit plaintiffs challenged reproductive policy from outside of the feminist movement. Although none of these women defined themselves as feminist, they expressed feminist ideas in that they sought to empower women and give them greater control over their reproduction. Some plaintiffs hoped their struggles would make it so that other women did not suffer as they had, but securing their own sterilization trumped the feminist impulses of most plaintiffs. When faced with a decision whether to continue their lawsuit and set a precedent or accept a settlement that included their own sterilization, most chose their own sterilization, sometimes with regret, sometimes with resignation, but always because they were unwilling to risk losing access to the much desired surgery. Plaintiffs' commitment to principles of reproductive autonomy reflected the extent to which such ideas—upheld in the recent decisions of *Griswold v. Connecticut* (1965), *Eisenstadt v. Baird* (1972), and *Roe v. Wade* (1973)—had filtered into mainstream society. Operation Lawsuit plaintiffs advanced ideas of reproductive autonomy that were feminist at their core and that had been advanced recently by white feminists in their struggle to legalize abortion.[8]

A "Forest Fire of Lawsuits across the Nation"

According to a 1972 study sponsored by the Commission on Population Growth and the American Future, 80 percent of Americans viewed voluntary sterilization as a legitimate method of contraception.[9] Leading medical and public health organizations revised their policies to reflect this change, as did a minority of states, which began to address the ambiguous legal status of voluntary sterilization at this time. The American College of Obstetricians and Gynecologists (ACOG) amended its sterilization guidelines in 1969 and 1970. In the first revision, ACOG replaced the 120 rule with the consent of two senior obstetrician-gynecologists and the patient. One year later, in August 1970, ACOG revised the consent requirement again, this time to eliminate the second opinion. Now, only a patient and her physician had to agree upon the surgery.[10] The 1970 policy essentially removed all institutional barriers to contraceptive sterilization, but did not constitute a victory for the AVS and other voluntary sterilization advocates because ACOG could only recommend policy changes; it could not force its members to adopt them. ZPG surveys of local hospitals found that few institutions actually amended their guidelines to reflect the change in ACOG policy, demonstrating ACOG's limited effect on medical practice.[11] Likewise, in 1972 the American Public Health Association (APHA) Executive Board adopted and promoted a Recommended Program Guide for Voluntary Sterilization to reflect Americans' increasing acceptance of permanent contraception (especially vasectomy), the increased availability of sterilization via new federal family planning funds, and the introduction of laparoscopic procedures. Developed by a task force with representatives from the American Medical Association, the American Urological Association, the AVS, the Office of Population and Family Planning in the Department of Health, Education, and Welfare (HEW), and the Centers for Disease Control (CDC), this policy also functioned as a guide, not a mandate for local hospitals to adopt.[12] The same year, the federal Commission on Population Growth and the American Future announced that "in order to permit freedom of choice," it "recommends that all administrative restrictions on access to voluntary contraceptive sterilization be eliminated so that the decision be made solely by physician and patient."[13] Like ACOG and the APHA, the commission could issue policy recommendations, but it did not have the power to force hospitals, clinics, and other medical institutions to implement them. Public attitudes, leading medical organizations, and a federal commission supported contraceptive sterilization, but the policy changes they recommended did not translate into changes in medical practices that granted women increased access to tubal ligation.

Hospital administrators resisted liberalizing their sterilization policies in accordance with the new guidelines because the legal status of sterilization remained ambiguous in the early 1970s. For example, according to the chairman of its Legal Committee, Peekskill Community Hospital in New York refused "to permit voluntary sterilization procedures at the hospital in the absence of either a statutory authorization for the same or a judicial determination that such procedure is not in violation of the criminal law."[14] A lawyer who sued the hospital on behalf of a woman denied tubal ligation described the policy as "absurd" when read in the context of New York's recent legalization of abortion. Yet the hospital held firm, insisting on explicit authorization from the state before it changed its policy, which caused the woman's husband to wonder, "Are we going to have doctors or politicians?" "If a woman decides not to have more children," he held, "that should be the end of it."[15]

A few states, like North Carolina and Virginia, passed statutes in the early 1960s that explicitly legalized voluntary sterilization, and by 1972 the last states with explicit prohibitions against permanent contraception, Connecticut and Utah, had updated their laws to reflect the changing status of the procedure. But these changes did not add up to a full legal mandate in favor of contraceptive sterilization. Most states continued to remain silent on the issue, neither explicitly criminalizing nor legalizing the surgery. The APHA read the lack of laws criminalizing the procedure to indicate its legality, as did ACOG, but the continued use of 120 rules suggests that hospital administrators and physicians did not share this interpretation.[16]

In early 1971, the AVS and ZPG joined together to challenge hospital barriers to voluntary sterilization and to clarify the legal status of the surgery across the nation by filing lawsuits on behalf of women who had been denied the surgery. Operation Lawsuit had three primary goals: obtain sterilization for its clients, force hospitals to revise their sterilization policies to comply with the recent ACOG guidelines, and secure damages for plaintiffs for the "suffering or injuries incurred" as a result of their failed requests for surgery.[17] The campaign's planners predicted a domino effect: one court would recognize women's right to contraceptive sterilization, and judges in other states would follow this lead, knocking down hospital barriers to contraceptive sterilization across the nation.

Lacking the requisite legal expertise to pursue their goals, the AVS and ZPG solicited the aid of the ACLU. The ACLU proved more receptive to the AVS's outreach in 1971 than it had to the AVS's attempts to recruit its support for the organization's campaign to promote contraceptive sterilization a few years earlier. Concerned about backlash an alliance with the AVS might generate, in the mid-1960s the ACLU kept its distance from the former eugenics group, insisting that sterilization was not a "civil liberties concern."[18] By 1971, when the AVS and ZPG approached the ACLU for help with Operation Lawsuit, the ACLU had established a policy against compulsory sterilization, but had not yet "adopted a national policy on voluntary sterilization." Given the lack of established policy on the voluntary surgery, the national ACLU decided not to join the campaign. Instead, it delegated the decision to become involved with Operation Lawsuit to its local affiliates.[19] State chapters around the country complied with many requests to support the campaign. The New York chapter was especially active.

Reliance on state affiliates was common practice for the ACLU, even after it established the Reproductive Freedom Project in March 1972. Led by director Ruth Bader Ginsberg and assistant director Brenda Feign Fasteau, the Reproductive Freedom Project was dedicated to protecting women's reproductive rights to abortion and contraceptive sterilization as well as women's right to be free from coercion related to forced sterilization and parental and spousal consent for abortion. The organization coordinated lawsuits brought by state affiliates, raised money to fund these suits, and engaged in public education campaigns designed to raise women's awareness of their reproductive rights and the resources the ACLU could provide to help women defend these rights if they were threatened or violated.[20] The Reproductive Freedom Project focused the majority of its attention on protecting women's right to abortion in the wake of *Roe v. Wade* and the backlash that this decision provoked. In a late 1970s publication, "The ACLU's Campaign for Choice," the Reproductive Freedom Project cited itself as the first organization to call "for the right of all women to obtain abortions" in 1965 and chronicled its continued commitment to preserving women's right to the procedure.[21] The ACLU's commitment to abortion rights extended beyond the Reproductive Freedom Project. In 1977, the ACLU board elected to make "restoring the right to abortions to all women" the group's "top priority" and launched a national campaign on this initiative.[22]

The ACLU's participation in Operation Lawsuit was clearly shaped by its commitment to abortion rights and to ensuring that women's reproductive decisions remained free from medical or legal interference. So, too, was its participation in lawsuits on behalf of victims of coercive sterilization. The ACLU's approach to reproductive freedom centered upon its commitment to women's right to make their own reproductive decisions—about abortion, sterilization, and contraception—without restriction or coercion. Writing about abortion in August 1973, seven months after the Supreme Court decided *Roe v. Wade*, the organization declared, "It is the ACLU's intention to mount an all-out-grassroots effort to persuade the people of the nation to keep the course charted by the Court and, in keeping it, to reach for a society in which children are born wanted, women are given control over their reproductive systems, and the religious and moral views of a minority are not forced upon the majority."[23] It applied these politics to both voluntary and forced sterilization.

Although the AVS functioned as a powerful and persistent advocate for its clients, its formal announcement of Operation Lawsuit revealed hints of its neo-eugenic agenda, which were at odds with the ACLU's position on reproductive freedom. "Is it any wonder that the uneducated and indigent mothers continue to produce children in larger-than-desired and unwanted numbers," it asked, before answering condescendingly, "they simply do not know how not to have offspring."[24] Although the AVS used the language of women's rights to advocate the overturning of restrictive hospital sterilization policies, its continued concern with the reproductive fitness of Americans suggests that its chief motivation was to make sterilization accessible to those who "needed" it. The AVS remained preoccupied with the quality of citizens and viewed the legalization of contraceptive sterilization as a means of increasing its availability. Concerned about overpopulation and especially about Mexican immigration (not surprising given its California roots), ZPG also used the language of reproductive freedom to advance its population control agenda by making sterilization available on demand. While the ACLU viewed sterilization within a larger set of struggles to secure and maintain women's reproductive rights, the AVS and ZPG viewed increased access to permanent contraception part of their agenda to reduce dependency and the reproduction of "unfit" Americans. Direct conflict between organizations never occurred, in large part because the national ACLU never committed to the campaign. The ACLU's involvement occurred on a case-by-case basis rather than through a broad commitment to the politics of its partners.

ACLU offices, ZPG, and the AVS played distinctive yet complementary roles in Operation Lawsuit. The AVS provided administrative support, dictated policy, and supplied funding; it donated $10,000 annually to the project. The AVS channeled these monies to ZPG, which coordinated and funded the campaign on a grassroots level.[25] ZPG affiliates monitored their local hospitals' compliance with the revised ACOG guidelines, requested that those institutions not in compliance with the new policy update their regulations accordingly, and identified and recruited potential clients. They also advertised campaign resources in local periodicals and petitioned state ACLU chapters for legal assistance when they encountered what they believed to be a good test case. Before approaching the ACLU, officials from both the AVS and ZPG wrote letters of support to hospital administrators on behalf of women whose requests for tubal ligation were denied.[26] When this failed, they contacted the state ACLU for support.

Operation Lawsuit followed a general sequence of actions that began when a ZPG chapter surveyed its local hospitals' sterilization policies. The ZPG chapter sent congratulatory letters to institutions in compliance with the new ACOG policy and issued written reprimands to noncomplying institutions that hinted at the possibility of legal action if the policy remained unchanged. Once the campaign won its first few lawsuits, ZPG affiliates began to append a list of successful cases to these letters to strengthen the threat of litigation.[27] If a hospital continued to refuse ZPG's request to revise its policy, a ZPG representative met with hospital administrators and issued an ultimatum: comply with our request within a designated period of time (usually a month) or risk litigation. During this interim period, the local ZPG chapter contacted the local ACLU to secure representation and undertook (sometimes with the assistance of the ACLU) the search for a plaintiff. ZPG members probed seven sources in this search: local legal aid societies, welfare departments, HEW units, ZPG chapters, ACLU chapters, doctors, and nurses. They also dispensed literature like that shown in figure 4.1 to raise awareness of their issue. Guided by neo-eugenic

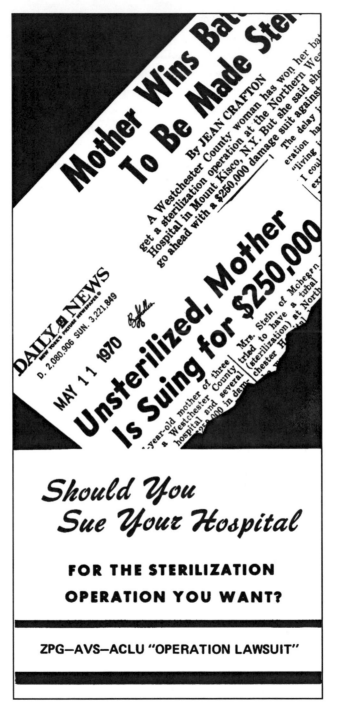

Figure 4.1 ZPG-AVS-ACLU Operation Lawsuit, "Should You Sue Your Hospital for the Sterilization Operation You Want?" Courtesy of the Association for Voluntary Sterilization Records, Social Welfare History Archives, University of Minnesota Libraries.

values, ZPG targeted public, secular hospitals for potential lawsuits because they served the largest indigent population—those individuals most "in need" of sterilization. "These institutions are completely supported by public funds and have the highest probability of serving the low-income group," the San Gabriel Valley, California, chapter proclaimed. "They are therefore top priority."[28] The AVS hinted at similar motivations in press releases and internal memos.[29]

Courtland Hastings, the AVS official who coordinated Operation Lawsuit, described the ideal plaintiff as "of sturdier-than-normal character and probably of above-average intellect, to withstand the slings and arrows and fanatical criticism almost certain to be thrown at her." "Above all," he maintained, "she must have made up her mind fully, and be determined, to go through with the lawsuit."[30] Sometimes the AVS and ZPG financed counsel for plaintiffs who subsequently dropped their suits. With limited resources, Operation Lawsuit sought to minimize its expenses by recruiting committed and determined plaintiffs. Neither the AVS nor ZPG used racial qualifications to determine if a woman was an appropriate plaintiff, but they may not have had to. Operation Lawsuit plaintiffs' complaints show that age/parity restrictions disproportionately affected white women across region, and appear to have had no effect on southern women of any color. Nationally, black women had a higher birth rate than white women (making it easier for them to qualify for sterilization under age/parity guidelines), but the gap decreased significantly in the late 1960s. Between 1957 and 1960, the black birth rate was 24 percent higher than the white birth rate, but this gap shrunk over the decade, so that between 1967 and 1970 the national black birth rate was only 7 percent higher than the white birth rate. Although blacks living in the rural South continued to have a higher birth rate than urban whites and blacks living in the urban South, the black birth rate between 1967 and 1970 had fallen below the white baby boom levels.[31] Black women would have scored higher than white women on age/parity equations, but not enough to account for the differential rates of sterilization between the races. In 1965, 14 percent of black women had undergone surgical sterilization whereas only 6 percent of white women had. Five years later, both groups of women had increased their use of contraceptive sterilization, but the racial differential remained significant: 20 percent of black women were sterilized in comparison to only 9 percent of white women.[32]

The national statistics obscure the regional component of access to voluntary sterilization. Not a single white plaintiff resided in a southern state, suggesting that hospitals in the region with the highest population of black women did not employ age/parity restrictions or did not employ them as rigidly as in other regions. CDC statistics indicate that southern women across race underwent sterilization in higher numbers than women in other regions. In 1970, 76,000 southern women (between the ages of fifteen and forty-four) were sterilized, as opposed to 47,000 women in the Northeast, 50,000 women in the north-central states, and a mere 2,800 women in the western states.[33] In all likelihood, southern hospital administrators and physicians chose not to adopt age/parity restrictions for voluntary sterilization in order to encourage covert forced sterilization. Operation Lawsuit received complaints from white women in all regions except the South, but not from women of color from any region. The AVS and ZPG did not need to make race a qualification for their choice of plaintiff; only white women appealed for assistance.

In announcing the creation of Operation Lawsuit, the AVS proclaimed its goal was to ignite "a forest fire of lawsuits across the nation."[34] But this grand proclamation conflicted with the economic reality of the campaign's financial constraints. The AVS's annual donation of $10,000 could only be stretched so far. This left the brunt of the financial burden of litigation to local ACLU chapters, which did not always possess the resources necessary to undertake suits on behalf of the women who contacted the AVS and ZPG for assistance. Although ZPG, the AVS, and the ACLU threatened noncompliant hospitals with litigation, they knew that they could not follow through on all of their threats. With their financial limits in mind, campaign officials hoped that the threat of litigation was sufficient to persuade most offending institutions to revise their policies. "A lawsuit is costly and time consuming, and therefore, it will only be filed if no other agreement can be reached," the San Gabriel Valley Chapter of ZPG admitted in an internal report dated July 1971. Thus, before taking legal action, ZPG chapters exerted pressure on resistant institutions through "mailings to the hospital, derogatory press releases and news conferences, appearances on local radio talk shows, public lectures on the issues, advertising for the plaintiff and picketing."[35] As of December 1974, Operation Lawsuit had resolved five cases, counted seven pending cases, and listed three cases as withdrawn. Its legal docket indicated notable success, but hardly constituted a forest fire of complaints.[36]

Igniting Operation Lawsuit

An examination of two of the earliest lawsuits reveals plaintiffs' commitment to women's reproductive autonomy. Both Janet Stein and Linda McCabe insisted that reproductive decision making was a fundamental right and a right that should be exercised privately, without the interference of the medical profession or government. "As a woman," Stein declared in an affidavit, "I feel

I should be free to decide what course my life should take. . . . I believe I have a right to plan my life and my family's life without the quixotic interference . . . by the defendant."[37] Both women refused to drop their lawsuits once defendant hospitals granted their requests for sterilization and insisted on collecting damages for the stress and inconveniences they endured as a result of hospital policies. These plaintiffs were distinctive in that they refused to concede even after their hospitals accepted their requests for surgery. They established precedents that other Operation Lawsuit plaintiffs drew upon when making similar claims.

On May 11, 1970, twenty-seven-year-old Janet Stein filed a $250,000 suit against Northern Westchester Hospital in Westchester, New York; its chief of obstetrics, Dr. Joseph Blanchard; its chairman of the board, Arthur W. Huguley Jr.; and its administrator, Jerome F. Peck Jr., for refusing to sterilize her after the birth of her third child. Stein's was the first Operation Lawsuit case. Stein sought sterilization for medical reasons: she had been pregnant four times, during which she had suffered a miscarriage, toxemia, hemorrhages, kidney infections, and high blood pressure. Pregnancy threatened Stein's health. Her physicians supported her decision to undergo sterilization and agreed to perform the surgery after she delivered her third child. When admitted to the hospital for delivery, Stein signed a consent form authorizing her sterilization the following morning. Stein recalled being prepared for surgery that night. "I was shaved and I was not permitted to have any food—altho I was famished. But when morning came I was told that the hospital would not permit my doctors to perform the tubal ligation because I didn't fit within the hospital's rules."[38] Northern Westchester Hospital enforced a 150 rule, which required sterilization patients to be at least thirty years old with five or more children in order to qualify for sterilization. It authorized surgery for younger women with lower parity only if pregnancy constituted a serious health risk. Stein also believed the hospital operated according to a quota system and that she was denied the surgery "solely because of the day and month" on which she requested it. Hospital administrator Jerome F. Peck Jr. denied this charge.[39]

Stein's case demonstrated the effectiveness of the Operation Lawsuit strategy to use litigation to force changes in hospital policy. Stein filed suit in May 1970, and by the first week of July the hospital had amended its policy to permit the sterilization of any adult who submitted a request in writing and obtained the consent of her spouse and physician. It also waived its spousal consent requirement for divorced or separated individuals and permitted the sterilization of minors with parental consent. The hospital claimed that the lawsuit had not prompted the policy change, that medical staff had submitted the new rules "independently" of Stein's case, and that the change was meant to reflect "less restrictive practices in respect to sterilization becoming more common in the medical field."[40] The timing of this revision and the hospital's sudden willingness to authorize Stein's request strongly suggest otherwise.

Stein continued to press for damages after securing her tubal ligation. Her perseverance signaled her desire to force the hospital to recognize the detrimental effects caused by its restrictive policies, which she believed violated her fundamental rights. In October 1973, Northern Westchester Hospital settled the case for $2,000, a payment meant to compensate Stein for the "mental anguish, invasion of privacy and denial of Constitutional rights" caused by its policy.[41] Her case set a precedent that Operation Lawsuit organizers hoped would be used and reinforced by subsequent plaintiffs.

Like Stein, Linda McCabe also successfully forced her local hospital to change its policy to reflect the new ACOG guidelines. In 1970, McCabe and her husband decided that they had completed their childbearing. A thyroid condition prevented McCabe from taking birth control pills, and like other Operation Lawsuit plaintiffs, she distrusted less effective methods of temporary contraception. She and her husband opted for her sterilization, and in August they signed a series of consent forms authorizing the surgery at the Family Planning Clinic at Nassau County Medical Center in Long Island, New York. But on August 26, 1970, the hospital denied McCabe's request. Nassau County Medical Center required its surgical candidates between the ages of twenty-five and twenty-nine to have at least five living children. (Essentially, the hospital employed a 125 rule.) McCabe was twenty-six and the mother of four living children, although she had been pregnant six times. Determined to undergo sterilization, McCabe contacted the ACLU and sued the hospital in November 1970.

Represented by Jeremiah Gutman and the New York Civil Liberties Union, McCabe sought an injunction restraining the hospital from enforcing its sterilization policy and compelling it to perform her surgery. She also asked the court to declare the policy unconstitutional and to order the hospital to award her monetary damages for the pain, suffering, and anxiety she suffered as a result of the institution's denial of her request. As the appeals court later explained, McCabe believed that she had the right "to decide for herself how many children she wanted."[42]

In a September 1970 letter to Gutman, Dr. Stewart L. Marcus, chief of obstetrics at the Medical Center, explained that the institution denied McCabe's request because she failed to meet the its sterilization requirements, which he said were based upon ACOG guidelines. Marcus clearly intended for his letter to protect the hospital, but instead it actually implicated it because the policy to which he referred was outdated, and his letter exposed his ignorance of the

1969 policy change.[43] Clearly at fault, the hospital quickly reversed its policy and performed McCabe's sterilization in January 1971.

Like Stein, McCabe refused to drop her damages claim after she underwent sterilization, believing that although she had received her desired surgery, she deserved monetary compensation because the hospital's policy violated her fundamental rights. Initially, the U.S. District Court for the Eastern District of New York dismissed McCabe's claim for damages as moot because McCabe had undergone sterilization. But McCabe appealed this ruling on the grounds that she remained uncompensated for the inconveniences the policy had caused: a second hospitalization, unnecessary exposure to anesthesia, and child-care expenses incurred during her hospital stay. Such claims were common among plaintiffs who pressed for damages after undergoing sterilization. McCabe also demanded damages for the pain, suffering, and mental anguish caused by anxieties about becoming pregnant that she endured in the interim between the hospital's denial of her request and its decision to grant her petition.[44] Stein and another plaintiff attempted to persuade the court of the damages the surgeries had caused to their marriages by introducing (or continuing to introduce) anxiety into their sexual relationships.[45] That women who did not affiliate themselves with radicalism or feminism employed such blunt language in their lawsuits demonstrates the changing social context in the last years of the sexual revolution. Not only did these women want their sexual relationships to be healthy and pleasurable, they also wanted to be compensated for interferences to these relationships caused by restrictive hospital policies. By demanding compensation for the damages suffered as a result of their hospitals' outdated sterilization policies, plaintiffs pushed the courts to recognize how denial of sterilization services affected areas of women's lives in the bedroom and beyond.

The Second Circuit Court of Appeals validated McCabe's claims and ruled in her favor in December 1971. Writing the majority opinion, Justice Feinberg maintained that the original complaint and supporting affidavits had sufficiently demonstrated that in the time between the hospital's denial of the petition and her surgery, McCabe "was in constant fear of becoming pregnant, which caused great pain and suffering and increased the likelihood of further irreparable injury." He also reinforced the arbitrariness of the hospital's policy when he wrote, "this rule is as constitutionally odious as a rule prohibiting voluntary sterilization of blacks," a declaration that surely made McCabe's legal counsel proud.[46] The Second Circuit's decision delivered a serious message to hospitals that continued to advance arbitrary policies: you can and will be held liable for the mental and financial costs resulting from denying a woman access to contraceptive surgery. Nonetheless, not all hospitals were listening, and many continued to insist on age/parity formulas. Thus, although these first few cases established important precedents, they did not go far enough to compel hospitals across the country to abandon their outdated sterilization rules. Operation Lawsuit still needed a landmark decision.

Plaintiffs Defend Their Reproductive Rights

A 1972 *Good Housekeeping* article on Operation Lawsuit plaintiff Florence Caffarelli described her as "the last person you would expect to find in the eye of a storm." But, the article continued, in 1971 this Peekskill, New York, housewife, who said she "grew up married," placed herself at the center of a legal battle over her right to voluntary sterilization because, as she explained, "I happen to think that what you do with your own body is your own affair."[47] Although her case would not provide the landmark decision Operation Lawsuit organizers hoped for, it generated considerable press and publicity for their cause.

At age twenty-six, this white mother of three children (then ages eight, seven, and three) asked her doctor to sterilize her. Caffarelli had experienced three difficult births, and when her son Michael was born, she and her husband decided that they had completed their childbearing, a decision that she believed to be "none of anybody else's business."[48] Caffarelli could not take the Pill because of the appearance of a breast tumor and had conceived Michael while using an IUD, which had caused her to cramp and bleed uncomfortably. By 1971, Caffarelli had experienced such difficulties with temporary contraception that she had come to believe that "all contraceptives seemed to be designed to make people miserable."[49] Extremely dissatisfied with her current birth control options and committed to limiting her family size, Caffarelli chose contraceptive sterilization.

The state of New York had legalized abortion in 1970; Caffarelli knew that if she became pregnant unexpectedly, she would have the option to terminate the pregnancy safely. She believed in a woman's right to choose abortion, stating, "I think every woman should be able to have an abortion if she wants one." But she did not want to confront such a decision herself, admitting, "I don't think I could decide to have an abortion."[50] Sterilization offered her the assurance that she would not experience another unplanned pregnancy; temporary methods of contraception could not do the same. Caffarelli learned about voluntary sterilization from a television appearance by AVS president H. Curtis Woods. The surgery he described seemed "fantastic" to her.[51]

Although her doctor supported her decision, believing future pregnancies to constitute threats to her health, Peekskill Community Hospital denied her request. The institution provided legal abortions but prohibited sterilization unless the life or health of a patient was threatened. Hospital administrators recognized that Caffarelli had many counterindications to pregnancy, but did not believe that they were sufficient to make her eligible for surgery. Caffarelli countered by accusing the hospital of discriminating against her on socioeconomic grounds. She did not work outside of her home, and her husband was a truck driver; the family was most likely middle to lower middle class. Her lawyers argued that the Peekskill Community Hospital's restrictive sterilization policy discriminated against "the economically disadvantaged," who could not afford to search private institutions until they could find one willing to sterilize them, and, as a result, created a situation whereby women with financial resources possessed greater reproductive freedom than women without them.[52] Caffarelli was not alone in these allegations. "If I had the money," Janet Stein claimed, "I would go at once to New York City and find a doctor connected with a hospital which would not bar me from becoming sterile."[53]

Upper-middle-class and wealthy women had greater access to contraceptive sterilization because they had the resources necessary to visit several physicians until they located one willing to perform the surgery. This is not surprising; historically, women with money have had greater access to abortion and birth control, especially when these services were illegal. Many middle- and working-class plaintiffs like Caffarelli could not afford to "shop around" for a doctor willing to sterilize them. They argued that the hospital policies created a discrepancy between themselves and wealthier women that granted women of means more reproductive rights than women without considerable financial resources. Notably, poor plaintiffs and plaintiffs receiving welfare approached the issue of access to sterilization differently. Instead of demanding equal rights, they drew upon neo-eugenic ideas to claim that sterilization was a cost-efficient way for the state to help them limit their family size. In both instances, women drew on their class status to argue against restrictive hospital policies, but their approaches varied depending on their reproductive "fitness." White middle-class and working-class women were "fit" because of their whiteness and their economic independence; they did not need to appeal to neo-eugenic sentiments. Instead, they demanded equal rights under the law. Poor women, however, played upon public preoccupation with the "dangers" of their reproduction and requested access to sterilization in order to reduce the threats their unchecked reproduction generated.

The hospital's rejection of her request for voluntary sterilization enraged Caffarelli. "How dare they? How dare they tell me and my doctor that I can't have this operation unless I'm in danger of imminent death?" she exclaimed. "I could cry to them about medical reasons—I might really die with another pregnancy—but why should I have to?"[54] Here Caffarelli articulated ideas about reproductive autonomy similar to those expressed by white feminists campaigning to legalize abortion, although she did not identify herself as such. Instead, she identified herself to *Good Housekeeping* as a "natural" wife and mother. Caffarelli was one of the most politically active of the Operation Lawsuit plaintiffs. She wrote letters of support to New York legislators in favor of legalizing abortion and was a member of ZPG. Her husband told a reporter that she was "for women's liberation 'to a certain extent,'" but insisted that his wife was not "one of those radicals."[55]

Other plaintiffs also believed that a woman should have complete control over her reproductive decisions; no paternalistic physician or arbitrary hospital policy should obstruct her right to choose voluntary sterilization. When Paska Ivezaj filed suit against Fordham Hospital in New York City in February 1971, she explained her desire for the surgery. "My first and basic reason for wanting sterilization is that I already have a family of 10, and that is enough—no other reason should be required," she maintained.[56] Similarly, after being denied sterilization by a Catholic hospital in Lorain, Ohio, an angry woman wrote to AVS executive director John R. Rague. "It just burns me," she began, that in order to undergo sterilization, "I have to leave my baby and the other 3 children, make arrangements for them to be cared for, and be worried all the time I am away, when I should be able to get it done right after I have my baby. . . . I should not have to go through all this aggravation, when sterilization is legal."[57] The women here expressed a firm belief that they bore the inherent right to determine the type of birth control they used and that they should not have to justify their decision to any physician, hospital administrator, or lawmaker. As another patient explained to the court, "I should be the one who decides on the risks to take. Since I am not a gambling woman and since I want to be the woman who raises my children I need to be sterilized."[58]

Caffarelli was one of only a few plaintiffs who viewed her lawsuit as part of a larger effort to expand women's reproductive rights. Robbie Mae Hathaway was another, albeit more reluctant, advocate for women's rights to voluntary sterilization. She sued Worcester City Hospital in Massachusetts in 1971, and her case became the landmark decision that forced hospitals across the country to abandon their age/parity restrictions. This mother of eight could hardly be called a feminist, though, and she certainly did not engage in any feminist activism. "I figure if this is what all the other women have to go through I might as well stand up and go through it all right now," she explained.[59]

Caffarelli, however, was more adamant than most plaintiffs that her lawsuit result in both her own sterilization and in a change of hospital policy in other institutions. Her case went to trial, and the judge helped arrange an agreement between the parties that would allow her to be sterilized at Peekskill Community Hospital provided she reapply for a medically necessary tubal ligation and secure written consultations in support of her surgery from two physicians. Caffarelli was reluctant to accept this agreement because it did not change hospital policy; it only ensured that she would be sterilized. At this rate, she predicted, "each individual hospital will have to be sued" before a change in policy occurred.[60] In the end, Caffarelli agreed to drop her damages claim in exchange for sterilization at the suggestion of her lawyer, who worried that if she refused the offer and continued to demand that the policy be overturned "on principle," she might lose her opportunity to be sterilized. Florence Caffarelli was sterilized at Peekskill Community Hospital on December 17, 1971.[61]

Plaintiffs' personal motivations for filing suit were underscored by their lack of collective organization. Although united in shared struggle through Operation Lawsuit, no evidence suggests that individual patients attempted to organize among themselves. In fact, no evidence indicates that patients even communicated with each other or attempted to do so. Plaintiffs' self-interest is also visible in their willingness to drop their lawsuits—including their damages claims—once the hospital agreed to change its policy or once it granted a plaintiff's request for surgery. Their actions annoyed Operation Lawsuit planners who wanted plaintiffs to continue to press for damages even after undergoing surgery in order to punish resistant institutions for their failure to comply with ACOG policy and to establish a precedent that would scare other hospitals into compliance. But having secured their desired outcome, plaintiffs dropped their suits because they had achieved their primary goal of obtaining sterilization. The precedents they could have possibly set disappeared.[62]

Although plaintiffs did not conceive of their suits as a feminist action, the AVS attempted to characterize its campaign as such in order to capitalize on growing public support for women's reproductive rights. When it launched Operation Lawsuit in 1971, the AVS solicited the assistance of feminist groups, which it asked to function in the same capacity as ZPG chapters, by surveying local hospitals' policies and bringing suits against noncompliant institutions. The AVS's mailing list of feminist organizations proved fairly comprehensive. It included radical groups like the Redstockings, Women's International Conspiracy from Hell (WITCH), and Seattle Radical Women; socialist groups like the Women's Caucus of Young Socialist Alliance and Bread and Roses; and liberal organizations like the National Organization for Women (NOW). Internal memos from the AVS reveal its strategy for courting feminists: executives hoped to capitalize on the popularity of the women's movement to gain publicity for their cause.[63] Predictably, the organization omitted references to its eugenic heritage in its correspondence with feminist groups.

In 1971, AVS executives toyed with the idea of coordinating a National Conference on Voluntary Sterilization and Women's Rights through which they intended to place voluntary sterilization in the context of other reproductive rights issues and persuade feminist leaders to include access to voluntary sterilization in their various platforms. No evidence suggests the AVS received any response to their requests for assistance. Preoccupied with their struggle to legalize abortion, white feminists ignored the AVS's solicitations. Abortion was—and continues to be—the central reproductive rights issue for most white feminists, and in the early 1970s these activists focused on legalizing the procedure. Sterilization rarely appeared on their radar, in large part because the single young women involved in the feminist movement were not considering permanently ending their fertility. It is possible that white feminists learned of the AVS's eugenic history and chose to ignore its requests for that reason. It is more likely, however, that white feminists did not associate with the AVS because they viewed sterilization-related activism as less important than abortion activism, especially before *Roe v. Wade*. The records of NOW and the National Abortion Rights Action League (NARAL, called the National Association to Repeal Abortion Laws from 1969 to 1973 and the National Abortion Rights Action League from 1973 to 1993), for example, hold few references to sterilization and the AVS, but are overflowing with strategies and efforts to legalize abortion.

The lack of organized feminist response did not, however, prevent the AVS from characterizing Operation Lawsuit victories as feminist. For example, when the Second Circuit Court of Appeals ruled in favor of Operation Lawsuit plaintiffs in *McCabe v. Nassau County Medical Center* (1971), John R. Rague, executive director of the AVS, declared, "The new court ruling shows that the concept of women as chattels is fading fast. The pro-natalist cult that interdicts, as if by holy writ, the rights of women to the use and control of their own bodies, must now be prepared to pay heavily if they persist in their folly."[64] Ira Glasser, executive director of the New York Civil Liberties Union, also declared the *McCabe* decision "a . . . victory for women's rights and women's liberation in the most vital and constructive sense of the word." "Doors long closed will now be open to women seeking sterilization," he predicted.[65] His use of this language seems less suspect as his organization was involved in advocating for women's rights beyond sterilization.

Hathaway v. Worcester City Hospital

The landmark voluntary sterilization decision came with *Hathaway v. Worcester City Hospital* in 1973. In this decision, the First Circuit Court of Appeals explicitly extended the reproductive freedoms granted to abortion and contraception in *Roe v. Wade* and its companion case, *Doe v. Bolton*, to sterilization. "While Roe and Doe dealt with a woman's decision whether or not to terminate a particular pregnancy," the court wrote, "a decision to terminate the possibility of any future pregnancy would seem to embrace all of the factors deemed important by the Court in Roe in finding a fundamental interest, but in magnified form."[66]

Thirty-six-year-old Robbie Mae Hathaway was a poor woman with eight children who lived in Worcester, Massachusetts. Although both Hathaway and her husband were employed, their combined yearly income amounted to approximately $7,500, a figure below the federal poverty level for a nonfarm family of ten. Despite their meager incomes, the Hathaways did not receive welfare, a point Robbie Mae made clear during a 1973 interview with the *Boston Globe*, which reported that "her dad taught her that welfare was bad and church was good."[67] At the time of the lawsuit, the Hathaways' insurer, Blue Cross and Blue Shield, covered childbirth but not sterilization, and their income classified them as medically indigent. The *Boston Globe* reported that because of her poverty, Hathaway had delivered her previous children as a ward patient, meaning that the state had covered her delivery expenses. Although she did not receive welfare payments, Hathaway had received free medical care from the state. Because her insurance did not cover sterilization and because her local hospital was obligated by law to finance the health care of indigent patients (Massachusetts law and Worcester city ordinances obligated the Worcester City Hospital to treat medically indigent patients), when Hathaway petitioned the Worcester City Hospital for a tubal ligation, she also asked the acute-care facility to fund the surgery.[68]

Hathaway's obesity, high blood pressure, umbilical hernia, and bleeding kidney made her pregnancies high risk; in fact, physicians had hospitalized Hathaway prior to several deliveries because of these difficulties. By the time she gave birth to her eighth child (Hathaway had been pregnant twelve times and bore eight children), Hathaway's doctors had become increasingly concerned about the health risks associated with additional pregnancies and encouraged her to employ contraception. But, like other Operation Lawsuit plaintiffs, Hathaway experienced difficulty finding a method of temporary contraception that she could use safely and comfortably. Doctors refused to prescribe the Pill because of her high blood pressure, and Hathaway was "scared" of the diaphragm. She had tried a contraceptive foam, but "it just didn't work" for her. So Hathaway began to consider sterilization. She recalled thinking, "This is pretty silly. I keep having all those children and not feeling good. . . . There's a way to have no more children."[69] Notably, Hathaway did not publicly discuss the possibility of her husband undergoing sterilization.

Like many other women, Hathaway learned about sterilization from her relatives. "The way I know about having no more children is from my niece," she explained to the *Boston Globe*. "She had a lot of trouble with her babies and so she got sterilized."[70] After the birth of her eighth child, Hathaway visited the local Planned Parenthood clinic, where she discussed alternative methods of contraception and chose sterilization. "I figured that I could go and get it done when I had my baby and nobody would know about it and they'd just think I did a good job of having no more children. But it just didn't work out that way," Hathaway remembered.[71]

In early 1971, Hathaway petitioned Worcester City Hospital for a postpartum sterilization, which her doctors classified as therapeutic given her medical problems and high parity. But the hospital denied Hathaway's request, citing a June 1970 ban on the procedure, again, further evidence of the limits of ACOG's ability to change medical practice with its new sterilization policy. Unlike the hospitals that Stein, Caffarelli, and McCabe challenged, which maintained outdated age/parity rules, Worcester City Hospital banned the procedure altogether. Hathaway was one of about thirty-five women referred by Planned Parenthood to Worcester City Hospital whose requests for surgery had been denied.[72] Frustrated at patients' inability to obtain the contraception they desired, Planned Parenthood contacted an attorney for the Massachusetts Civil Liberties Union, Mel Greenburg.

Greenburg chose Hathaway to be his test case because "she had the most acute physical problem and because she represented persons not on welfare."[73] It is not clear whether Greenburg adhered to neo-eugenic ideas personally. His statement here indicates that, professionally, he believed it important to find a client who could generate public and judicial sympathy rather than contempt. Hathaway's physical ailments offered Greenburg a measure of protection against opposition to contraceptive sterilization, as pregnancy constituted a threat to her health. More important, Hathaway embodied the AVS's argument for voluntary sterilization of the poor, especially those with larger families, at the same time her relative financial independence and marital status granted her a measure of reproductive fitness. Hathaway was a poor woman with eight children who wanted to prevent future pregnancies by employing sterilization. She was an ideal sterilization candidate because, although poor, she did not receive welfare and thus could not be criticized for bearing children she could not support, and because she was white, she did not fit the welfare queen stereotype. Greenburg's comment suggests that he believed Hathaway's marital status would protect her from critics who might attack her sexual appetite. Hathaway's frequent pregnancies revealed her sexual activity, but her marital status and commitment to her family should have shielded her from accusations of promiscuity. While these factors kept her insulated from public criticism, they did not protect her from sharp judicial reprimand.

Judge Charles Wyzanksi repeatedly dismissed Hathaway's case. He dismissed her first petition, and Hathaway appealed. The Massachusetts Circuit Court of Appeals ordered that the case be tried in federal district court, and returned it to Wyzanski's courtroom, where the judge dismissed it a second time. Hathaway recalled the judge's attitude during the proceedings: "He was saying about how his grandmother had 15 children and he figured as how the state could afford a few more Hathaways. The man didn't even know we weren't on welfare. Then he said something about how me and my husband didn't have to have intercourse anymore. Well now, I'll tell you—then they'd have a real case on their hands. He wouldn't stand for that. Leastways I hope he wouldn't."[74] The judge read Hathaway's high parity as indication of an "excessive" sexual appetite, which she should learn to control herself rather than rely upon permanent contraception to support her activity without the consequences of pregnancy. "What the plaintiff seems to regard as significant is that her appetite for sexual intercourse is so fundamental and so like an appetite for food that she is being denied equal protection if she is not permitted freely, and without risk to enjoy such intercourse with her husband," the judge wrote.[75]

The judge's rationale for dismissal blatantly contradicted centuries of legal tradition that protected the right of married couples to engage in sex without undue state interference. The judge inserted himself into Hathaway's marriage, the one site that the law has historically considered appropriate for sexual relations, the one place in which heterosexuals could freely express their sexual desires without state inference or religious condemnation.[76] The Supreme Court had upheld married persons' right to employ contraception without state interference in *Griswold v. Connecticut* (1965) and even extended this right to single persons in *Eisenstadt v. Baird* (1972). In this context, the judge's rationale for dismissal appeared outdated, a personally motivated protest of the recent liberalization of contraceptive policy.

When the Second Circuit ruled in favor of Linda McCabe in 1972, Hathaway's attorney saw one more opportunity to convince the judge of the constitutional merit of his client's case. Greenburg applied for yet another hearing, and predictably Wyzanski dismissed the case yet again. Greenburg appealed (again) to the Massachusetts Circuit Court of Appeals. The appellate court remanded the case to a lower court for clarification, but not before it ordered

Wyzanski off of it. Another judge handled the hearing, and the higher court subsequently ruled in Hathaway's favor on March 23, 1973. Two weeks after she
won her case, Worcester City Hospital approved the performance of abortions
and sterilization at its facilities. Hathaway scheduled her tubal ligation for July
1973.[77] Operation Lawsuit had won the landmark precedent it so desired.

Hathaway's case centered upon two key questions. First, could the hospital
ban sterilization but not other comparable procedures? Second, did the law compel a public hospital to provide sterilization services for the medically indigent?
In determining whether the Worcester City Hospital sterilization policy was
discriminatory, the First Circuit relied upon recent Supreme Court rulings
involving abortion and contraception. The Supreme Court developed a "rational
relationship" test in *Eisenstadt v. Baird* that compared the issue in question with
a comparable one to determine if discrimination had occurred. One year later, the
Court applied this test to Georgia's abortion code in *Doe v. Bolton*, the companion case to *Roe v. Wade*. Here the Court found no medical procedure comparable
to abortion prohibited by law, which led it to strike it down. Following the
High Court's lead, the First Circuit Court of Appeals applied the "rational relationship" test to Worcester Hospital's sterilization guidelines and concluded
that "once the state has undertaken to provide general short-term hospital care,
as here, it may not constitutionally draw the line at medically indistinguishable
surgical procedures that impinge on fundamental rights. . . . Doe . . . requires that
we hold the hospital's unique ban on sterilization operations violative of the
Equal Protection Clause of the Fourteenth Amendment."[78] Using recent precedents in reproductive rights policy, the First Circuit determined that as a public
institution, Worcester City Hospital could not arbitrarily discriminate in the
services it chose to perform at its facility. Declaring "Worcester City Hospital's
policy against the use of its facilities in conjunction with sterilization operations
unconstitutional," the court ordered the hospital to rescind its ban on sterilization and to provide sterilization to the medically indigent as it would any other
in-patient procedure.[79] With this ruling, the First Circuit extended the right to
privacy and substantive due process already established for contraception and
abortion to voluntary sterilization. In doing so, it reaffirmed Hathaway's and
other Operation Lawsuit plaintiffs' claims that women held the fundamental
right to control their reproduction in matters related to sterilization.

Spousal Consent Lawsuits and Conscience Clauses

Hathaway v. Worcester City Hospital established an important precedent
for individuals seeking voluntary sterilization, but like *Roe v. Wade*, it also
ushered in new legal questions and potential challenges to women's reproductive

freedom. The development of voluntary sterilization policy directly followed that of abortion policy. After courts found each procedure to be legal, opponents used spousal/parental consent and conscience clause claims to challenge this new status.

Immediately after the Supreme Court legalized abortion, some men tried to undermine this victory by claiming that they held as equal a stake in pregnancy as the women who carried the pregnancy, and, as a result, women should not be allowed to undergo abortion without first obtaining spousal consent. Courts overwhelmingly denied such claims. In most cases, courts recognized that male partners bore a responsibility for a pregnancy and many were invested in it, but this investment, courts determined, did not equal that of a woman, who had to bear the risks associated with pregnancy and childbirth and in whose body the pregnancy developed.[80] At the same time that husbands sought a greater say in their wives' reproductive decisions, some state politicians sought to "protect" minors from abortion and instituted parental consent laws that required girls under eighteen years old to obtain parental consent before abortion, except in emergency situations. Both spousal and parental consent laws aimed to take the abortion decision out of the hands of women and girls and mandate that they share this decision with a partner or parent, regardless of the health of such relationships. Supporters of abortion rights as well as pregnant women under attack challenged these restrictions in court. Their victories once again created precedents that supported Operation Lawsuit plaintiffs' claims.

One of the first spousal consent for abortion cases to reach trial was *Coe v. Gerstein* (1973), in which a federal court ruled Florida's spousal consent statute unconstitutional. While the court emphasized the importance of spousal agreement on the decision to undergo abortion, it determined that "the failure of the Florida 'spousal or parental consent' requirement is that it gives to husbands and parents the authority to withhold consent for abortions for any reason or no reason at all."[81] Similarly, in *Jones v. Smith* (1973), another Florida man attempted to prevent his girlfriend from having an abortion. The twenty-seven-year-old intended to marry his nineteen-year-old partner and assume the financial responsibilities of fatherhood. His girlfriend, however, wanted to terminate the pregnancy. The Florida Fourth District Court of Appeals denied Jones's claim and upheld his girlfriend's right to choose abortion. "The initial decision to terminate a pregnancy . . . *is one that is purely personal to the mother*," the court determined. Granting judgment in favor of the potential father would constitute "unreasonable governmental inference" in the defendant's privacy.[82] Courts in Massachusetts and Illinois handed down similar decisions, reaffirming the primacy of women in the decision-making process.[83]

The Supreme Court reaffirmed these lower court decisions in *Planned Parenthood v. Danforth* (1976), when it struck down, among other things, the spousal and parental consent components of a Missouri abortion statute. "No marriage may be viewed as harmonious or successful if the marriage partners are fundamentally divided on so important and vital an issue," the Court wrote, "but," it continued, "it is difficult to believe that the goal of fostering mutuality and trust in a marriage, and of strengthening the marital relationship and the marriage institution, will be achieved by giving the husband a veto power exercisable for any reason whatsoever or for no reason at all." The Court also held that "the state did not have the constitutional authority to give a third party an absolute, and possibly arbitrary, veto over the decision of a physician and his patient to terminate the patient's pregnancy."[84] Three years later, in *Bellotti v. Baird* (1979), the Supreme Court further delineated the constitutional boundaries of parental consent laws. "If a state decides to require a pregnant minor to obtain one or both parents' consent to an abortion," it asserted, "it also must provide an alternative procedure whereby authorization for the abortion can be obtained."[85] This decision authorized parental consent laws provided that the minor maintained the right to petition a court and be declared competent to consent to her own surgery.

Men who filed suits in favor of spousal consent for abortion sought to have the courts determine that their reproductive rights equaled or exceeded those of women. But the courts overwhelmingly found that women's right to reproductive self-determination trumped that of men because abortion and pregnancy occurred within women's bodies, not men's. Spousal consent suits for voluntary sterilization appeared in two forms, and both rested upon the precedents set in related abortion cases. First, only a minority of husbands sued their wives' doctors for sterilizing their partners without their permission. Operation Lawsuit played no part in such suits, as it wanted to increase women's access to sterilization, not restrict it. Instead, Operation Lawsuit endorsed the second type of case, which was far more common. In these, women filed suit against their hospitals and/or physicians in an effort to strike down spousal consent requirements for voluntary sterilization. Like women who challenged age/parity restrictions, these plaintiffs objected to the paternalism of spousal consent requirements. They contended that women, not their husbands, or their hospital, or their government, possessed the right to choose voluntary sterilization. Similar to plaintiffs who challenged age/parity restrictions, those who filed suits in opposition to spousal consent policies proved largely successful.

Although most hospitals withdrew their age/parity guidelines after *Hathaway* in order to comply with the decision, many still did not make sterilization available upon demand. Instead, they conditioned tubal ligation on the presence of spousal consent. In part, this insistence reflected the continued legal ambiguity of sterilization. For example, a physician from West Virginia, which legalized contraceptive sterilization in 1974, explained that he used spousal consent as a defensive strategy. "Regardless of the law you should have both signatures," he maintained. "I think the physician should take every precaution to protect himself."[86] According to the ACLU Reproductive Freedom Project, this physician's fear was totally unfounded. In its report "Spousal Consent for Voluntary Sterilization," the ACLU analyzed the possible causes of action against a physician or hospital that sterilized a woman without her husband's consent and concluded that women's reproductive rights had been shown to trump spousal interests in almost every instance.[87] Furthermore, to date, no husband had ever successfully argued a complaint against a physician for sterilizing his wife without his consent, and no evidence suggested that a wife ever brought such a claim against the doctor who sterilized her husband. Despite these conclusions, many doctors remained fearful of litigation from angry husbands and continued to insist upon spousal consent before performing surgery.

After the *Hathaway* victory, the Operation Lawsuit docket contained an increasing number of cases involving spousal consent. Judith Ponter of New Jersey filed one of these spousal consent lawsuits in 1975. Ponter and her husband had separated in 1969, and in 1975 Judith was pregnant with another man's child. She planned to be sterilized the day after her delivery and had the support of her physicians. In a novel alliance, Ponter and her doctors filed suit together against her husband, John Ponter, who refused to consent to his wife's surgery. In *Ponter v. Ponter*, Judith Ponter challenged the constitutionality of her hospital's spousal consent policy while her physicians sought an injunction to prevent John Ponter from bringing charges against them for sterilizing his wife. Citing *Roe v. Wade*, *Doe v. Bolton*, and *Coe v. Gerstein* (as well as *Murray v. VanDevander*, another spousal consent case), the New Jersey Superior Court ruled that "Judith Ponter has a constitutional right to obtain a sterilization operation without the consent of her husband." Firmly linking a woman's right to control the terms and conditions of her reproduction with her social equality, the court concluded, "Women have emerged in our law from the status of their husband's chattel to the position of 'frail vessels' and now finally to the recognition that women are individual persons with certain and absolute constitutional rights. Included in those rights is the right to procure an abortion or other operation without her husband's consent."[88]

Nonetheless, women's actual experiences with spousal consent requirements did not quite reflect the evolution from "chattel" to "frail vessel" to individuals with "absolute constitutional rights" that the *Ponter* decision outlined because many spousal consent policies remained in place. In one especially petty instance, Lawrence General Hospital in Lawrence, Massachusetts, barred a mother of two from surgery because she had not obtained notarized consent from her husband—who had left her three years earlier and whom she could not divorce because she lacked the resources to instigate the proceedings. This woman believed that her husband was living with another woman in New York at the time and had actually secured his consent to her surgery. But the hospital rejected the estranged husband's consent because the document was not notarized. The plaintiff petitioned the court to order her hospital to accept the nonnotarized consent and perform her surgery. In doing so, she expressed her belief that she was entitled to reproductive self-determination. "Why can't I make my own decisions," she asked. "I'm 30 years of age. I have two children. I haven't seen my husband in over three years."[89] Why should she have to receive the permission of a man who abandoned her, she wanted to know, when the decision to become sterile was hers and hers alone?

Helen Marie Brink filed a similar lawsuit. Jeff Davis Hospital in Texas refused to sterilize this mother of seven because she could not comply with its spousal consent requirement. Her husband had abandoned the family years earlier, just after she gave birth to her last child. Brink suspected that he resided in Ohio, but could not locate him. Once more, "even if I could contact him," she declared, "I know he would be opposed to the sterilization. He's hungup on this manhood thing and all he wants to do is pump women full of babies. . . . But I want out."[90] Unable to effectively use temporary methods of birth control (birth control pills made her dizzy and caused her to faint, and she became pregnant with the IUD, diaphragm, and foam), unwilling to become pregnant again, and unable to care for the children she already had, Brink wanted to be sterilized. "Everytime I would have sex, no matter what I tried to do, I would get pregnant," she complained exasperatedly. "My children are with the welfare department because I can't afford to feed them all and take care of them anymore. I'm weak after this last baby. . . . I'm just tired."[91] Brink, who lived in a "rescue mission" with her youngest child, a baby two months old, viewed sterilization as a means to reduce her dependence on welfare. When the hospital refused to perform the surgery after the birth of her last child, she filed suit, insisting that the hospital provide her with access to the contraception she desired.[92]

The Texas ACLU heard about Brink's situation and sued Jeff Davis Hospital on her behalf. Politicizing the suit, an ACLU attorney drew upon neo-eugenic sentiments to garner public support for Brink's case. Mel Greenburg had chosen Robbie Mae Hathaway because her marriage and lack of dependence on welfare granted her a measure of reproductive fitness that he hoped would protect her from criticism. This ACLU attorney did the reverse; he pointed to his client's dependency and contraceptive failures to make a case for her sterilization. Instead of rebutting negative images of poor women, the Texas attorney used them to declare his client "unfit" and in need of sterilization. "You often hear people who are against welfare say women who can't afford to support their children should be sterilized," he stated. "Well, even if some of those women want to be sterilized, it's often difficult in Harris County." Brink's attorney blamed physicians, not women, for promoting the reproduction of "social undesirables." How, he asked, could physicians complain about the "excessive" and "costly" reproduction of this population when they prevented women like Brink from obtaining sterilization?[93] This attorney cast his client as a social undesirable and played upon public resentment of women like her to generate public support for her sterilization. As with Greenburg, it is unclear whether the Texas attorney personally accepted neo-eugenic ideas about reproductive fitness and parenthood. It is possible that he did and that his sentiments motivated him to advocate for Brink. But it is also possible, given the national ACLU's commitment to women's reproductive rights, that the attorney adopted neo-eugenic language in an effort to gain the sympathies of the court and public. There is not enough evidence to indicate which theory is correct. Either way, Brink's case highlights the popularity of neo-eugenic sentiment in American culture.

As the ACLU Reproductive Freedom Project had predicted and as abortion precedent dictated, the few husbands who filed suits against physicians for sterilizing their wives without their consent lost their cases. In the most prominent case (not filed by Operation Lawsuit), in 1974 J. C. Murray filed suit against Dr. D. C. VanDevander of St. John's Hospital and Hillcrest Medical Center, both located in Oklahoma, for performing a hysterectomy on his wife, Artie, without his consent and with the knowledge that he "strenuously objected to the performance of such surgery." He alleged that the surgery interfered with both his and his wife's marital rights, and he sought damages in the amount of $100,000 for the loss of his right to consortium and "the right to reproduce another child." The Oklahoma Court of Appeals found that "the right of a person who is capable of competent consent to control his body is paramount."[94] Because Artie Murray was competent to consent to her hysterectomy and had done so willingly, the court ruled that neither the operating physician nor the hospital needed to secure the consent of her husband. It also denied J. C. Murray's loss of consortium claims and held that this doctrine did not include the right to a fertile wife. Sterilization had not altered Artie

Murray's ability to engage in sex; it simply prevented her from becoming pregnant.[95]

Unlike those men who chose to undergo vasectomy when their wives could not obtain tubal ligations, husbands who filed spousal consent lawsuits sought to usurp the reproductive freedoms recently accorded to their wives. Men who chose vasectomies acted on behalf of the couple and shared their wives' reproductive interests. But men who objected to their wives' sterilization, especially individuals like J. C. Murray, who claimed that his marriage contract entitled him to a fertile wife with whom he could consort at his will, sought to impose their reproductive values upon their wives. Their suits articulated an outdated understanding of American gender roles and of the rights of women in relation to men in marriage—rights that were increasing steadily in the 1970s as feminists pressed for equality under the law and an end to sexual discrimination.

Plaintiff Peter Gilbert offers a unique exception to this trend. In 1974, he filed suit against Nassau County Medical Center (the same hospital involved in the McCabe case) for refusing to perform a vasectomy without his wife's consent. Elona Gilbert was unable to use the Pill because of diabetes and had been advised not to undergo sterilization because of surgical risks associated with her obesity. Unwilling to rely upon other methods of contraception, Elona and Peter turned to vasectomy.[96] Elona, however, refused to provide spousal consent for the surgery—not because she did not want her husband to be sterilized, but because she objected to the principle behind spousal consent. Sterilization, she declared, was "purely private and personal in nature."[97] Peter Gilbert contacted the ACLU and went to court. Seeking to avoid public controversy, U.S. District Judge Jack B. Weinstein sidestepped the issue of spousal consent by submitting that Elona Gilbert's affidavit served as sufficient evidence of her consent and dismissing the case. Nassau County Medical Center preserved its spousal consent policy.[98]

Peter Gilbert was an exception because of his sex and because he lost his case. In most other spousal consent suits filed by Operation Lawsuit or by independent attorneys representing women whose access to voluntary sterilization had been blocked by spousal consent regulations, judges turned to the precedent set in related cases involving abortion, specifically *Roe v. Wade* and the notable spousal consent cases, to rule in favor of plaintiffs and to strike down spousal consent policies as arbitrary and in direct violation of women's rights under the Ninth and Fourteenth Amendments. Like the first group of Operation Lawsuit plaintiffs who sued to overturn age/parity restrictions, the second group of plaintiffs who challenged the legality of spousal consent policies also articulated the belief that they held the right to make their own reproductive decisions without the inference of the state, the medical profession, and their husbands. Most of the women who filed these claims had been abandoned by their spouses or were estranged from these men. That hospitals would require these women to consult with their former partners and ask their permission for surgery caused great anger among plaintiffs, who believed that they alone held the right to choose permanent contraception. In their suits and in interviews with the press, they stressed what they believed to be their inherent right to make reproductive decisions on their own behalf. Again, their claims were feminist in nature, but none of these plaintiffs identified with the formal feminist movement.

The second type of suit Operation Lawsuit undertook after scoring a major victory with the *Hathaway* decision involved conscience clauses and centered largely on challenges to the constitutionality of the Church Amendment to the Health Programs Extension Act of 1973. This act, named after its sponsor, Senator Frank Church (D-Idaho), created a policy that allowed hospitals and medical personnel to refuse to perform abortions and/or sterilizations if the performance of these procedures conflicted with their moral or religious beliefs. It also protected the medical personnel who refused to perform these procedures from employment discrimination as a result of their refusal. While the Church Amendment covered both public and private hospital employees, it only applied to private, religious facilities, as the separation of church and state prevented secular, public hospitals from operating according to a religious code of ethics. Congress restricted public hospitals from prohibiting sterilization or abortion on ethical grounds, but legislators in twenty states overcame this limit by adopting twenty-five similar laws—nineteen of which were constructed broadly enough so as to be applied to public facilities. Only two of the twenty-five laws specifically repeated Congress's provision that the clauses apply only to private hospitals.[99] These new laws governed practices not covered by earlier sterilization precedents and became the target of proponents of voluntary sterilization.

Proponents of voluntary sterilization fiercely opposed the passage of the Church Amendment, a law they interpreted as policy makers' attempt to erode women's right to voluntary sterilization and which they feared would significantly reduce women's access to the surgery. According to the *Congressional Record* of March 1973, there were 4,838 private hospitals and 2,159 public hospitals—more than twice as many private hospitals as public ones. Where would women go to receive tubal ligations if the majority of hospitals in the country refused to provide the surgery, voluntary sterilization proponents wondered?[100] In the December 1973 *Family Planning/Population Reporter*,

New York Civil Liberties Union attorney Jeremiah Gutman declared the amendment to be unconstitutional, in violation of the equal protection clause, and predicted (incorrectly) that it would not survive legal challenge.[101] The AVS also vehemently protested the passage of the Church Amendment. A. S. Holmes, the Kentucky physician active in the Hartman Plan (the AVS's pilot sterilization program in Appalachia), called the Church Amendment an egregious violation of the separation of church and state. Holmes wrote to Kentucky senator Harley O. Staggers, "In the interest of freedom, and to help keep America a Democracy, please let me beg you to reflect heavily on this 'Church Amendment,' which ironically, has a name which reflects precisely what it is—an amendment being promoted by the Church."[102] Similarly, John R. Rague, former executive director of the AVS and now president of Negative Population Growth, declared on behalf of his organization: "We oppose efforts to subvert the U.S. Constitution. . . . We oppose sectarian medicine, and uphold the right of American physicians to practice medicine without religious fiat against them."[103]

In previous cases, Operation Lawsuit plaintiffs relied on precedents set in abortion rights cases to support their claims. But few abortion rights advocates challenged the constitutionality of the Church Amendment, probably because most abortions occurred at private clinics designed specifically to provide the surgery. One abortion-related challenge arose, but the Supreme Court refused to hear the case. In *Greco v. Orange Memorial Hospital Corporation* (1975), a Texas physician brought suit against his hospital for prohibiting the performance of nontherapeutic abortions. The Fifth Circuit Court of Appeals ruled against him, determining that a private hospital funded by the state and federal government and partially controlled by the state government could refuse to perform elective abortions.[104] In the absence of supportive precedents, voluntary sterilization plaintiffs were on their own to prove that the Church Amendment violated their fundamental rights. That they failed time and again reinforces the importance of abortion-related precedents to the success of age/parity and spousal consent cases.

Conscience clauses lawsuits were distinct in another way from other voluntary sterilization lawsuits. Whereas age/parity and spousal consent suits involved women accusing hospitals and physicians of violating women's fundamental rights by obstructing their access to sterilization, conscience clause suits involved a battle of constitutional rights between hospitals, hospital employees, and women. Conscience clause suits pitted women's Ninth Amendment right to reproductive privacy (established in *Griswold v. Connecticut*) and the Fourteenth Amendment right to substantive due process (established in *Roe v. Wade*) against hospitals and hospital employees' First Amendment right to exercise their religious beliefs without state interference. Most courts ruled in favor of hospitals, arguing that as private religious institutions not directly affiliated with the state, they could not be made to perform a procedure that violated their code of ethics.

Operation Lawsuit plaintiffs argued that any hospital that received Hill-Burton funds (federal grants for hospital construction), whether public or private, functioned as an arm of the state, and in this capacity could not refuse to provide sterilization on religious grounds without violating the separation between church and state.[105] For example, Claudia Ann Kransky sued Holy Rosary Hospital in Montana for refusing to sterilize her when she delivered her third child via cesarean section in December 1972. The court dismissed her case "for want of jurisdiction," holding that the state had no involvement in the hospital's policy despite its receipt of Hill-Burton funds. Kransky's physician, James Ham, appealed the decision and asked the court to restrain "from enforcing its sterilization rules insofar as Mrs. Kransky was concerned."[106] In his suit, Ham raised an important issue regarding women's access to sterilization services. Holy Rosary Hospital was the only hospital in the area; it held a monopoly on local medical services. If this hospital refused to allow its physicians to treat women in a specific manner, the doctor argued, then its policy functioned to deny physicians the ability to treat their patients effectively, as no other alternative facility existed for doctors to use to provide tubal ligations. The Supreme Court of Montana, however, did not agree with Ham. Instead, the court ruled that although the hospital received federal funds, it remained a private entity that could not be compelled to perform the controversial surgery. That it held a monopoly on medical services in the area did not change this fact.[107]

Many women, however, thought otherwise. Most women who filed suit against hospital bans on sterilization resided in rural communities, in areas with only one local hospital, much like Claudia Kransky. Conscience clauses forced these women to travel, sometimes great distances, to facilities that would perform the procedure, and plaintiffs complained bitterly about the inconveniences this entailed: time spent away from their families, child-care expenses, travel expenses, and, for women who had sought postpartum sterilizations, a second hospitalization (and additional surgery for women who had undergone cesarian sections). A woman from Lorain, Ohio, viewed her local hospital's ban on elective sterilization as a violation of her own religious freedom. "Why should I have another's religious beliefs forced on me in this manner?" she asked. "Sure, I can go to Cleveland or Columbus or elsewhere to have it done, but that means I will have to be re-admitted to another hospital, to be away from my baby and family for another period of time—when I should have it done when I have my baby and not have to leave it later. My baby is due in exactly one month—and I have to run around like a nut from doctor to doctor because I live in a Catholic town."[108] These plaintiffs argued that their hospitals' bans on sterilization rendered *Hathaway* irrelevant, as they remained unable to obtain the desired surgery without considerable inconvenience, which constituted a violation of their reproductive rights.

Operation Lawsuit plaintiff Nery Padin presented a similar argument in her case against Fordham Hospital. Padin was married with seven children and received public assistance. She entered Fordham Hospital, a publicly funded institution run by the city and state of New York, to give birth to her seventh child in May 1972. She and her husband requested that a tubal ligation be performed after her cesarean section, and the hospital agreed to perform the surgery. But the anesthesiologist who treated her during delivery refused to participate in the second surgery, claiming that it violated his Roman Catholic beliefs. Padin received her tubal ligation months later, in September of the same year. She filed suit claiming that the hospital violated her fundamental rights "of privacy and liberty in matters relating to marriage, family, sex, and the right of every individual to control her own person" by failing to comply with her request for sterilization upon delivery.[109] Padin complained that by failing to sterilize her upon delivery, the hospital treated her differently than it would have treated a patient not dependent upon state aid, and, as a result, she experienced anxiety regarding possibly pregnancy and was subjected to a second surgery and the additional medical risks it entailed. A district court disagreed and dismissed her suit in 1975. "Plaintiff's constitutional rights clearly were not violated," the court wrote. "A public hospital may not be able constitutionally to maintain a policy of refusing to perform tubal ligations [here it referenced the *McCabe* decision], but it surely is able to schedule tubal ligations at its convenience so long as scheduling does not operate to effectively establish a policy of not performing such procedures."[110]

Public policy related to sterilization and conscience clauses was determined primarily by three federal cases—*Chrisman v. Sisters of St. Josephs of Peace* (1974), *Taylor v. St. Vincent's Hospital* (1975), and *Watkins v. Mercy Medical Center* (1975)—none of which went in favor of plaintiffs. In each case, women accused the hospitals of violating their constitutional rights while acting as agents of the state when they refused to provide the requested surgeries. (All of the hospitals involved received Hill-Burton funds.) In all three cases, the Ninth Circuit Court of Appeals ruled that the receipt of Hill-Burton funds alone did not make a hospital an instrument of the state.[111] The appellate court determined that the state had to be actively involved in the institution's operations in order for a religious hospital to be found guilty of acting under color of law and ordered to perform a surgery that violated its code of ethics. Although successful in overturning age/parity restrictions and spousal consent policies, voluntary sterilization plaintiffs failed in their challenges to conscience clauses. Private, denominational hospitals retained the right to refuse to perform sterilizations on the grounds that the surgery violated the institutions' code of ethics. Women who resided in communities served only by such institutions continued to have to travel great distances to receive tubal ligations, and those who delivered in these private hospitals and wanted postpartum sterilizations had to submit to a second surgery months later at a public institution a distance away. Those like Nery Padin who confronted medical personnel who refused to assist with postpartum surgery on ethical and religious grounds also had to submit to a second surgery. When women's reproductive rights were pitted against hospitals' and individuals' religious freedom, women lost.

Chapter 5

"Unfit" Women Fight Too

On April 24, 1973, Valerie Cliett gave birth to her third child, a son, at the Hospital of the University of Pennsylvania. The next day, the twenty-three-year-old black mother was sterilized. The *New York Times* reported that Cliett "had not requested the surgery, does not know who ordered it, did not know in advance that it was to be done and did not learn until six months later that the effect of the tubal ligation . . . was virtually always permanent."[1] In 1976, Cliett had surgery to reverse her sterilization. "The doctors [at the hospital's infertility service] told me that I didn't have good odds, but if that's what I wanted, that's what they would do," she told the *Times*. "I told them that being that the first operation was done without my consent, this operation would be done *with* my consent."[2] Doctors told Cliett that the surgery was successful, but almost two years later, she still could not conceive. In June 1978, with the aid of the American Civil Liberties Union (ACLU), she filed suit against the physicians and hospital responsible for her forced sterilization. Cliett insisted that she did not want to sue the hospital, instead she "just want[ed] them to put me back like they found me."[3]

Victims of forced sterilization and Operation Lawsuit plaintiffs shared the belief that women possessed a fundamental right to reproductive self-determination, but they envisioned the application of this right in distinct ways that reflected their different socioeconomic, racial, and ethnic positions. Victims, who were poor women and almost always women of color, filed lawsuits in order to secure the right to be free from coercion, and some of these plaintiffs requested financial compensation for the loss of their fertility and the hardship this caused. Those who used lawsuits to change public policy advocated the establishment of regulations designed to create a protective space between vulnerable women and coercive surgeons in order to reduce the incidence of sterilization abuse. Operation Lawsuit plaintiffs, on the other hand, were white women whose socioeconomic status ranged from middle class to quite poor. They went to court to remove administrative obstacles that obstructed their access to contraceptive sterilization. Like victims, some Operation Lawsuit plaintiffs pursued damage claims, but instead of asking for compensation for the loss of fertility, these women requested compensation for the anxiety that being denied permanent contraception caused them.

The claims put forth by both groups of women reflected their politics of reproductive freedom. When compared, these lawsuits reveal the extent to which race and class shape women's notions of reproductive rights. Operation Lawsuit plaintiffs defined reproductive rights as unrestricted access to reproductive health services, a definition that reflected both the racial privilege that their white skin afforded them and their own experiences with restrictive hospital policies like the 120 rule. Operation Lawsuit plaintiffs' ideas about reproductive freedom corresponded with those articulated by white feminists in the early 1970s who sought to legalize abortion. Because white feminists, Operation Lawsuit plaintiffs, and white women in general lacked access to abortion and voluntary sterilization but rarely experienced coercion, they tended to frame reproductive rights as a struggle to access health care services. They aimed to break down barriers—legal and/or medical—that blocked their access to abortion, contraception, and sterilization. Overturn restrictions, their thinking went, and gain reproductive freedom. Victims of forced sterilization, women of color, and feminists of color, however, viewed access to reproductive health services as only one part of their agenda to secure their reproductive rights. These women insisted that the right to restrict one's reproduction had to be accompanied by the right to bear and raise children without interference. Their definition of reproductive freedom revealed that they faced a very different set of reproductive health issues than white women did. To begin, they responded to discrepancies in the health and health care of their community. In this period, women of color experienced higher maternal mortality rates, higher rates of poverty-related diseases that complicated their ability to become pregnant and carry a pregnancy to term, and higher rates of death from illegal abortion than white women.[4] In addition, they placed struggles for reproductive control within the context of contemporary social movements, including the Black Power movement, the Puerto Rican independence movement, the Chicano/a movement, the welfare rights movement, and the feminist movement. Women who filed lawsuits against those physicians and institutions complicit in their infertility incorporated their demand.to be free from coercive sterilization within a broad philosophy of social justice that included the right to equal access to health care services, decent housing, adequate nutrition, and safe work environments as well as the right to choose contraception and abortion without interference. Keenly aware that sterilization abuse inscribed the triple oppressions of racism, sexism, and poverty onto their bodies, these plaintiffs incorporated their demands for reproductive freedom within the larger struggles for racial equality and economic opportunity.

Operation Lawsuits plaintiffs proved generally successful in their attempts to challenge restrictive hospital sterilization policies, but victims of forced sterilization were not so lucky. Out of thirty-three cases filed by victims against the individuals and institutions responsible for their sterilization in the 1960s and 1970s, only one yielded a verdict favorable to the plaintiffs, and even this verdict had its limits. Women who filed lawsuits complaining of forced sterilization faced three main barriers. First, the contraception, sterilization, and abortion cases brought by white feminists and Operation Lawsuit plaintiffs had created a legal definition of reproductive freedom that emphasized women's access to reproductive health services, but did not address their right to be free from coercion. Operation Lawsuit proved so successful, in large part, because it built upon a rapidly developing body of reproductive rights law that could be applied directly and easily to voluntary sterilization. But victims of forced sterilization had no such precedents to draw upon. Second, when the practice of forced sterilization changed during the late 1960s and 1970s in response to the development of federal family planning and the legitimization of contraceptive sterilization, physicians involved in coercion began to record coercive surgeries as voluntary. When women went to court to protest their abuse, they found the validity of their claims questioned by defense attorneys who pointed to the presence of signed consent forms to argue that women knowingly and willingly submitted to surgery. Defense attorneys sometimes painted plaintiffs as unstable women who regretted their choice and blamed their regret on their physicians instead of assuming responsibility themselves. In doing so, attorneys stigmatized plaintiffs as mentally ill and untrustworthy, demeaning their testimonies and offering an alternative explanation for their traumatizing experiences. Finally, evolving but unclear definitions of informed consent stymied plaintiffs' efforts to win their lawsuits. Sterilization abuse victims came forward with their claims precisely when bioethicists, legislators, judges, hospital administrators, and some doctors began to standardize definitions of informed consent and to formalize the consent process. Because definitions of informed consent remained in flux at the time of their trials, victims struggled to establish violations of rights that had not been explicitly recognized by medicine and the law at the time of their surgeries.

Victims of forced sterilization articulated their definitions of reproductive rights through their lawsuits, but the courtroom was not the only forum through which victims and their advocates demanded reproductive freedom. Grassroots coalitions of black, Chicana, Puerto Rican, and Native American women also called attention to new forms of forced sterilization and demanded an end to the practice in the form of the development of protective safeguards for women at risk. Minnie Lee and Mary Alice Relf, the two Alabama girls who were sterilized without their knowledge in June 1973 and whose case brought sterilization abuse into the national spotlight, filed the first forced sterilization lawsuit that same summer, while Congress tackled legislation involving standards of informed consent for research subjects and regulation of medical experimentation. The girls became a cause célèbre for the issue of sterilization abuse, and their case acted as a catalyst for the development of a loosely organized sterilization abuse movement that developed in the mid-to-late 1970s.

Forced Sterilization Plaintiffs

At least thirty-three lawsuits involving coercive sterilization were filed in the late 1960s and 1970s, along with other informal complaints of the practice.[5] These lawsuits constitute a small minority of those women touched by forced sterilization, but they offer insight into plaintiffs' backgrounds, their experience with forced sterilization, the repercussions that followed surgery, and women's understanding of their rights under the law, specifically their reproductive rights.

Several differences exist between plaintiffs in voluntary and involuntary sterilization lawsuits, most notably their race. All Operation Lawsuit plaintiffs were white, and it appears that all forced sterilization plaintiffs were women of color.[6] Some poor white women were sterilized without their knowledge or informed consent during this era, but they constituted a minority of victims and do not appear to have filed lawsuits. All forced sterilization plaintiffs were poor; some received welfare, others did not. Financial independence did not protect poor women from abuse. In contrast, Operation Lawsuit plaintiffs spanned the socioeconomic spectrum, from poor to middle class. (Upper-class women possessed the resources necessary to "shop around" for a doctor willing to provide the controversial surgery and thus did not participate in Operation Lawsuit.) That poor white women filed suits to gain access to surgery but not to protest sterilization abuse indicates that poor women of color were far more at risk for forced sterilization than their white counterparts.

Poverty did not prevent forced sterilization victims from defending their reproductive rights in court. The nonprofit Southern Poverty Law Center, a firm established in 1971 in Montgomery, Alabama, that was committed to civil rights, and the ACLU's Reproductive Freedom Project provided legal counsel for plaintiffs.[7] Theoretically, funding should not have influenced whether a woman filed suit, especially because both organizations maintained connections with the communities in which plaintiffs resided. But access to legal aid was not the only factor influencing a woman's decision to challenge her sterilization in court. Lawsuits involved public exposure, something that many victims of forced sterilization did not want, as many women reported feeling shamed by the experience, and some went so far as to hide their infertility from family and friends. The experiences of the women who filed the thirty-three lawsuits are fairly representative of forced sterilization in this era, but their determination to file suit set them apart from their peers.

Plaintiffs resided in rural and urban communities across the United States, including cities in California, South Carolina, New York, North Carolina, Arizona, Georgia, Washington, Indiana, and Maine. The diversity of locales indicates the rapidity with which sterilization abuse proliferated beyond southern states following the development of federal family planning and the legitimization of voluntary sterilization in the late 1960s and early 1970s.

Victims' suits exposed the number of government institutions and employees complicit in forced sterilization. Most involved local and state governments, whose failure to police their employees suggests a silent endorsement of the practice. For example, in *White v. Druid City Hospital*, a Selma, Alabama, woman accused her city hospital and the Department of Pensions and Security of forcing her to undergo sterilization in order to regain custody of one of her children. Three months pregnant at the time of the tubal ligation, the woman delivered a stillborn fetus one month later.[8] In *Johnson v. City of New York*, Rosalind Johnson accused the city of forcing her to submit to sterilization under false pretenses while a prisoner at Rikers Island Penitentiary. A physician punitively sterilized Johnson when she underwent a late-term abortion at Kings County Hospital Center in March 1976 without her informed consent. According to Johnson's lawyer, the attending physicians informed Johnson, who was twenty years old at the time, "if you become a normal citizen you can have your tubes untied."[9] Filed in 1977, the case closed in 1983 after being brought to trial and "settled after discussion with the trial judge." Johnson received $22,500 in compensation for her forced sterilization, and the judge settled the case without the recommendation of the plaintiff's attorney, which suggests the possibility that Johnson's interests were not entirely protected.[10]

In *Harris v. Karam*, two Arizona women filed a class action suit against Pinal County for denying them maternity care on the grounds that their benefits only covered abortion and sterilization. They argued that the policy encouraged poor women to end their reproduction by refusing to support prenatal care but funded the termination of pregnancy and fertility.[11]

Most forced sterilization lawsuits were brought by individuals, although few class actions were filed and tried. Once sterilized, plaintiffs lacked standing as representatives of the class of women at risk of abuse. In addition, forced sterilization victims sought damages for injuries already sustained, damages that could not be divided easily among plaintiffs like class actions require. Courts refused these plaintiffs class standing on these grounds. Class actions are expensive undertakings and require resources that most small law firms do not possess, as well as attorneys with experience with what in the 1970s constituted a new form of litigation. The ACLU Reproductive Freedom Project and the Southern Poverty Law Center had experience and funding to undertake such suits, but local ACLU chapters likely did not, which helps explain why Operation Lawsuit cases were filed on behalf of individuals rather than classes. It is likely that the individualized nature of medical claims also contributed to the lack of class action claims filed by women seeking access to surgery.

Forced sterilization victim Nial Ruth Cox failed in her attempt to represent women vulnerable to abuse. In 1965, at age eighteen, she agreed to undergo a sterilization that she believed to be temporary after a welfare worker threatened to revoke the family's funding if Cox did not accept the sterilization. The welfare worker petitioned the state eugenics board to sterilize Cox, using her poverty and illegitimacy as evidence of her lack of reproductive fitness. Five years later, Cox learned the truth: her sterilization was permanent. With the help of the ACLU, Cox sued to have the North Carolina eugenics law overturned and asked for $1 million in damages for the emotional and physical injuries she sustained as a result of her surgery. In *Cox v. Stanton*, Cox sought to represent the class of women susceptible to similar forced sterilization, but the lower court determined that she lacked standing because she could no longer prove that she was threatened by the eugenics law, as she had already been sterilized. After dismissing her class action claim, the court found in favor of the defendants (which included not only state officials but also the physician and hospital administrators responsible for her surgery) after it determined that the three-year statute of limitations had expired. Cox was sterilized in 1965; she learned her surgery was permanent in 1970. Cox believed the clock should begin when she learned of her sterilization, not when she was sterilized, as the defense argued. The lower court sided with the defense and ruled against Cox.

Cox appealed, and a year later an appellate court upheld the statute of limitations, although it did note that the district court had "incorrectly applied" the law. This portion of Cox's case was essentially lost on a technicality.[12]

Although most victims could not serve as plaintiffs in class actions, they could use the courts to demand compensation for the damages caused by their forced sterilization. They asked the courts to award them millions of dollars in compensation for their stolen fertility and the pain and suffering that resulted. Through their suits, victims of forced sterilization challenged stereotypes like the "welfare queen" and "pregnant pilgrim," which rested upon the notion that women of color's reproduction was inherently costly, destructive, and unworthy of government support. By demanding significant compensation for their losses, victims insisted that the courts recognize the value of their reproductive labor and protect their right to determine the terms and conditions of their reproduction just as it protected middle-class white women's access to abortion, birth control, and voluntary sterilization.

Impediments to Victims' Lawsuits

Operation Lawsuit plaintiffs drew upon recent precedents in reproductive rights law to make their claims. The right to reproductive privacy recognized in *Griswold v. Connecticut* (1965) protected married couples from government intrusion into their contraceptive practices. *Eisenstadt v. Baird* extended this same right to unmarried individuals in 1972. One year later, the Supreme Court legalized women's right to reproductive autonomy in the context of abortion in *Roe v. Wade*. That same year, in *Hathaway v. Worcester City Hospital*, the First Circuit Court of Appeals ruled that public hospitals could not arbitrarily refuse to provide sterilization to patients, effectively extending the right to privacy already granted to temporary contraception through *Griswold* and *Eisenstadt* to permanent contraception. These landmark decisions granted women unprecedented access to abortion and contraception, but did not afford the most vulnerable women protection against coercive medical practices. White feminists' struggles to legalize abortion and birth control involved creating a zone of privacy around a woman's body upon which the government could not infringe. In theory, this zone could have protected against coercion. But in practice, as the lawsuits explored here demonstrate, the zone encompassed only women's access to abortion and contraception.

Griswold, *Eisenstadt*, and *Roe* reflected the reproductive rights philosophies of middle-class white women and, to a lesser extent, middle-class women of color (who possessed the resources to hire physicians to carry out their reproductive decisions, but whose skin color kept them somewhat vulnerable to medical racism). Most forced sterilization plaintiffs filed suits asking the court to recognize that their fundamental rights had been violated during their surgeries, and in doing so, called upon judges to expand the boundaries of reproductive freedom further to protect the interests of some of the most vulnerable women—poor women of color. With one exception, *Relf v. Weinberger*, the judges rejected these claims. In part this is because victims could not use recent abortion and contraception precedents to support their claims. *Griswold* and other precedents involved access to surgery, not protection from coercion. Most forced sterilization lawsuits were based upon civil rights precedents and U.S. Code 1983, which prohibits states and state employees from discriminating against citizens.[13] As a result, these cases did not directly impact existing reproductive rights precedent, although at least one judge recognized the right to reproduce as fundamental.[14] With successful litigation, Operation Lawsuit plaintiffs gained access to voluntary sterilization, and white women's definition of reproductive rights became inscribed into law. Poor women of color, however, generally lost their cases, remained vulnerable to forced sterilization, and had to look beyond the courts for protection. Despite plaintiffs' efforts, race continued to shape and define women's reproductive rights and experiences, and the courts' recognition of white women's demands but not poor women of color's regarding sterilization ensured that differential levels of reproductive freedom would endure in the United States in the 1970s.

News of the Relfs' sterilization occurred at a moment when policy makers began to insert themselves into medical decision-making processes and the public learned of earlier medical abuses, especially those directed toward people of color. The Relfs' story broke during a series of congressional hearings about human experimentation that was dominated by the Tuskegee Syphilis Study. Between 1932 and 1972, the Public Health Service (PHS) undertook a study of syphilis in Tuskegee, Alabama, that monitored the effects of the disease when left *untreated* in roughly 600 African American men. PHS researchers went so far as to instruct draft boards not to conscript participants in order to prevent subjects from being treated by Armed Services doctors and to withhold penicillin after the antibiotic's introduction in 1945. Public outrage over the Tuskegee study erupted in July 1972 when an Associated Press journalist, Jean Heller, exposed the story. To many, especially those involved in the civil rights and Black Power movements, revelations of the unethical treatment of black research subjects confirmed not only the continued secondary status of blacks in America but also reignited concerns about medical racism.[15] News of the Tuskegee Syphilis Study emerged one year before the Relf case, and when the second story broke, the public, the media, and the politicians quickly linked the two together. For example, the author of an article published in the *Peabody (Mass.) Times* in July 1973 bluntly concluded, "I don't think it's a coincidence that the victims of these federally-funded experiments were black. Time and again people in power have abused their office by victimizing black people and by seeing them as sub-human objects."[16] An article in the *Boston Globe* published the same month was titled "Blacks Major Victims of Medical Experiments." It pointed to the Tuskegee study, the Relfs' sterilization, and a third study involving medical racism to argue that "there is particular reason for blacks to maintain a certain amount of paranoia, even today, because they continue to be the brunt of these cruel jokes, all in the name of medical science."[17] For black women, this history of abuse extended back to the days of slavery when slave women became the subjects of early gynecological research, in the years before anesthesia.[18]

News of the Tuskegee study compelled policy makers to confront the history of American medical research, most of which went unregulated for over a century. For most of the twentieth century, American physicians conducted experiments with human subjects without the presence of specific protocols or standards of consent and without judicial oversight or interference. Although not hampered by explicit policies, physicians in the first half of the century "observed limits in their experiments with human subjects."[19] These limits included engaging in therapeutic experiments, which could benefit patients, rather than nontherapeutic experiments, which could only harm patients; benevolent deception, whereby physicians disclosed a limited amount of information about a given experiment or treatment believing that full disclosure could lead to depression or discouragement in a patient; the attainment of written consent (in the absence of a clear definition of what constituted consent); and compensating patients monetarily for their time and effort. Physicians who generated positive outcomes that improved the health of their subjects or that yielded new medical innovations without harming patients received the greatest support from their colleagues and from the press and general public. Physicians also tended to avoid public condemnation for their human subject experiments when they first tested a given substance on themselves, their families, and/or their medical students. The medical profession cast these individuals as heroes (if they survived) and martyrs (if they succumbed to disease). Although antivivisectionists (those opposed to nontherapeutic human and animal experimentation) attacked physicians involved with human subject experiments in the first decades of the twentieth century, by the 1930s organized medicine had accumulated enough status through recent advances related to insulin, sulfa drugs, and treatments for pernicious anemia to rebuff critics' claims and to ease public concern about human experimentation.[20]

Doctors functioned with internal mechanisms of control in the first half of the twentieth century, but without clear, established standards that defined the line between consent and coercion, without a definitive framework to judge risk levels, and without hospital or university oversight boards to govern the ethics of experimentation, experiments sometimes injured human subjects, often those with the fewest legal rights and financial resources. It was not uncommon, for example, for physicians in the first few decades of the century to use orphans as subjects of their experiments. In 1921, a New York journalist exposed studies of scurvy being performed on orphans at the Home for Hebrew Infants that involved the withholding of orange juice from infants until they developed signs of the disease. Wondering if it was possible for the orphans to develop the disease a second time, researchers repeated the experiment on the same subjects. Similar experimental methods were used to study rickets.[21]

The fuzzy line between consent and coercion is visible in a 1915 study of pellagra. A PHS investigator wanted to prove that pellagra was caused by poor nutrition, not a bacterium. He planned to place prison inmates on a pellagra diet to demonstrate this and approached the governor of Mississippi with a request for human subjects. The governor complied and offered inmates a pardon in exchange for their participation in the study, an offer that generated a sizable group of volunteers, twelve of whom were chosen for the experiment. Although antivivisectionists characterized this quid pro quo—participation for pardon—as coercion, the majority of critics expressed concern not about the ethics of the experiment but rather about the leniency of the law. This response points to the ways in which contemporary cultural beliefs and trends shape public response to medical experimentation. In a similar instance, during World War I military physicians recommended the removal of the gall bladders of chronic typhoid carriers. Military physicians could force soldiers to accept surgery in a way that civilian physicians could not, which raises the question, to what extent then, did soldiers who were carriers have a choice as to their medical treatment?[22]

Government regulation of human experimentation emerged in the 1970s, spurred on by calls from within the medical profession for reform. In 1966, Henry Beecher, a medical professor at Harvard University, published an exposé of abusive research practices in the *New England Journal of Medicine*, which demonstrated the regularity and commonality of practices like the injection of live cancer cells into subjects as part of a study examining immunity to cancer.[23] Beecher's piece began a decade of public, legal, and medical discussions of medical ethics and the limits of human subject research that occurred during the golden age of medicine in which such experiments had led to huge medical innovations, such as the development of penicillin and cortisone. During World War II, medicine and the government cast experiments on "marginal" citizens as patriotic and necessary. Although the war ended in 1945, the practice of using individuals confined to mental institutions and prisons, or enlisted in the armed forces, did not stop, as federal monies poured into hospitals and medical schools. In fact, one of the first trials of the Pill involved psychiatric patients at the Worcester State Hospital.[24] At midcentury, the practice of medicine was in a period of transition as the profession experienced its golden age. The local doctor who made house calls was replaced by the large, impersonal hospital and medical specialists, creating a gulf between patients and physicians. During this period, physicians retained their professional authority despite the fact that they no longer shared a common bond or worldview with their patients—a bond that had previously helped patients to feel comfortable permitting physicians to make their health care decisions. Research physicians maintained this decision-making authority and actively withheld information from their subjects. Most often they did not believe that subjects could fully understand the inner workings of a given experiment, and some researchers feared that if patients knew about all of the risks involved in the experiments, they might become frightened or want to pull out of the study. Unwilling to lose subjects and committed to medical innovation and advancement, many physicians experimented on subjects who could not refuse treatment or who did not have the information necessary to make an informed decision about their participation.[25]

Beecher's article launched a period of investigation by journalists, scholars, and federal investigators, who uncovered scandalous incidents of medical abuse between 1968 and 1973. The most disturbing example was the Tuskegee Syphilis Study. Beginning in 1968 with Senator Walter Mondale's bill to establish a Commission on Health Science and Society, federal legislators inserted themselves into the medical decision-making process. Mondale's bill failed, but in 1973 Senator Edward Kennedy conducted hearings on human experimentation that resulted in development of the National Commission for the Protection of Human Subjects the following year. Kennedy devoted one day to involuntary sterilization and the Relfs' experience, but the Tuskegee Syphilis Study dominated the hearings.[26] Other reproductive abuses came out during these hearings, including those related to contraceptive uses of Depo-Provera and DES (diethylstilbestrol), which had been approved by the Food and Drug Administration (FDA) for noncontraceptive purposes. Kennedy's hearings exposed the story of a Tennessee clinic that injected fifteen women on welfare with Depo-Provera without informing them that it had been found to cause cancer in beagles. (The same family planning workers that sterilized the Relfs had also given the girls and their sister Depo-Provera before permanently sterilizing them.) In addition, the Kennedy hearings also revealed that fifteen university health care centers had been prescribing DES as a "morning after treatment." In the 1940s, doctors began to prescribe DES for pregnant patients in order to reduce miscarriage. Despite the fact that no clinical trials ever demonstrated its effectiveness, by 1971, 500,000 to 2,000,000 pregnant women had taken DES. In the early 1970s, researchers identified a link between DES and a rare cancer of the vagina, and subsequent studies found DES children were at risk for other health effects and their mothers were at increased risk for breast cancer. The FDA warned against prescribing DES for pregnant women soon after the first study was published. Given the clear evidence of risk from reputable sources (the first article published citing the dangers of DES appeared in the *New England Journal of Medicine* by doctors from Massachusetts General Hospital), why was it being used on young female college students who presumably would want to have children in the future, Senator Kennedy and the public wanted to know.[27]

Although the Kennedy hearings and the establishment of the 1974 commission signaled the government's concern about medical abuses directed at the poor and people of color, they did not offer victims of sterilization abuse any tangible protection against coercion or precedents that could be used in a court of law. The regulations and committees established to govern human subjects were related to experimentation and research; they did not cover forced sterilization recorded as voluntary. They helped raise awareness of medical racism, but they did nothing to prevent sterilization abuse or to compensate victims for their suffering. Once again, women forcibly sterilized fell outside the bounds of government protection.

Patients in hospital and clinic settings confronted different issues of medical ethics than patients involved in medical experiments, and these entered public conversation in the 1960s and 1970s with the rise of the consumer movement, the women's health movement, and the welfare rights movement. The women's health movement challenged the dynamics of the doctor-patient relationship and sought to redistribute power between patient and physician by educating women about their bodies and by informing them that while their physician had medical expertise, they were experts about their own bodies. The publication of *Our Bodies, Ourselves* in 1971 reflected this thinking, as it encouraged its readers to use the information it provided to assert their authority in medical situations, challenge their physicians, and advocate on their own behalf. Production of this book and subsequent editions was a collective effort that involved not only members of the Boston Women's Health

Book Committee but also readers who wrote into the collective to share their stories, their knowledge, and their comments about the book. This collaboration represents the democratization of medical knowledge central to the women's health movement.[28]

Hospital administrators shared federal legislators' commitment to curbing medical abuses and responded to health activists' calls for greater patient protection. The American Hospital Association (AHA) adopted a Patient Bill of Rights in 1973, which theoretically should have protected against forced sterilization, but which in practice did not. First published in 1970 by the Joint Commission on the Accreditation of Hospitals (JCAH) and inspired by the National Welfare Rights Organization (NWRO), the published policy provided that patients should be treated equally regardless of race, class, or ethnicity and mandated that medical staff respect patients' rights to privacy and "considerate and respectful care."[29] The AHA policy indicated hospital administrators' commitment to patients' rights and reflected the influence of contemporary social movements. But like the establishment of the National Commission for the Protection of Human Subjects, the AHA policy offered victims of forced sterilization no tangible basis upon which to rest their legal claims. The Patient Bill of Rights was not public law, and it was not adopted by all hospitals. Indeed, as *Madrigal v. Quilligan* (a case involving ten Chicanas forcibly sterilized at the University of Southern California, Los Angeles County Medical Center [USC, L.A. County Medical Center]) showed, some hospitals adopted patients' bills of rights and standards of informed consent only after patients complained of sterilization abuse. Further, a major flaw existed in these policies: they lacked enforcement mechanisms to ensure physicians' compliance. In fact, some critics charged that administrators designed the policy to reduce the potential for litigation rather than to protect patients' rights.[30]

The absence of hospital policies standardizing informed consent coupled with the lack of enforcement mechanisms in the polices established during the years of peak sterilization abuse (1970–1974) left patients interested in filing lawsuits in a predicament. Their abuse had occurred in the interim between the time that medical professionals, legislators, hospital administrators, feminists, and consumer activists began to openly discuss issues of informed consent, but before they could effect change. With no explicit policies on the books at the time of their sterilization, plaintiffs could not successfully argue that their surgeons had deviated from the national standards of obtaining consent. In fact, in *Madrigal v. Quilligan*, the testimony of the plaintiffs' expert witness on informed consent conflicted with the testimony of the defendant physicians, signaling the transitional nature of the issue. Medical professionals and policy makers created commissions to investigate medical abuses and proposed policies to protect patients' rights in the early-to-mid-1970s, but these efforts yielded no enforceable rules that victims could use in court to argue that their fundamental rights had been violated.

Walker v. Pierce

"I feel that sterilization is a necessity in patients showing an unwillingness to not provide [an] adequate environment in which to bring up a child," Dr. Clovis Pierce wrote to the commissioner of the South Carolina Department of Social Services on October 1, 1973.[31] Pierce had become the subject of a local controversy earlier that July when Carol Brown, a white mother of four who received welfare, complained that the physician refused to deliver her child unless she consented to sterilization—which she declined. Brown had enrolled in welfare in February of that year, after her husband went to prison to serve an eighteen-month sentence for grand larceny. Pierce wrote to the commissioner in defense of his policy, which required that Medicaid patients with two or more children submit to sterilization upon delivery. "At no time is there any manner in which this (the policy) can be misconstrued as being mandatory as no patient is ever forced to come to this office for medical care," he insisted, before concluding that women "certainly have the free choice of not coming to this office."[32]

But in fact, poor women in Aiken, South Carolina, did not have the freedom to choose an obstetrician who respected their reproductive autonomy. Pierce was one of only three obstetricians in Aiken County. It seems all three physicians enforced similar sterilization policies, while two of the three obstetricians refused to see Medicaid patients. This made Pierce the only available provider for pregnant women on welfare. Carol Brown had to travel twenty miles to Augusta, Georgia, in order to locate a physician willing to deliver her child without requiring that she submit to sterilization.[33]

Shortly after Pierce's policy had become the subject of public debate, Virgil Walker and Shirley Brown (not related to Carol Brown, who complained but did not sue) filed suit against the physician for forced and attempted forced sterilization, respectively. Both plaintiffs were black and welfare recipients. Walker and Brown used a report on Pierce's practice conducted by the commissioner of the Department of Social Services in the wake of Carol Brown's complaints to reinforce their claims.[34] The investigation revealed that Pierce had sterilized eighteen welfare recipients between January 1, 1972, and June 30, 1973. Sixteen of the eighteen women were black, and Medicaid paid the doctor $60,000 for his services.[35] When the commissioner received the results of his investigation, he requested that Pierce sign an affidavit promising not to discriminate against Medicaid patients. Pierce refused, and the department imposed nonpayment sanctions against him on September 27, 1973.[36]

Virgil Walker consulted Pierce twice in January 1972 for prenatal care while pregnant with her fourth child. She repeatedly refused to submit to Pierce's stipulation that she undergo sterilization—even after he threatened to have her welfare benefits withdrawn. Unwilling to accept Walker's decision, Pierce contacted a Department of Social Services caseworker and requested that he convince Walker to consent to the unnecessary and unwanted surgery. The caseworker testified that he offered to locate another physician for Walker, but Walker countered that the caseworker told her that he could do nothing to remedy her situation. She then unsuccessfully attempted to locate an alternative provider, but the doctor she contacted was not accepting new patients. Feeling defeated and rapidly approaching her due date, Walker surmised that continuing to resist Pierce "would have been futile," and agreed to sterilization.[37] She delivered her fourth child on April 6, with the aid of a different physician who secured yet another consent to sterilization. Pierce sterilized Walker on April 17, 1973.

The second plaintiff, Shirley Brown, consulted Pierce during her third pregnancy in 1973. Because Brown did not receive welfare at the time of this appointment (Brown's insurance covered a portion of her fee, and she paid for the remainder herself), Pierce did not request that she comply with his policy. By August of the same year, though, Brown had separated from her husband and taken maternity leave from her job at Seminole Mills. As a result, she qualified for medical assistance. She delivered on September 2 with the assistance of another physician. Upon learning that Brown had given birth, Pierce sent his nurse to obtain her consent for sterilization because Brown now qualified for sterilization under his policy. When Brown refused to submit to Pierce's demand, he ordered her discharged from the hospital—less than twenty-four hours after delivery. Concerned about her daughter's health, Brown's mother offered to pay the hospital bill, but "afraid something might happen to her," Brown instead chose to leave the hospital. When she complained about her treatment to a hospital administrator, he replied that he lacked the requisite authority to interfere with doctors' discharge orders and suggested that she file a complaint with the board of trustees. Brown later named this official as a defendant in her lawsuit.[38]

Two other patients corroborated plaintiffs' accounts of coercion but did not join the lawsuit. Both women were black. In the summer of 1973, Marietta Williams told her story to the *New York Times*. Pierce sterilized Williams after the birth of her third child in 1973. She was only twenty years old. Williams claimed that Pierce threatened to take her to court if she refused to sign a consent form. Fearful of such action, she consented despite her desire to retain her fertility. Her new son suffered from an "intestinal disorder that keeps him from retaining any oral nourishment." He remained hospitalized at the time the article appeared. Williams worried about the health of her child and lamented her sterility. "I wouldn't marry again," she confessed, "who would want me, knowing that I cannot have any children?"[39] The *Washington Star News* published another patient's story the same summer. Dorothy Waters claimed that two weeks prior to delivering her fifth child, Pierce "informed her that he would not deliver the child" unless she consented to sterilization.[40]

With the aid of the ACLU Reproductive Freedom Project and the Southern Poverty Law Center, Virgil Walker and Shirley Brown filed suit against Pierce for his discriminatory policy and the injuries it caused them and sued the local government officials and hospital administrators involved in their surgeries for conspiring with Pierce to deprive them of their fundamental rights. A lower court judge found in favor of the government officials, and a jury fined Pierce $5.00 in nominal damages for his treatment of Brown. Nominal damages are meant to validate a plaintiff's claims in cases in which the plaintiff suffered no real harm.[41] The jury's ordering of Pierce to pay $5.00 in nominal damages indicates that jurors recognized that Brown was mistreated, but that they did not believe that she suffered real harm. The jury decided that Walker had consented to her surgery and found in favor of Pierce. Both parties appealed the decision, and the Fourth Circuit Court of Appeals heard the case in March 1977. The appeals court reversed the lower court's judgment against Pierce (the $5.00 nominal damages) and affirmed its finding in favor of the government officials and hospital administrators in July. Walker and Brown appealed the decision to the Supreme Court, but the Court refused to hear their case.[42]

The issue of where and how to negotiate a balance between women's right to reproductive autonomy and physicians' right to practice their politics lay at the center of this case. Patients claimed that they were forced to consent to surgeries that they did not want in order to receive medical care. Pierce claimed that he had a right to practice medicine according to his own politics, to establish the conditions of medical care he provided without interference, and to maintain two standards of care—one for patients on welfare, one for patients not receiving aid. He insisted that women on welfare who objected to his policies were free to seek another provider. But his patients complained that they did could not locate another provider willing to treat them because either no other local doctors accepted Medicaid or the other doctors employed the same policy as Pierce did. In their suit, plaintiffs claimed that because he accepted Medicaid, Pierce acted as an agent of the state and could not discriminate against his patients when serving in that capacity. Pierce denied that he functioned as a government agent when he accepted Medicaid payments and patients, and he defended his right to practice medicine according to his personal politics. The majority on the Fourth Circuit agreed with him.[43]

As was common in forced sterilization suits, the majority in *Walker v. Pierce* pointed to the presence of signed consent forms as evidence of defendants' innocence. "At no time is he [Pierce] shown to have forced his view upon any mother," the court determined. "Indeed, quite the opposite appears . . . in this case . . . not just one but three formal written consents were obtained." Here the court referred to the consent forms Shirley Brown signed before and after her delivery—after she had determined that resisting Pierce "would have been futile." The majority ruled that because Medicaid did not cover Walker's delivery fee (although it did cover her hospital and physicians' bills), Pierce had not functioned as a representative of the state and therefore was not guilty of discriminating against Brown and Walker in this capacity. "We perceive no reason why Dr. Pierce could not establish and pursue the policy he has publicly and freely announced," the court wrote.[44]

This ruling illuminates a critical set of issues raised by forced sterilization plaintiffs. Should women who receive welfare be granted less reproductive freedom than women who can afford medical care? Does the government have a responsibility to ensure that women on welfare possess the same reproductive freedom as women who do not receive state assistance? Pierce conditioned his treatment of women on welfare upon their acceptance of sterilization and received government funding for the services he provided. Plaintiffs in *Walker v. Pierce* asked, was this practice legal? Should women who accept welfare relinquish their reproductive rights as a condition of receiving aid?

Pierce testified that his "policy was with people who were unable to financially support themselves, whether they be on Medicaid or just unable to pay their own bills, if they were having a third child, to request they voluntarily submit to sterilization following the delivery of the third child. If they did not wish this as a condition for my care, then I requested that they seek another physician other than myself."[45] The majority upheld his right to do so. But the problem was that women could not always choose an alternative provider. Most poor rural women lacked the resources necessary to search for another doctor, and because not all doctors accepted Medicaid, women found their search limited to those physicians willing to accept their payment plan. The time limitations of pregnancy also handicapped women's attempts to locate a cooperative physician. And as Shirley Brown's experienced showed, even those women who managed to avoid Pierce during delivery could fall victim to his postpartum harassment.

Notably, Pierce removed race from the debate. His defense of his policy did not include a reference to race, even though the report issued by the commissioner of the Department of Social Services showed that 89 percent of the patients sterilized under this policy were black and Pierce's own statements reflected his distain for "welfare queens."[46] This raises the questions, To what extent were race and neo-eugenics factors in this verdict? Did the judges look at the plaintiffs as "welfare queens" like Pierce did, and if so, did this perception influence their ruling? Did the judges believe that women on welfare should forfeit their reproductive decision making as a condition of receiving aid? While theoretically judges are objective, in reality, personal opinions sometimes shape judges' rulings. Nancy Hernandez's sentence to sterilization for the misdemeanor of occupying a room with marijuana demonstrates this, as does Judge Sprankle's sentencing of Miguel Vega Andrade to undergo a vasectomy for failure to pay child support. Although the majority rejected plaintiffs' accusations of discrimination, the minority opinion highlighted the neo-eugenic assumptions implicit in Pierce's policy and called them and the majority's endorsement of Pierce's behavior into question in its dissent.

Appellate Judge John D. Butzner Jr.'s dissent illuminated the prejudices implicit in the majority ruling. Butzner concluded that Pierce's policy privileged his politics over the health of his patients and that the doctor's actions constituted a clear violation of his patients' fundamental rights—not to mention the code of medical ethics. This liberal judge and advocate of civil rights appointed to the Fourth Circuit Court of Appeals by President Lyndon B. Johnson in 1967 wrote: "It is clear that he [Pierce] undertook to grant or deny Medicaid benefits for reasons unrelated to his patients' health." South Carolina did not act as an intermediary between Medicaid patients and their physicians as many states did. Instead, it allowed recipients to contact Medicaid providers independently and thus granted doctors the right to accept or reject these patients freely. The state did not involve itself in the doctor-patient exchange until the physician submitted for reimbursement. Therefore, the dissenting judge determined that Pierce had assumed an administrative responsibility for the Medicaid program and that, as such, the doctor had discriminated against the plaintiffs while acting as a state agent. "Had Dr. Pierce's decisions to sterilize his patients been based on their medical needs," Butzner wrote, "he would not have acted under color of state law." But because the judge conditioned his treatment of welfare recipients upon sterilization, Butzner believed him to be guilty of administering a policy that "was based on economic factors instead of the health of his Medicaid patients," and doing so while acting on behalf of the state.[47]

Judge Butzner reviewed the plaintiffs' claims in the context in which they occurred, moving beyond the presence of consent forms to examine the nature of the consent process. He determined that Pierce's politics had contaminated his medical practice and that because the doctor acted as an agent of the state, he implicated the state in his social engineering agenda. Butzner's dissent validated the victims' claims and pointed to Pierce's guilt.[48] Although the majority ruled in favor of Pierce, the debate within the appellate court shows that judges did not unilaterally endorse forced sterilization and suggests that neo-eugenic sympathies influenced the majority's support of Pierce's policy.

The local medical community proved less divided than the Fourth Circuit on the issue of Pierce's policy. Thousands of citizens, the South Carolina Medical Association, and hospital administrators stood behind Pierce and defended his right to practice medicine according to his own social politics. "I have no quarrel with that policy," Aiken County General Hospital Administrator J. Sam Nesbitt told reporters for the *Charlotte Observer*. "It is well within accepted standards." A New Ellenton pharmacist circulated a petition that collected 5,279 signatures in support of Pierce's right to practice medicine according to his own politics. And the South Carolina Medical Association announced its support for Pierce by passing a unanimous motion in January 1974 that supported a doctor's right "to insist upon sterilization permission before accepting a patient," provided the doctor articulate his or her stipulations "at the initial visit." Requiring doctors to explain their policies to patients during the initial visit offered patients no protection against abuse; the policy was designed to support physicians' right to reduce the number of children on welfare.[49]

Madrigal v. Quilligan

On June 18, 1975, ten Chicanas filed a civil lawsuit against the USC L.A. County Medical Center for coercively sterilizing them during delivery. All of the women were poor and eligible for medical assistance, but none received welfare.[50] All were sterilized between 1971 and 1974. In January 1970, the USC L.A. County Medical Center terminated its age/parity policy, which required women to be at least twenty-five years old and the mother of four children in order to be considered eligible candidates for sterilization, and sterilization became far more accessible as a result. But it took four years before the hospital enacted a policy to monitor the consent process. In February 1974, the chairman of the Department of Obstetrics and Gynecology, Dr. Edward James Quilligan, issued a memo in response both to new federal sterilization guidelines developed by the Department of Health, Education, and Welfare (HEW) and to concerns reported by one of his residents, Dr. Bernard Rosenfeld, that "patients were not getting adequate counseling as to their sterilization procedure." The 1974 policy stated: "Effective immediately, patients will not be approached for the first time considering sterilization when they are in active labor. All patients should be aware of the methods of family planning prior to entering the hospital in labor and should they wish some form of permanent sterilization, this should have been recorded in the chart prior to the admission to the hospital in labor. If a patient has had no prenatal care and has high parity, she should then be informed after her labor and delivery of the methods of family planning available, and should she wish sterilization, she should be scheduled for elective surgery at a future date on the gynecologic service. This includes individuals undergoing a Caesarean section."[51]

Plaintiffs in *Madrigal v. Quilligan* argued that the absence of a clear policy governing informed consent for sterilization encouraged sterilization abuse. Nine of the ten plaintiffs were sterilized in the interim between when the hospital lifted its age/parity policy and when it established the consent policy. That one plaintiff was forced to accept sterilization one month after the hospital instituted its protective policy demonstrates its limited effectiveness in preventing coercion. According to her lawyers, when Estela Benavides was admitted to the USC L.A. County Medical Center in March 1974, she "found herself in the labor room in pain, hemorrhaging, being confronted by several doctors—several doctors came to her bedside, spoke to her, told her several times that she needed to be sterilized. Fearing for her life, believing that if she did not have the operation that she would die, Mrs. Benavides signed the consent."[52] Seven of the ten plaintiffs signed consent forms while under duress and/or under the influence of pain medication. The remaining three patients were sterilized without their written consent.[53] Plaintiffs' lawyers sought to prove that their clients had been pushed into accepting surgery during labor when they lacked the power to resist effectively or else consented to the procedure without fully understanding its permanence. In a few instances, patients left the hospital after birth and sterilization without knowing that they could no longer have children.

The *Madrigal v. Quilligan* trial began on May 31, 1978, and lasted two and a half weeks. Plaintiffs were represented by a young lawyer who was just two months out of law school, Antonia Hernandez, with the Model Cities Center for Law and Justice. Hernandez and another attorney, Charles Nabarrete, prepared and tried the lawsuit with considerable assistance from Gloria Molina, a member of Comisión Femenil Mexicana Nacional, a Chicana activist group established in 1970 to address employment-related issues.[54] Molina helped with fund-raising, media relations, and office space, in addition to organizing demonstrations against forced sterilization and in support of the plaintiffs. The Southern Poverty Law Center also helped finance the suit.[55]

During the trial, Hernandez and Nabarette provided strong evidence of abuse, most notably through the affidavits of victims themselves and the testimony of one former medical student (who graduated from USC Medical School in 1971), Dr. Karen Benker, willing to testify against her colleagues.[56] They also called expert witnesses to support their claims that their clients had not provided their informed consent for sterilization. Anthropology professor Dr. Carlos Velez-Ibanez, of the University of California, Los Angeles (UCLA), studied the women and presented his findings, which showed the women to have been deeply scarred physically and mentally by the surgery. Dr. Don Sloan, a New York physician with experience testifying in court on issues of informed consent, concluded that "a woman, while in labor undergoing emotional and psychological stresses which accompany labor, and being in the labor room, and being approached for the first time regarding sterilization, cannot give a valid and informed consent." Plaintiffs' attorneys also brought in a psychologist to testify that the surgery caused "emotional trauma" and led to depression, as well as a handwriting specialist to examine the signatures on the consent forms, who determined that the writers experienced distress while signing.[57]

Benker's testimony exposed the neo-eugenic attitudes of her colleagues, which plaintiffs' affidavits and testimonies supported. In addition to attending medical school at USC, Benker worked at the hospital as an obstetrical technician, so she had considerable exposure to the hospitals' obstetrical culture and practices. During her tenure at the hospital, Benker witnessed Dr. Quilligan make derogatory remarks about the fertility of poor Mexican and black women. She recalled that on her first day on the obstetrics ward, her class met Dr. Quilligan. When asked about the new equipment in his ward, Quilligan allegedly said, "We just got a federal grant . . . to show how low we can cut the birth rate of the Negro and Mexican population in Los Angeles County."[58] Here Benker accused Quilligan of accepting federal funds with the goal of evaluating the effectiveness of using sterilization to reduce the birth rates of black and Mexican women in order to reduce welfare costs. Benker also testified that many doctors "would express very prejudiced remarks about patients who didn't speak English—Mexican-American patients" and referred to Mexican American women as "beans."[59]

Benker's testimony proved quite damning, as evinced by the repeated objections of defendants' attorney, William Maskey. Judge Jesse W. Curtis's own pessimistic views of Mexican women's fertility emerged during Benker's testimony. Interrupting Benker's testimony, the seventy-year-old Nixon appointee postulated, "Suppose he [a doctor] does favor sterilization at every chance he can get. . . . There is a big segment of the people in this country . . . who believe that one of the prime causes of our social and economical problems are big families where the parents are not able to socially or economically support them." The judge continued, "I do not think it is surprising that you might find a doctor who believes that people who are inclined to big families shouldn't, and particularly for good medical reasons, undertake to persuade a person not to have a large family. And if that person agrees and is willing to be sterilized, then I cannot see anything wrong with the doctor having suggested it or having convinced the patient, so long as he does not use his powers, his ability, his circumstances to override what would be a *reasonable* decision on the part of the patient."[60]

But plaintiffs' affidavits and testimonies demonstrated that the physicians on trial had in fact exploited their professional authority and forcefully compelled some women to consent to the unwanted surgery on the basis of their own prejudicial ideas about Chicanas' reproductive fitness.[61] Consuelo Hermosillo, sterilized at age twenty-four after the birth of her third child, testified that during her prenatal visits, hospital staff repeatedly requested that she consent to postpartum sterilization. "They told me that there was a limit of only three cesareans by law; that the limit was three cesareans," she testified.[62] Of course, no such law existed. In fact, the nurse who attended Hermosillo during her prenatal exams told her that the three cesarean rule was not true. "Don't be crazy," the nurse told Hermosillo, "I have had five cesareans and I do not need that." The same nurse also warned Hermosillo of coercion, telling her "not to pay any attention to the doctor, that all they wanted was to cut the person's tubes, even though they could have another cesarean."[63] Hermosillo resisted signing the consent form before labor, but after fearing that she would not be allowed to have her baby via cesarean until she consented to sterilization, she relented and signed the consent form while in labor and under the influence of pain medication.[64]

Several Chicana patients at the USC L.A. County Medical Center not named in the lawsuit submitted affidavits that supported plaintiffs' claims. One patient shared Maria Figueroa's experience. In labor with her sixth child, a doctor approached her while in the labor room. Unable to deliver naturally after several hours because the baby was breach, physicians decided to operate. "The doctor asked how many children I had," she recalled. When she told him five, "he said that I had too many children, also that having future children would be dangerous for me." She stated that "a nurse brought forms for my signature, no one explained the contents or meaning of the forms nor did I read the forms." She signed because she was "in considerable pain" and was desperate to have her baby "as soon as possible." She learned of the permanence of her sterilization three to four months after her surgery.[65]

Dr. Benker corroborated patients' accounts when she testified that physicians routinely threatened to withhold treatment from patients until they consented to tubal ligation. "Once it became clear that a C-section was going to be necessary the resident staff was extremely aggressive in pushing for sterilization, virtually without exception," she explained. Describing abuse that she witnessed "on an almost daily basis," Benker said that "the doctor would hold a syringe in front of the mother who was in labor pain and ask her if she wanted a pain killer; while the woman was in the throes of a contraction the doctor would say, 'Do you want the pain killer? Then sign the papers. Do you want the pain to stop? Do you want to have to go through this again? Sign the papers.'"[66]

Plaintiffs' lawyers hired Velez-Ibanez to evaluate the cultural impact of sterilization on the plaintiffs. Days before Velez-Ibanez's scheduled testimony, the judge questioned the relevance of this expert's opinion, again revealing his own personal prejudices. "The court knows, and everybody knows, the Mexican people have strong feelings about a big family, and how they have an intense love and affection for children and that sort of thing," the judge lectured plaintiffs' attorneys, before condescendingly adding, "I do not anticipate anything that he will tell me that I don't already know." Curtis's comments expressed a widely held stereotype about Mexican women's hyperfertility. Judge Curtis expressed such confidence in the validity of these ideas that he chided plaintiffs' attorneys for hiring Velez-Ibanez, saying, "If you are paying any real money to get him here, I think it is a waste of money."[67]

Curtis ultimately allowed Velez-Ibanez to testify. Velez-Ibanez's study consisted of "participant observation, unstructured interviews, and questionnaires." It concluded that the women placed an extremely high value on motherhood consistent with their rural Mexican origins, and thus their forced sterilizations proved immensely devastating to their gendered identities and social standing. "Motherhood lay at the center of plaintiffs' personal, social, and cultural identities," the anthropologist maintained, "to be *una mujer* [a woman] was to have children."[68] Forced sterilization had violently and fundamentally undermined victims' social and cultural identities. The anthropologist claimed that each plaintiff's "sense of continuity with the past had been fractured, her sense of self-worth had been shattered." In short, "each woman is in fact now stigmatized."[69] Ashamed of their infertility, six of the plaintiffs hid their surgeries from their siblings, and three hid their victimization from their mothers.[70] Plaintiffs' attorneys also hired New York psychiatrist Terry A. Kupers to examine the plaintiffs, evaluate their mental health after surgery, and determine whether they had provided informed consent to sterilization. Kupers examined nine of the ten plaintiffs (the tenth was in Texas at the time). The psychiatrist reiterated much of Velez-Ibanez's findings that patients experienced physical ailments and mental stress as a result of their surgery.[71]

The anthropologist also attributed an increase in family tensions to forced sterilization. As a direct result of the surgery, eight marital relationships "suffered irreparable damage," three of which resulted in divorce (before the trial had begun), and two of which involved physical violence.[72] Plaintiffs themselves articulated these problems to journalist Claudia Dreifus. One woman reported that "to this day, he [her husband] is very angry. There are constant problems. Fighting. He says 'Surely we will part. You never lacked a home. You never lacked food. Why did you let them do this to you?'"[73] Another victim's common-law husband of eight years abandoned her and their two children because of her infertility.[74]

Judge Curtis filed his opinion on June 30, 1978. He found entirely for the defendants and dismissed all charges against Dr. Quilligan and another administrator at the hospital, Dr. Roger K. Freeman, on the grounds that plaintiffs had "failed to show that either of these defendants participated personally in the sterilization operations."[75] In a rather cruel twist, the judge manipulated Velez-Ibanez's findings and used them to blame the victims for their own sterilization, which he deemed a result of "miscommunication" between patients and their physicians caused by the victims' cultural background. The judge determined that plaintiffs had characterized themselves as "victims of a concerted plan by hospital attendants and doctors to push them, as members of a low socioeconomic group who tend towards large families, to consent to sterilization in order to accomplish some sinister, invidious, social purpose." He found no evidence of such a plot administered by the defendants. Instead, the judge found that "whenever a sterilization procedure was suggested or advised, it was done on the initiative of the individual employee," and that hospital administrators were not accountable for their physicians' actions, especially because "no hospital rule of instruction directed to these employees" encouraged them to push sterilization on poor Chicanas.[76]

In the final opinion, Judge Curtis reviewed each plaintiff's case and concluded that each had failed to provide sufficient evidence to support her claims of coercion. He further determined that each physician who performed a sterilization "was acting in a bona fide belief" that the patient "had consented to the operation and that such belief was reasonable."[77] After disregarding plaintiffs' accounts as flawed, the judge attacked the evidence provided by plaintiffs' expert witness, the New York psychiatrist specializing in issues of informed consent who maintained that women in labor could not give actual informed consent because of the duress labor caused. "Such a statement," Judge Curtis declared, "completely defies common sense." Instead, the judge found defendants' testimony that informed consent "depended on many facts, and that a judgment could best be made by someone present at the moment the decision is made" more convincing. This someone, of course, was a physician; patients themselves were there too, but Curtis rejected their "non-expert" opinions. The judge believed that the power to determine when informed consent could and could not be given rested with the attending physician, "since he would be acutely aware of the necessity of having the patient's consent."[78] When confronted with conflicting expert testimony about contemporary medical ethics and regulation of the consent process, the judge endorsed the one that better upheld physicians' authority.

The judge concluded his opinion by declaring, "There is no doubt that these women have suffered severe emotional and physical stress because of these operations. One can sympathize with them for their inability to communicate clearly, but one can hardly blame the doctors for relying on these indicia of consent . . . which are in constant use in the Medical Center." Yet no clear policy regarding informed consent, specially related to sterilization, existed between 1970 and 1974, when nine of the ten plaintiffs' surgeries occurred. Instead, the judge preferred to grant physicians continued control over the consent process and allowed them to disregard the latest trends in medical practice related to standards of informed consent, which the New York psychiatrist brought to the court's attention. In fact, while plaintiffs testified repeatedly that they spoke Spanish fluently but had been given consent forms in English—and were rarely provided a translator—and thus were unable to understand the permanent nature of the surgery, the judge concluded the plaintiffs bore responsibility for their own sterilizations. It was their fault that they could not "communicate clearly" with their physicians in English, not the fault of the physicians who failed to communicate with their patients in Spanish. That only two of the ten women understood English "even a little," according to their lawyer, did not influence the judge's ruling.[79] Curtis's emphasis on English as the required language hints of anti-immigrant attitudes.

Soon after the decision came down, plaintiffs' lawyers announced that they would file a Notice of Appeal of the decision, and Nabarrete indicated that "a main issue to be raised on appeal would be the failure of the court to discuss the issue of informed consent." Nabarrete was especially concerned that the judge disregarded his expert witness on informed consent, whom he maintained represented the views of the medical community.

It is unclear what actually happened to the appeal, as the legal and archival records stop with Curtis's decision.

Madrigal v. Quilligan was one of the largest forced sterilization lawsuits of the 1970s. It received national media attention, and considerable coverage by local newspapers, most notably the *Los Angeles Times*. The lawyers, community activists, and physicians who worked on the case uncovered considerable evidence of abuse at the USC L.A. County Medical Center. Dozens of affidavits and depositions from women who ultimately did not join the suit, could not represent the class for logistical reasons, or chose not to move forward with it corroborated plaintiffs' claims of mistreatment. But the court refused to recognize the abuse plaintiffs experienced, blaming patients for their victimization and upholding physicians' rights to impose their politics on their patients.

Early Sterilization Abuse Activism

In the summer of 1973, news of Minnie Lee and Mary Alice Relf's forced sterilization shocked the nation and prompted both an outpouring of sympathy and heated condemnations of the state and federal agencies involved in the abuse. The timing of the announcement, on the heels of public exposure of the Tuskegee scandal and during congressional hearings on biomedical abuses, ensured that the story would attract media attention. In a statement to the Senate Health Committee on July 13, the Urban League denounced the incident as a "horrific action" that illustrated the extent to which "racism is still an underlying factor with many of the agencies providing family planning services to the poor."[80] Four days earlier, fourteen social and religious organizations had issued a collective statement expressing their contempt for the government's role in the Relfs' sterilization and calling for the establishment of federal and state laws to protect women from sterilization abuse, especially minors and individuals mentally incompetent to consent to surgery. This diverse coalition demonstrates the range of activists concerned about forced sterilization. Led by the National Council of Negro Women, the alliance included the United Methodist Board of the Church and Society, the Church Women United, the National Council of Jewish Women, the National Organization for Women (NOW), Zero Population Growth (ZPG), the American Ethical Union, the American Humanist Association, the Church of the Brethren, the Citizens Committee on Population and the American Future, the National Women's Political Caucus, the Unitarian-Universalist Fellowship, the United Church of Christ's Division of Health and Welfare, and the Women's Equity Action League.[81]

In an interesting twist, the Relfs' sterilization prompted the Association for Voluntary Sterilization (AVS) to form a partnership with the NWRO.

The NWRO, established in 1967, developed and promoted the first succinct ideology that linked issues of racial justice with reproductive rights and economic freedom. Black women dominated the ranks of this grassroots organization of welfare recipients, accounting for roughly 85 percent of members by one estimate.[82] Initially, the NWRO privileged poverty-related issues, but by 1972 it assumed a more overtly feminist position, broadening its commitment to mothers' rights and personal choice to one of women's rights and reproductive choice. Although many historians have claimed that welfare rights activism brought gender into existing struggles for racial equality, more recent scholarship argues the inverse: that welfare rights activists "attempted to define welfare and poverty as women's issues."[83] Securing reproductive freedom, defined by the right to bear and raise children with dignity and to have unrestricted access to reproductive health services, became a central goal of the NWRO.

Welfare rights activists strove to empower poor women and grant them access to the resources necessary to achieve autonomy. Characterizing welfare as an entitlement rather than a privilege, the NWRO sought to push the government to recognize the labor involved in child care and housework and to level the myth of the welfare queen. By supporting a guaranteed annual income, NWRO members hoped that to ensure welfare recipients' financial independence from men and help these women to avoid being forced to work in the lowest paid and most humiliating jobs. By demanding that the government validate their reproductive labor with a guaranteed annual income, welfare rights activists enjoined the state to invest in their families to the same extent that it invested in white middle- and upper-class families. Since the earliest days of mothers' pensions in the second decade of the twentieth century, the welfare system "rewarded" mothers who complied with white middle-class codes of conduct and imposed harsh, invasive regulations to force those women who challenged these norms into submission. In the first decades of the century, reformers denied black women access to welfare services on the basis of their race, and in the postwar era policy makers created punitive rules like "man-in-the-house" and "suitable" home policies with the same intent. In both instances, policy makers demeaned black women's reproductive labor, deeming it not valuable enough to warrant a government subsidy. The NWRO, like the other welfare rights groups it inspired, argued that the government bore a responsibility to help all poor women provide for their children by ensuring them access to living-wage jobs, child care, public housing, and medical assistance. Poor people, NWRO members maintained, deserved to live decently and with dignity.[84]

Reproductive choice played a critical role in the NWRO's materialist politics of entitlement.[85] In welfare activists' minds, living decently and with dignity involved guaranteed access to quality medical care, including reproductive health services, and the right to birth control and abortion must be accompanied by the right to purchase these services without fear of coercion. Years before white feminists would define their movement to defend the right to abortion as pro-choice, women on welfare organized around their right to choose when and under what conditions to bear children. "Nobody realizes more than poor women that all women should have the right to control their reproduction," NWRO leader Johnnie Tillmon stated.[86] Countering neo-eugenicists' claims that poor women could not reproduce responsibly and opposing punitive sterilization bills that mandated the sterilization of welfare recipients with two or more illegitimate children, welfare rights activists argued that all women possessed the right to bear as many children as they desired, and insisted that regardless of its level of financial support, the state could not interfere with women's reproductive decisions. "Ain't no white man going to tell me how many babies I can have. . . . And ain't nobody in the world going to tell me what to do with my body, 'cause this is mine," Doris Bland of the Mothers for Adequate Welfare in Boston proclaimed.[87]

The NWRO and the AVS issued a "Joint Statement Against Forced Sterilization," just five days after the Relfs' surgery, which branded coercive sterilization "a violation of inalienable human rights and an unreasonable assault on human dignity."[88] The AVS did not explicitly explain its motivation for joining with the NWRO to protest the Relfs' surgery. Most likely, the AVS allied itself with the NWRO as part of its effort to recast itself as an organization committed to voluntary sterilization on demand and to distance itself from its eugenic past. With medical and scientific abuses coming under congressional and public scrutiny, the AVS needed to emphasize the voluntary nature of its goals in order to avoid backlash and accusations of social engineering. Establishing an alliance with the organization that represented women who could be characterized as "welfare queens" constituted a clever strategy to achieve this outcome.[89] Sterilization abuse like the Relfs' threatened to undermine the AVS's efforts to bring sterilization to the masses and to taint public perception of the surgery. Speaking out against forced sterilization put the AVS on the "right" side of the issue and helped the organization to delineate its goals from medical abuses.

Government agencies and lawmakers responded to the Relf scandal by ordering investigations into the incidence of sterilization abuse in other states and issuing protective guidelines. On July 3, the *New York Times* reported that three federal agencies had begun inquiries into the matter. Most notably, the Civil Rights Division of the Justice Department opened an investigation to determine if the girls' civil rights had been violated, and if so, whether the violations warranted civil or criminal charges. The Senate also investigated the Relf case. Nearly one month after the girls' sterilization, Senator Edward Kennedy invited Mr. and Mrs. Relf to testify at a Senate Health Subcommittee Hearing on the Status of Healthcare in America and Human Experimentation. Kennedy devoted one day of the lengthy hearings to the Relf case. He continued to lobby for an end to sterilization abuse after his committee hearings concluded. The senator appeared before the House Subcommittee on Public Health and the Environment in September 1973 to urge representatives to endorse a bill designed to protect patients from medical abuses and to safeguard research subjects' rights. In his testimony, he pointed to the Relfs' story as a "crystal illustration of the problems that surround the issue of adequate informed consent or lack of it."[90]

Charged with the distribution and monitoring of federal family planning funds, HEW formulated the most comprehensive and active response to the Relfs' accusations. Previously, HEW shared its responsibility for financing and monitoring federal family planning with the Office of Economic Opportunity (OEO) (the Relfs were sterilized by a clinic that received OEO funds). But the OEO transferred its family planning initiatives to HEW on June 1, 1973; thus, when the Relfs' story broke in July, HEW was the sole agency responsible for federal sterilizations. "Deeply disturbed" by the incident, Secretary of HEW Casper W. Weinberger issued an immediate moratorium on all federally funded involuntary sterilizations. Weinberger defined involuntary sterilizations as those involving individuals unable to consent to their own medical care, generally minors and people mentally incompetent under the law, and ordered the moratorium to continue until his department could develop guidelines to cover these surgeries. "My purpose in directing the preparation of guidelines is to insure that the rights of the individual are always observed and always secure," the secretary professed.[91] The agency also began to develop a series of guidelines to protect sterilization patients from coercion.

Despite the policy changes, HEW refused to concede that the absence of regulations may have contributed to the girls' abuse. Instead, Assistant Secretary of Health Dr. Charles C. Edwards blamed physicians. "It has been the Department's belief that professional judgment and ethics should govern the practice of medicine in health service projects," he contended, implying that the burden rested with providers, not the government. His statement stands in sharp contrast to the rulings in *Walker v. Pierce* and *Madrigal v. Quilligan*, which privileged physicians' judgment over patients' rights. Shifting the burden away from HEW and onto physicians, Edwards implied that the government lacked control over its providers, which made the department appear callous, not to mention incompetent. Moreover, Edwards's comment ignored the fact that the OEO had prepared its own sterilization guidelines in January 1972. The White House and a leading OEO official had prevented the guidelines from taking effect, but their existence signified that the antipoverty agency recognized a clear need for regulation.

The Relf case brought forced sterilization to public attention and inspired the formation of a loosely organized coalition of sterilization abuse groups. But these activists were not the first to protest forced sterilization. They built upon earlier traditions developed by black women within the civil rights, Black Power, black feminist, and welfare rights movements that linked the fight for reproductive freedom to existing struggles for racial and economic justice. Since slavery, white men had used black women's bodies to assert their racial supremacy and economic power. Black women in the 1960s and 1970s had grown up with the legacy of rape, especially in the South, and many black women lived with the continued threat of sexual assault that white supremacists used to punish them for challenging the prescribed racial hierarchy. They knew from personal experience and community history that the politics of race could not be disentangled from the politics of reproduction. Forced sterilization constituted a new manifestation of a much older tradition of white resistance to black equality.

Civil rights leader Fannie Lou Hamer was the first activist to speak out against sterilization abuse in 1964. Sterilized in 1961 via a "Mississippi appendectomy" when she entered a Mississippi hospital for uterine surgery, Hamer exposed the prevalence of sterilization abuse in southern hospitals in a conference on racism sponsored by the Council of Federated Organizations (COFO). "One of the other things that happened in Sunflower County, the Northern Sunflower County Hospital, I would say about 6 out of the 10 Negro women that go to the hospital are sterilized with the tubes tied," Hamer testified. Referring to a proposed law punishing illegitimacy among welfare recipients, Hamer continued, "They are getting up a law [that says] if a woman has an illegitimate baby and then a second one, they could draw time for 6 months or a $500 fine. What they didn't tell is that they are already doing these things, not only to single women but to married women."[92] Hamer's testimony points to pervasive abuse early in the decade. There is no way to confirm Hamer's statistics, as no such figures exist, but her claim surely represented black women's perception of widespread abuse. Hamer's decision to testify about sterilization abuse during a conference about racism indicates that she considered this reproductive rights issue to be a civil rights issue and suggests that she sought to push the movement to take direct action to expose and combat forced steril-ization. Her testimony is even more significant given that Hamer "consciously distanced herself from feminists and a feminist agenda."[93]

In the late 1960s and early 1970s, a black feminist movement developed in response to sexism within the Black Power and civil rights movements and racism within the white feminist movement.[94] Black feminists addressed race, gender, and class oppressions simultaneously, refusing to privilege one over the other because in their experiences, the three were intimately intertwined. Black women "find it difficult to separate race from class from sex oppression because in our lives they are most often experienced simultaneously," wrote the Combahee River Collective.[95] Similarly, black feminist Toni Cade Bambara articulated the need to link reproductive rights to economic and racial equality in her essay about the Pill. "It may liberate her sexually," she declared, "but what good is that if in other respects her social role remains the same?"[96] The revolutionary potential of the Pill rested in its ability to grant women control over their reproductive decisions, and Cade Bambara astutely argued that achieving the right to abortion could only take black women so far if society continued to discriminate against them on the basis of their race and gender, and, in the instance of poor women, class. Black congresswoman Shirley Chisholm, who represented the Bedford-Stuyvesant neighborhood of Brooklyn, risked alienating her black constituency when she became an advocate of legal-izing abortion in the early 1970s. Highlighting the differential dangers of illegal abortion for women of different races and classes, Chisholm declared, "Rich white women somehow manage to obtain these operations [abortions] with little or no difficulty. It is the poor Black and Puerto Rican women who are at the mercy of the local butcher."[97] For Chisholm and other black feminists, reproductive polices and practices were race issues.

Black feminists spoke out against sterilization abuse in position papers, public demonstrations, and workshops in the early 1970s, before the Relfs had been sterilized. In 1971, the Third World Women's Workshop identified an intersection between members' demands for legal abortion and their struggle to end forced sterilization, something white radical feminists would not do for at least five more years. "The campaign to get rid of the abortion laws is one of the best ways to fight forced sterilization because the lack of legal abortion has been used for years to force women to undergo sterilization," activists wrote.[98] Black feminists also publicized the effects of forced sterilization on black women's health in the years before the Relfs were sterilized. Their words reached local communities and like-minded activists, but did not become heard nationally until after the Relf story broke. In her 1970 essay "Double Jeopardy," Frances

Beale argued that sterilization abuse contributed to black women's poor health, as fear of sterilization abuse prevented many women from seeking necessary medical care. "Black women are often afraid to permit any kind of necessary surgery," she wrote, "because they know from bitter experience that they are more likely than not to come out of the hospital without their insides."[99] Beale's reference to "Mississippi appendectomies" was strikingly similar to Hamer's COFO speech.

Black feminists were not the only ones to speak out against forced sterilization in the late 1960s and early 1970s. The Nation of Islam and the Black Panther Party also exposed sterilization abuse of poor black women. The Nation of Islam began speaking out against forced sterilization in the mid-to-late 1960s, describing abuse as a genocidal plot of population control. Leader Elijah Muhammad preached that black women's primary responsibility was to bear children and labeled those who could not reproduce as "non-productive." Elijah Muhammad did not trust women to make their own reproductive decisions and thus issued many warnings about the dangers of birth control. While the Nation of Islam clearly did not articulate a feminist ideology, it did raise awareness of forced sterilization within black communities. Contributors to *Muhammad Speaks*, published by the Nation of Islam, "were some of the first to outline the dual demands for an end to reproductive abuses and improvement of total healthcare in poor communities."[100]

Initially, the Black Panther Party opposed the use of birth control and abortion by black women and accused federally funded family planning clinics as advancing a genocidal plot to reduce the black population. It changed its position in the early 1970s, as women in the party simultaneously challenged prohibitions against birth control and gained power within the organization. Much of the change in Black Panther policy toward abortion and birth control reflected the influence of black feminist thought.[101] Despite its changing position on birth control and abortion, the Black Panther Party remained steadfastly opposed to forced sterilization. It opposed a Tennessee bill that would authorize the state to sterilize all women on welfare with two or more children (women who refused to submit to surgery would lose their benefits and their children). And it condemned the practice of Dr. Clovis Pierce, of *Walker v. Pierce*. The Panthers called Pierce's policy (that women on welfare with two or more children undergo sterilization) "a racist, genocidal extermination directed at poor, Black girls and women," and pledged to oppose it and similar policies. "Every evidence of such a policy, in every corner of this country must be exposed, condemned and destroyed," the Black Panthers maintained.[102] By 1975, the Panthers had adopted some policies related to women's liberation, and although these were never the organization's central goals, they were situated alongside a series of other issues like access to decent health care, housing, employment, and child care, as well as increasing welfare entitlements and ending police violence.[103] This comprehensive view partially reflected the complicated definition of reproductive freedom that black feminists advanced.

Relf v. Weinberger

In response to news of the Relf girls' sterilization, HEW formally proposed guidelines for federal sterilizations in August 1973. On February 6, 1974, it issued the first federal sterilization regulations. This new policy required that all legally competent adults undergoing federally funded sterilization provide their informed consent to the procedure. It prohibited the sterilization of any individual under eighteen years old who did not obtain permission for surgery from a review committee (in addition to submitting her or his own informed consent), as well as the sterilization of any individual declared mentally incompetent to consent to her or his own medical care without the authorization of an external review committee and a court, as policy makers deemed the substituted consent of a parent or guardian insufficient to guarantee that the patient's best interest remained paramount.[104] HEW never actually activated the guidelines, which were scheduled to take effect upon publication in February 1974, because the NWRO and the Relfs filed separate class action suits challenging the constitutionality of the new rules, and the lawsuits forced HEW to defer their implementation and ultimately to withdraw them entirely. The court certified the NWRO to represent the class of women at risk for sterilization, maintaining that the "NWRO clearly has standing to bring this action since it has an organization interest in the rights of its welfare recipient members, many of whom may be directly subject to involuntary sterilizations as authorized by the challenged restrictions." Minnie Lee and Mary Alice Relf, along with the two other plaintiffs, were denied standing because they had already been "subject to federally funded sterilization," but the court determined that Katie Relf, their seventeen-year-old sister who narrowly escaped a social worker's attempt to sterilize her, could accurately represent the class of women at risk of forced sterilization.[105] The two other plaintiffs were Dorothy Waters and Virgil Walker, both patients of Pierce. Walker was the lead plaintiff in *Walker v. Pierce*. In early 1974, Washington, D.C., District Judge Gerhard Arnold Gessell consolidated the two lawsuits and tried the cases together.[106] The Southern Poverty Law Center represented the plaintiffs.

In *Relf v. Weinberger*, the NWRO and Katie Relf challenged the constitutionality of HEW's February 1974 guidelines. "Plaintiffs do not oppose the voluntary sterilization of poor persons under federally funded programs," Judge Gessell explained in his opinion. "However, they contend that these regulations are both illegal and arbitrary because they authorize *involuntary* sterilizations." Plaintiffs described the guidelines as weak and ineffective, citing the absence of any regulatory mechanism to ensure providers' compliance. They also deemed the new policy unconstitutional because it authorized the involuntary sterilization of minors and people who were mentally incompetent, who could never legally provide their informed consent, and argued that HEW lacked both the congressional mandate and constitutional privilege to authorize the involuntary sterilization of any individual. Plaintiffs sought to prevent the guidelines from going into effect and asked the court to order HEW to develop a more comprehensive sterilization policy.[107]

Secretary Weinberger insisted that HEW only funded voluntary procedures.[108] But the Relfs' sterilization, as well as the testimonies of other victims and affidavits from Dr. Bernard Rosenfeld and Dr. Sidney M. Wolfe, authors (along with Robert McGarrah Jr.) of the 1973 *Health Research Group Study on Surgical Sterilization*, directly contradicted this pronouncement, as did HEW's attempt to have the lawsuit dismissed. Charging the plaintiffs with filing premature charges, HEW maintained that the plaintiffs had to wait for abuse to occur under the new guidelines before they could seek to have them declared ineffective. Judge Gessell rejected this motion to dismiss, holding that the defendants' argument held "no legal or realistic merit." "One does not have to forfeit fundamental rights before he or she may complain," the judge maintained, "so long as the threat is real, as it is here."[109] Validating victims' claims and holding the right to be free from sterilization to be fundamental— essentially adopting the plaintiffs' inclusive concept of reproductive rights—the judge rejected defendants' motion. Gessell was the only judge who presided over forced sterilization suits to explicitly hold the right to be free from coercion as fundamental, and he relied upon *Griswold*, *Eisenstadt*, and *Roe* to do so. Quoting from *Eisenstadt*, the judge wrote, "The Supreme Court has repeatedly stated that the right of privacy entails the right of the individual 'to be free from unwarranted government intrusion into matters so fundamentally affecting a person as the decision whether to bear or beget a child.' . . . Involuntary sterilizations directly threaten that right."[110] Gessell linked the right to reproductive health services with the right to be free to refuse the same services.

Plaintiffs in *Relf v. Weinberger* used federal investigations, government statistics, physicians' affidavits, patients' claims, and studies like the *Health Research Group Study on Surgical Sterilization* to argue that the absence of federal oversight condoned the practice of forced sterilization in government-funded institutions.[111] The most damning evidence of federal neglect, however, came from the discovery of 25,000 copies of sterilization guidelines printed but never distributed by the OEO in 1972 in a federal warehouse on Third Street in Washington, D.C. The existence of the guidelines indicated that the OEO had recognized the potential for sterilization abuse and that health officials within the agency had taken deliberate action to prevent coercive practices.[112] At least one OEO official, Dr. Warren Hern, branch chief in the Family Planning Division of the OEO and author of the guidelines, believed that publication of the guidelines could have prevented the Relfs' abuse. When asked by Senator Kennedy during Senate hearings on forced sterilization why he believed the guidelines were necessary, Hern replied, "We really had in mind the kind of situation that we have had down in Alabama."[113]

Judge Gessell ruled in favor of the Relfs and the NWRO on March 15, 1974, stating, "there is uncontroverted evidence in the record that minors and other incompetents have been sterilized with federal funds and that an indefinite number of poor people have been improperly coerced into accepting a sterilization operation under the threat that various federally supported welfare benefits would be withdrawn unless they submitted to irreversible sterilization." A well-known supporter of women's right to abortion, Gessell found that the February 1974 sterilization guidelines failed to protect indigent women from abuse, issued an injunction against them, and ordered HEW to revise its sterilization policy in accordance with a series of strict requirements he designed to protect poor women's fertility.[114] The judge agreed with the plaintiffs that individuals who could not legally consent to sterilization should not be sterilized because they could never provide true informed consent, and because he recognized women's right to be free from coercion, Gessell refused to grant any individual or agency the authority to substitute its consent for that of an individual, especially without a specific legislative mandate. In his opinion, neither the Social Security Act nor the Public Health Act authorized HEW to fund the sterilization of minors and people who were mentally incompetent. "The dividing line between family planning and eugenics is murky," the judge wrote, "and yet the Secretary [of HEW], through the regulations at issue, seeks to sanction one of the most drastic methods of population control . . . without any legislative guidance." Gessell ruled that the department had overstepped its prescribed authority when drafting the guidelines, which he characterized as "arbitrary and unreasonable" because they failed to "implement the congressional command that federal family planning funds not be used to coerce indigent patients into submitting to sterilization."[115]

Judge Gessell issued a moratorium on the sterilization of minors (defined as individuals under twenty-one) and those deemed mentally incompetent and ordered HEW to revise the guidelines so as to establish clear standards of informed consent for those individuals competent to provide it. He also ordered HEW to amend its consent process to mandate that patients be informed verbally that their refusal to consent to sterilization would not result in the revocation of their federal assistance and directed that this last statement appear at the top of the consent form in a clearly visible position. The judge then held that the regulations in question "fail to provide the procedural safeguards necessary to insure that even competent adults voluntarily request sterilization." "Even a fully informed individual cannot make a 'voluntary' decision if he has been subjected to coercion from doctors or project officers," Gessell surmised.[116] Here the judge articulated what would become a long-standing criticism of federal guidelines by antisterilization abuse activists, who argued that no amount of procedural safeguards could prevent abuse in the absence of effective monitoring and enforcement mechanisms. In order for government sterilization policy to be effective in curbing forced sterilization, those who violate the policy must be held accountable and punished.

In response to the ruling, HEW implemented new interim guidelines to govern federally funded sterilizations while it revised its February 6, 1974, regulations to comply with the court order. The interim guidelines established a moratorium on all nonemergency sterilizations of individuals under twenty-one or those unable to consent to their own medical care and required the informed consent of all individuals legally competent to submit to sterilization. In 1975, Judge Gessell rejected the revised guidelines that HEW submitted on the basis of their failure to establish a standard for voluntariness, ensure that providers obtain patients' informed consent, differentiate between therapeutic and nontherapeutic surgeries, require physicians to certify that consent to surgery was informed, and create a monitoring system to ensure that providers complied with the new law, among other things. "The Court is not satisfied that the complex program envisioned is susceptible to the careful, effective monitoring by the agency that would be essential to prevent abuse," Gessell asserted.[117] Unable to put new rules into effect with the case on appeal, HEW withdrew its revised regulations and began formal rule-making proceedings on a new series of regulations under an agreement acceptable to both sides.[118] The interim guidelines remained in effect until February 1979, when the second set of guidelines became active. While the guidelines HEW eventually drafted proved more comprehensive than those challenged in *Relf v. Weinberger*, they also failed to include an efficient enforcement mechanism, a policy that Gessell championed and may have insisted upon had he retained authority over their creation.

Chapter 6

Irreconcilable Conflicts

Women's race, class, and ethnicity clearly shaped their sterilization experiences, which in turn influenced their ideas of reproductive freedom. White women across class, free of medical racism, struggled to gain access to sterilization and to overturn age/parity, spousal consent, and conscience clause policies. This led many to define reproductive freedom as access to reproductive health services and some to use the courts to transform their personal reproductive politics into public policy. Poor women, especially women of color, found themselves the targets of coercive sterilization practices, which was for many yet another example of the continued prejudice they faced in America. Women of color tended to view coercive sterilization within the context of larger struggles for racial equality and economic justice. As such, they advanced a broader definition of reproductive freedom than white women did, insisting that all women possessed the right to determine when and under what conditions to become pregnant and that women who accepted government assistance should not be forced to give up their reproductive decision making in exchange for a welfare check.

Women's different definitions of reproductive freedom came into direct and irreconcilable conflict in the mid-to-late 1970s when community activists, radical feminists, and some concerned medical personnel began to promote a new type of sterilization policy designed to protect women from abuse. One of the first antisterilization abuse groups formed in New York City in 1975 and called itself the Health and Hospital Corporation (HHC) Advisory Committee on Sterilization. After investigating sterilization practices at local institutions and studying the 1974 federal sterilization rules, the group proposed a series of guidelines designed to eliminate sterilization abuse in New York City hospitals.

Advisory Committee members confronted fierce resistance from physicians, family planners like Planned Parenthood, and the Association for Voluntary Sterilization (AVS), which objected to the regulation of their medical and businesses practices. Perhaps the most surprising opposition came from white liberal feminist organizations like the National Organization for Women (NOW) and the National Abortion Rights Action League (NARAL). These groups opposed forced sterilization, but disagreed with the strategies for ending abuse that the Advisory Committee proposed. Specifically, they objected to a mandatory waiting period between consent and surgery, designed to prevent coercion during labor and delivery, and protested mandatory age minimums, designed to prevent the sterilization of minors, on the grounds that these policies interfered with women's right to sterilization on demand. NOW's, NARAL's, and Planned Parenthood's opposition to the guidelines reflected their privileging of abortion rights over other reproductive rights issues and their concern that if the government could prevent women from receiving sterilization on demand, it could use this precedent to prohibit women from accessing abortion on demand.

Advisory Committee members recognized that the policies they recommended to prevent sterilization abuse could interfere with women's ability to receive sterilization on demand. But, they argued, women's right to be free from coercion trumped women's right to have unrestricted access to sterilization services. Herein lay the conflict: in order to protect one group of women from forced sterilization, policy makers had to restrict another group of women's access to the procedure. If policy makers chose not to implement guidelines in order to maintain the second group of women's right to sterilization on demand, then they continued to allow the first group of women to be at risk for sterilization abuse. In either instance, public policy (or lack thereof) would infringe upon one group of women's reproductive freedom.

The New York City debate over sterilization guidelines sparked grassroots movements in cities across the country as feminists of color and radical white feminists teamed with community groups to pressure their local, state, and federal governments to support policies to prevent forced sterilization, like the one proposed in New York City. After the New York City measure passed, grassroots activists in many states, including Missouri, New York, Massachusetts, Connecticut, and Pennsylvania, joined together to pressure the federal government to develop a similar protective policy. In each of these instances, women's reproductive rights existed in irreconcilable conflict, as the guidelines designed to protect poor women from forced sterilization infringed upon middle-class and white women's access to surgery. Debates over sterilization policy reinforced the extent to which women held diverging ideas of reproductive freedom. No single policy could support the reproductive rights of all women because no single definition of reproductive rights existed.

The Push for Sterilization Guidelines

Established in the winter of 1974 in New York City, the Committee to End Sterilization Abuse (CESA) was the first grassroots organization developed to combat forced sterilization, emerging one year before the Advisory Committee was formed. (CESA members were involved in the creation of the Advisory Committee.) CESA began with about ten members, including several prominent reproductive rights activists like Dr. Helen Rodriguez-Trias, a Puerto Rican feminist and member of the Puerto Rican Socialist Party; Rosa Garcia, Maritza Arrastia, and Anna Maria Garcia, also of the Puerto Rican Socialist Party; Nancy Stearns, a lawyer who helped to topple abortion statutes in New York and Connecticut and who participated in Anne and Barton Yohns' suit to overturn age/parity policies; and Karen Stamm, a prominent feminist.[1] Originally, the group addressed forced sterilization in Puerto Rico, citing abuse as evidence of imperialism and population control politics. As it began working in communities across New York City, however, its members became aware of forced sterilization occurring at home. For example, during its first citywide meeting at St. Mark's Church in the Bowery, a nurse from King's Hospital in Brooklyn testified to having witnessed "violations of informed consent in the delivery room." She explained that physicians harassed black women in labor to consent to surgery. Awareness of abuse at home led CESA to shift its focus from Puerto Rico to New York City.[2]

CESA became a unique multiethnic organization that drew its membership from a diverse range of activists, including the Puerto Rican Socialist Party, the Marxist Education Collective, the Committee for the Decolonialization of Puerto Rico, the Medical Committee for Human Rights, and the Center for Constitutional Rights. Much of this diversity can be attributed to the original members' inclusive definition of reproductive rights. CESA subscribed to ideas of reproductive freedom like those articulated by black feminists and other women of color. Many opposed white feminists' single-issue approach to the legalization of abortion, arguing that privileging access to legal abortion above all other reproductive rights issues reflected a white middle-class bias. CESA members shared a commitment to understanding sterilization abuse within the context of the social and economic inequalities that fostered neo-eugenic attitudes and to challenging the institutions and forces that upheld them. "The lack of employment opportunities, education, daycare, decent housing, adequate medical care, safe effective contraceptive methods, access to abortion, combined with hysterical 'overpopulation' scare stories, have helped create an atmosphere of subtle coercion," CESA maintained in a pamphlet entitled *Sterilization: What You Need to Know before Making a Decision* (written in Spanish and English).[3] Many CESA members had experience with the civil rights, New Left, and Puerto Rican independence movements and had witnessed firsthand how reproductive abuses existed within the larger context of racial and ethnic inequality, economic injustice, and sexual discrimination.[4] Their own experiences shaped their philosophy of reproductive rights.

In its statement of purpose, CESA pledged to educate the public about the risks of forced sterilization and to publicize incidents of abuse.[5] When it joined the newly established HHC Advisory Committee on Sterilization, CESA became involved in an effort to develop sterilization policy for New York City public hospitals. Esta Armstrong, an employee in the New York City Office of Quality Assurance at HHC, the agency that governed the city's municipal hospitals, established the committee in January 1975. Armstrong first became aware of forced sterilization in 1971 while working at a city clinic involved with abuse. "Half the female patients who used the clinic had been sterilized," she said, and doctors (employed by the city) targeted women of color especially.[6] The Advisory Committee was an umbrella organization that included representatives from CESA, the Center for Constitutional Rights, HealthPac (Health Policy Advisory Center), the Puerto Rican Socialist Party, *Ms. Magazine*, the American Civil Liberties Union (ACLU), and the National Black Feminist Organization. It also drew from members of community health groups and institutions like the Lower East Side Neighborhood Health Center, Gouverneur Hospital Community Board, Morrisania Hospital, Bellevue Hospital Community Board, and the Family Planning Division of the Human Resource Administration.[7] Like CESA, the Advisory Committee was ethnically and racially diverse. Although members maintained their own political agendas, they came together to investigate incidences of forced sterilization in local hospitals and to devise a method for ending the abuse. This single goal helped minimize intergroup conflict.

Working from within the established HHC bureaucracy, the Advisory Committee examined sterilization abuse within HHC facilities and studied the 1974 Department of Health, Education, and Welfare (HEW) guidelines (the interim regulations put in effect during the Relfs' suit). It published the results of its study in a 1975 report entitled "Why Sterilization Guidelines Are Needed." The report identified "a number of causes for alarm," most significantly: a "dramatic" increase in the number of sterilizations performed in recent years, medical personnel's ignorance of existing federal guidelines, the routine performance of tubal ligations by inexperienced young physicians, and the lack of information regarding sterilization available to patients.[8] The report also expressed committee members' deep concern about the consent process and the lack of adequate protocol for obtaining informed consent, a central cause of abuse. Members specifically took issue with the language that doctors used to describe surgery. Terms like "belly-button" and "Band-Aid" surgery "minimized" the dangers and effects of the procedure, they charged. Committee members also found that doctors frequently failed to inform patients of the mortality and complication rates of tubal ligation, which further contributed to women's misperceptions about sterilization and, in activists' minds, violated the informed consent process. Finally, the report criticized the educational literature hospitals distributed to potential patients, which committee members believed painted a "rosy, trouble-free picture" of sterilization that glossed over its risks and consequences.[9]

In response to these findings, the Advisory Committee drafted a policy to prevent abuse, more aggressive than the national regulations. The Advisory Committee's proposed guidelines established a thirty-day waiting period between the time of initial consent and surgery, prohibited the obtaining of consent during abortion or delivery, and banned the sterilization of individuals under twenty-one years of age. The committee insisted that a thirty-day wait was "required" to prevent coercion and ensure that patients provided informed consent. The existing seventy-two-hour period (under the 1974 HEW guidelines) was "virtually meaningless as a protective device," the group concluded, insisting that "no woman should be expected to decide in such a brief period whether or not to permanently terminate her ability to have children, particularly if this period is post-partum or post-abortal, or when a hospitalized woman is in unfamiliar surroundings and lacks privacy for consultation with family and friends." To ensure that coercion no longer occurred during delivery, the guidelines specifically prohibited physicians from eliciting consent "during admission or hospitalization for childbirth or abortion or other medical treatment." They also mandated that women be counseled by someone other than a physician before consenting to the procedure, required that the counselor conduct the session in the patient's primary language, and instructed the counselor to explain alternative methods of contraception as well as the known risks and benefits of sterilization to the patient before soliciting her consent.[10]

After issuing its report, the committee confronted strenuous opposition from physicians within the HHC. All seventeen directors of obstetrics and gynecology departments governed by the HHC vehemently objected to the proposed policy, charging that the regulations interfered with the doctor–patient relationship. The doctors—all of them men—claimed that Advisory Committee members lacked the medical expertise required to develop medical policy, and many accused

HHC members of using the report as a means to impose their feminist politics upon city institutions. After the committee published a first draft of its proposed regulations, which the physicians rejected, the parties engaged in three months of negotiations that yielded twelve drafts of a revised proposal. They had finally reached an agreement on everything but the length of the waiting periods when the physicians withdrew their support at the last minute and ended all attempts to compromise.[11]

In order to gain public support for the guidelines, the Advisory Committee and CESA took their movement to the communities most vulnerable to forced sterilization. With the aid of newly established feminist health centers and radical health feminists, CESA activists gathered petitions in favor of the regulations, organized public meetings and demonstrations, collected victims' testimonies, conducted educational workshops, published informative pamphlets, and secured the endorsement of local organizations. Activists also lobbied hospital community boards, whose support Esta Armstrong deemed "decisive" to the HHC Board of Director's final vote. CESA's grassroots campaign proved successful because the organization defined sterilization abuse as a community problem rather than a feminist issue, as an issue bound up within the same forces of poverty, racism, and discrimination that community activists were already challenging.[12]

While CESA rallied community support for the proposal, the Advisory Committee worked within the existing HHC system to secure administrative approval. Their dual strategy proved successful. The HHC Board of Directors unanimously approved the Advisory Committee's proposed guidelines in September 1975, and the new regulations went into effect on November 1. Sterilization abuse activists attributed their success to their two-pronged strategy, a unique model of activism that linked hospital administrators and local communities in a collective struggle to defend the reproductive rights of poor women and women of color according to these women's philosophy of reproductive freedom.[13]

Refusing to Concede: Doctors Challenge the HHC Guidelines in Court

The HHC guidelines engendered more resistance after they became HHC policy than before they went into effect. Physicians, especially, expressed their opposition to the new policy. In January 1976, six chairmen of obstetrics and gynecology departments governed by the HHC filed a lawsuit to invalidate the new guidelines and overturn the interim federal regulations.[14] Gordon W. Douglas, Saul Gusberg, Irwin Kaiser, James Nelson, Martin Stone, and Raymond Vande Wiele charged that the regulations violated their First Amendment right to free speech by obstructing the privileged communication between doctors and patients and impeding their ability to practice medicine safely. The physicians also filed suit on behalf of two women who received welfare and sought sterilizations: a mentally challenged nineteen-year-old and a woman preparing to undergo her third caesarian section. The doctors claimed that the guidelines discriminated against the two women on the basis of their class. One opponent of the guidelines (but not a plaintiff in the lawsuit), Dr. Shuyler Kohl, acting chairman of the Obstetrics and Gynecology Department at Kings Hospital in Brooklyn, denied that sterilization abuse existed and questioned the need for regulations. "Show me one case of sterilization abuse here," he dared the *Medical Tribune*. "No one has come up with one single case. It's all a big lie," he exclaimed. The *Medical Tribune* rebutted him by citing several instances of abuse, including one in which a "20-year-old black woman with one child . . . was treated in the very hospital where Dr. Kohl and his colleagues do several hundred sterilizations a year." In this instance, doctors told the woman that her tubal ligation would be reversed when "she decided to become a 'good girl' once again."[15]

Physicians pleaded their case to liberal feminists outside of the courtroom. In an op-ed piece published in the *New York Times* on January 12, 1976, Dr. Irwin Kaiser described the regulations as condescending and patronizing, arguing that the guidelines implied "that women, of age and competent, are somehow uniquely unable to make rational decisions pertaining to their child-bearing."[16] Kaiser cast himself as a protector of women's right to sterilization on demand and used neo-eugenic ideas to support his medical authority. A member of the AVS, Kaiser was no stranger to neo-eugenics. (Not only was he a member of the AVS, he was also nominated to its board in February 1976, one month after publishing the editorial.) "There is no medical, moral, or legal reason for prohibiting sterilization of women under 21 years of age," Kaiser asserted, especially when young women exhibited a clear lack of reproductive fitness. To reinforce this point, Kaiser declared, "I have cared for a 20-year-old with five children!"[17] He suggested that patients like this one needed to be sterilized, and the guidelines would prevent him and other physicians from performing this public service. Kaiser's colleague Dr. Kohl also used neo-eugenic sentiments to defend his rejection of the guidelines. He contended that the guidelines interfered with physicians' ability to sterilize "unfit" women, telling the *Medical Tribune*, "Some people just don't have the 'gray matter' to handle the responsibilities of raising children or having more children."[18]

Like liberal feminists and family planners, the New York doctors cast themselves as guardians of poor women's reproductive rights, but tellingly, they did so by advancing a middle-class white definition of reproductive freedom that was premised upon preserving on-demand access to reproductive health services. "These regulations and their numerous burdensome restrictions operate solely against women on Medicaid or who otherwise seek medical care through the public hospital system," the six plaintiffs declared. They also complained that the regulations "discriminate invidiously against women Medicaid patients and their physicians," noting that no other comparable procedure was subject to similar restrictions.[19] What they did not mention, however, was the reason that the guidelines had been established: poor women, especially those receiving Medicaid, were being forcibly sterilized. Kaiser used the same tactic in his editorial when he wrote sterilization abuse victims out of the story, and, in doing so, made the contest about access to sterilization rather than the prevention of sterilization abuse. In the one instance in which he referred to forced sterilization, the doctor dismissed victims' testimonies. "The Health and Hospitals Corporation has not kept records of the number of female sterilizations . . . any assertion that excessive numbers are being performed is totally empty," he wrote.[20]

These doctors received the support of two large institutions: the American College of Obstetricians and Gynecologists (ACOG) and the City of New York Department of Health. Both organizations reiterated the six plaintiffs' claims that the guidelines interfered with doctors' medical practice and violated their right to free speech. In a letter to the HHC Board of Directors, ACOG described the guidelines as "prejudicial, inaccurate, and distorted," and claimed that the restrictions imposed by the new policy were so great that they made "sterilization unavailable to the patients." Planned Parenthood echoed similar sentiments, complaining that the regulations obstructed women's access to permanent contraception. The Department of Health argued that the guidelines discriminated against poor women who were subject to additional (and unnecessary) regulation because they received public assistance. CESA, however, believed that the Department of Health opposed the guidelines because they would be "too costly and burdensome to enforce."[21]

CESA responded to this "ferocity of opposition" by shifting the focus of the debate back to sterilization abuse victims. Doctors blamed activists for imposing "invasive" guidelines, but CESA reminded physicians and the public of the reasons that guidelines were necessary: to curb physicians' abusive behavior. "These guidelines were designed to protect, not abridge, the rights of the individuals involved, so as to insure that the procedure would indeed be voluntary and not coerced," CESA reiterated.[22]

Determined to defend the recently passed guidelines, CESA, the United Welfare League, and the Center for Constitutional Rights intervened in defense of the HHC guidelines. The case never made it to trial. In January 1977, one year after the doctors filed their lawsuit, a combination of public condemnation of forced sterilization and legal technicalities convinced five of the six physicians to drop their claims. "It was all too clear," CESA later recounted, "that the guidelines were essential to protect the rights of people who were most vulnerable to abuse, i.e., poor and Third World women." The following fall, the remaining physician withdrew his complaint, ending this specific challenge to New York City's sterilization guidelines, but by no means concluding the larger contest over regulations.[23]

The Burden Bill: Expanding the Reach of the HHC Guidelines

The physicians withdrew their lawsuit against the HHC guidelines during a heated battle over a bill designed to translate the HHC policy into city law. Sterilization abuse activists strove to make their new policy permanent, for while HHC policy could be altered by order of the mayor or by agency administrators, formal legislation could be repealed only by vigorous legal challenges or a legislative measure. New York City councilman Carter Burden proposed Intro 1105-A in the fall of 1976, a bill to extend the HHC guidelines to all public and private sterilizations performed in New York City hospitals. Like the HHC guidelines, Intro 1105-A established a thirty-day waiting period (that could be reduced to seventy-two hours in cases when a woman delivered earlier than her expected due date or underwent emergency abdominal surgery), a minimum age of twenty-one, and strict standards of informed consent that mirrored those proposed by the HHC committee. Burden's bill also went beyond the HHC guidelines to cover both male and female sterilizations and to hold individuals accused of violating the guidelines liable for "a penalty of not more than $1,000 to be recovered in a civil action."[24]

For three reasons, debate over the passage of Intro 1105-A proved more intense than that surrounding the HHC guidelines. First, both sides were prepared for this fight. Antisterilization abuse activists had already developed an organizational base and garnered community support for their efforts, and their opponents had also mobilized once before. Second, Planned Parenthood, the AVS, NARAL, and NOW intensified their opposition to the policy after this bill was proposed. Each of these groups had spoken out against the HHC policy, but they increased their efforts once the Burden bill threatened to extend the policy to private hospitals and men.[25] Third, the Burden bill held a national significance that the HHC policy did not. As the first local law governing sterilization, its passage or failure would establish a precedent for future sterilization policy, and activists on both sides of the guidelines debate endeavored to determine the critical vote. Burden's bill bore additional weight in the context of the physicians' lawsuit: if the court ruled in the plaintiffs' favor and invalidated the bill, it would prevent other lawmakers from proposing similar reforms.

Planned Parenthood and the AVS provided the greatest opposition to the bill.[26] In June 1977, representatives from Planned Parenthood New York (PPNY), Planned Parenthood World Population (PPWP), and the AVS met in New York City to discuss the Burden bill. Attendees were most concerned with the thirty-day waiting period, which they believed interfered with women's access to contraception. One participant went so far as to declare that the guidelines "run contrary to the general position of the Federation in spirit," and ran "afoul of the basic tenets upon which Planned Parenthood has traditionally operated." All "agreed that any waiting period would necessarily be arbitrary." Unlike the doctors who filed suit against the HHC guidelines, attendees did not debate the validity of sterilization abuse accusations. Their main concern, as Fred Jaffe of the PPWP expressed, was the effect that restrictions on sterilization would have on abortion, which he called "the more salient issue." Planned Parenthood feared that allowing government restrictions on sterilization would begin a slippery slope of government restrictions on other reproductive health services, such as contraception and abortion. As one attendee explained, if the Burden bill failed to elicit any "public outcry," then "the other side"—that is, the pro-life movement—"would be strengthened to impose greater regulation in the entire field."[27] The PPNY reinforced this connection between abortion and sterilization policy in a letter to New York City mayor Abraham Beame in which it declared that the proposed guidelines were "so fundamentally restrictive" that they "will seriously interfere with the constitutionally guaranteed rights of New Yorkers to decide when and whether to have a child and to use appropriate means to achieve that end."[28]

NOW and NARAL joined Planned Parenthood and opposed the Burden bill because they, too, believed abortion to be "the more salient issue." Like the AVS, these groups did not question the validity of women's claims of sterilization abuse; instead, they sought an alternative solution to the problem, one that did not interfere with women's right to sterilization on demand. They acted according to an ideology of reproductive rights that was based upon white middle-class women's experiences. Their position reflected a combination of self-interest, insensitivity, and racism. By rejecting the restrictions imposed by the bill, liberal feminists acted in defense of their reproductive rights agenda, which privileged defending women's abortion rights above all other reproductive health issues and ignored medical racism. NOW, NARAL, and Planned Parenthood objected to forced sterilization but refused to support the policies necessary to deter abuse for fear that doing so would compromise their abortion rights agendas. But by not championing sterilization guidelines, these groups effectively said that the reproductive rights of middle-class white women were more important than the reproductive rights of poor women and women of color. Whether they intended to put forth a racist policy or not, these organizations adopted a strategy that defended the reproductive rights of middle-class white women at the expense of poor women of color.

Although national NOW opposed sterilization guidelines, the New York chapter chose to position itself on the other side of the debate, in favor of the Burden bill. Conversations with a CESA delegation of feminist physicians, lawyers, and health care activists caused NOW New York to join with feminists of color and radical white feminists on this issue and to adopt a broad defini-tion of reproductive freedom that included the right to be free from coercion. "While we are weary of government interference in matters of fertility," NOW New York wrote in a letter to Councilman Burden, "certainly a distinction must be made between laws designed to insure freedom of choice and access to family-planning information and methods and laws which restrict choice or limit access. This bill seeks to increase freedom, not limit it."[29]

NOW New York's conversation breached the division between radical and liberal feminists at the local level and undermined physicians' and family plan-ners' lobbies by throwing the balance of feminist activism behind the regula-tions. The group's conversion and continued commitment to sterilization abuse activism during the federal debates provide a rare example of white liberal fem-inists adopting a broad philosophy of reproductive rights and teaming with ster-ilization abuse activists to support sterilization regulations. During the federal debates, the Middlesex and Boston chapters of NOW followed the New York model and sided with guidelines supporters on the opposite side of the debate from the national organization.[30] These local chapters' decisions to work with CESA on behalf of the guidelines demonstrates that in a few exceptional instances, liberal feminists cast aside their race and class privileges and adopted the inclusive definition of reproductive rights advocated by feminists of color.

Planned Parenthood and the AVS maintained another motivation for opposing the bill—a financial one. Both organizations had been involved in the development and financing of vasectomy clinics since the late 1960s and early 1970s, and in April 1977 they endeavored to expand their services to include female sterilization procedures. Planned Parenthood and the AVS aimed to create a network of outpatient clinics that used mini-laparotomy, a technique used fre-quently by private population control organizations and the federal Agency for International Development (AID). Population controllers lauded the "mini-lap" for its minimally invasive nature as well as its relative technical simplicity. In the mid-to-late 1970s, Americans working in international family planning increasingly used the mini-lap in their international programs, and Planned Parenthood and the AVS planned to introduce this technology to the United States and develop a series of mini-lap clinics in major cities across the country.[31] The central feature of these outpatient clinics was their promise of same-day surgery.

In 1977, Planned Parenthood and the AVS established a $700,000 loan fund for the creation and expansion of outpatient clinics for female sterilization. The fund administered loans to potential providers for up to thirty-six months and funded clinical training in mini-laparotomy. In 1978, the AVS and Planned Parenthood sponsored seminars in Syracuse, New York, and San Francisco to introduce doctors and family planning organizations to the new technique (which they actually demonstrated to seminar attendees) and to recruit participants for their loan program. Thirty-six family planning agencies and physicians attended these meetings. The Burden bill's prohibition of sterilization of individuals under twenty-one years old and its thirty-day waiting period threatened to undermine this joint initiative. Planned Parenthood was prepared to operate according to a seventy-two-hour waiting period established by the 1974 interim federal guidelines (applicable to Medicaid patients only), but believed the thirty-day wait would interfere with its business plan and therefore opposed the measure.[32]

CESA met opposition from physicians, family planners, and liberal feminists with a second grassroots drive to rally community support for sterilization regulations. As it had with the HHC guidelines, CESA coordinated community education projects and public demonstrations and lobbied city council members. Its members also took to the airwaves, urging radio listeners to attend the public hearings held in the fall of 1976 and the spring of 1977 and to direct their councilpersons to endorse the proposal. The city broadcast the Burden bill hearings on the radio, and CESA capitalized on this publicity by packing the proceedings with supporters and recruiting victims, health care professionals, and activists to testify in favor of the guidelines. Among those who testified were local women on welfare who had been victimized. The grassroots organization also marshaled endorsements for the bill from the New York Civil Liberties Union, the National Black Feminist Organization, the Medical Committee for Human Rights, the Brooklyn Council of Churches, Women United for Action, Physicians Forum, Committee of Interns and Residents, NOW New York, and the American Public Health Association. CESA's grassroots organizing paid off; the city council passed the bill thirty-eight to one (with three abstentions) on April 28, 1977.[33]

This victory, however, did not signal the end of opposition to sterilization regulations in New York. Even after the Burden bill became Public Law 37 (PL37),

guidelines opponents refused to concede defeat. Soon after the enactment of
PL37, Assemblyman and AVS member Mark Alan Siegel introduced a sterilization bill in the New York state assembly that purported to safeguard women
against sterilization abuse, but in fact it functioned to undermine PL37 by
replacing the thirty-day waiting period with a seventy-two-hour delay and
eliminating the prohibition of sterilization on patients under twenty-one.[34] The
AVS provided the prototype for Siegel's bill.

CESA and the newly established Committee for Abortion Rights and Against
Sterilization Abuse (CARASA) launched a grassroots educational campaign
against the bill, lobbied their local legislators, and again took to the streets to
gather public support against the measure. Established in 1977, CARASA constituted a new type of feminist reproductive rights organization, one that rejected
the single-issue politics of abortion advanced by NOW, NARAL, and Planned
Parenthood and adopted the broad ideas of reproductive freedom advanced by
feminists of color. CARASA members were predominately white. They had lis-
tened to the critiques feminists of color leveled against white feminists for their
failure to recognize the role of race and class in shaping women's reproductive
experiences and responded by appropriating their critics' notion of reproductive rights. CARASA aimed to bring "a wide range of other issues ranging from
women's health to sexuality to class and race" to the struggle for women's reproductive freedom. In its founding conference, CARASA defined reproductive
freedom as "the freedom to *have* as well as *not to have* children, with whatever
that takes—not just abortion rights and better birth control and women's health
care, but childcare and good public schools, adequate wages and welfare[,] gay
rights, and an end to the kind of oppressive definitions of women we grew up
with and the right-to-lifers were trying to enforce."[35] CARASA established two
simultaneous goals: to defend *Roe v. Wade* against a rising pro-life movement
and to protect women against sterilization abuse. Historian Jennifer Nelson dubs
this "a new reproductive rights agenda."[36]

CESA and CARASA also received the support of historian and activist Joan
Kelly of the Ad Hoc Women's Studies Committee against Sterilization Abuse,
who scored a major victory for antisterilization abuse activists when she publicly exposed Planned Parenthood's and the AVS's investment in the mini-lap
clinics. In a public letter to Assemblyman Siegel, Kelly revealed the assemblyman's ties to the AVS and accused him of proposing legislation designed to
advance the interests of the organization at the expense of his constituents'
reproductive rights. She alleged that Siegel intended for his bill to override the
city guidelines in order to facilitate the construction of outpatient sterilization
clinics across the state and to fulfill the AVS's neo-eugenic goals.[37]

Siegel's bill took another hit when liberal activists in the New York state campaign for abortion rights began to worry that the controversy surrounding the guidelines was detracting from their efforts to ensure that abortion remained "safe, legal, and accessible" in New York. A member of the New York Civil Liberties Union involved in this campaign requested that Siegel withdraw his bill.[38] Other women in New York City pressured the assemblyman to do the same, also in the interest of protecting abortion rights. Siegel agreed, explaining that he "did not want to split the abortion movement."[39] The assemblyman's statement demonstrated his misunderstanding of the conflict. Feminists were divided over the regulation of sterilization, not the defense of legal abortion. They aimed to preserve women's right to abortion, but they disagreed over how this right related to other reproductive rights.

Sterilization abuse activists sought to extend their local victory to the state level, and over the next year CESA and CARASA worked closely with Assemblyman Jerrold Nadler of Manhattan's Upper West Side to develop a measure that would strengthen and extend PL37 to the entire state. Nadler's bill broadened the New York law by establishing a statewide enforcement system to monitor providers' compliance and make violation of the code a criminal offense punishable by fines and possible incarceration. The Nadler bill never made it out of committee during either the 1978–1979 or the 1979–1980 legislative sessions. When questioned about their votes, dissenting legislators cited the lack of hard evidence of sterilization abuse. Legislators reiterated a common argument of guidelines opponents: in the absence of clear documentation of abuse, no significant rationale existed for passing legislation that trampled upon women's access to voluntary sterilization. Activists could not provide this type of evidence, however, because federal agencies did not begin to compile sterilization statistics until the early-to-mid-1970s. Once more, much of the evidence that lawmakers sought did not exist; the covert nature of forced sterilization ensured as much. Activists had to rely upon victims' and witnesses' testimonies, and in the instance of the Nadler bill, CARASA failed to recruit victims willing to testify at the hearings.[40]

Not all lawmakers rejected the Nadler bill. In its first committee vote, the bill failed by a vote of twelve to nine, and this narrow margin gave activists hope that, over time, they could marshal sufficient evidence of abuse to persuade dissenting assemblypersons to pass the measure. In 1981, sterilization activists vowed to continue to reintroduce the Nadler bill annually until lawmakers passed it. But this promise soon became overshadowed by a Supreme Court decision that upheld the Hyde Amendment, the third ruling on the controversial law. The Hyde Amendment eliminated Medicaid funding for elective abortion, and CARASA and other feminist groups feared that their opponents would use it to undermine all women's access to legal abortion. Although the organization remained committed to combating sterilization abuse, after the sterilization guidelines debate concluded in 1979, CARASA shifted the bulk of its resources to defending women's right to abortion.[41] By this time, federal sterilization guidelines had been established, reducing the need for specific state regulations.

Sterilization Regulations in California

Activists in New York City created CESA in 1974, and activists in other cities like St. Louis, Los Angeles, Boston, Northampton (Massachusetts), and Hartford (Connecticut) followed their lead. Some adopted the CESA name; others created their own title. Each group operated at the local level, addressing the specific forms of sterilization abuse that plagued its city. In Philadelphia, Women Against Sterilization Abuse spent most of its energy supporting Norma Jean Serena, the Native American woman sterilized in Pittsburgh without her informed consent. Activists in western Massachusetts addressed the issue of forced sterilization of low-income women in their community, especially Puerto Rican women. They also identified the forced sterilization of a white woman receiving welfare in Northampton and of a Native American woman from Holyoke. Feminists in Chicago formed their own CESA chapter after hearing "about abuses in Puerto Rico, New York, Los Angeles, and Alabama." Chicago CESA focused its activism in two areas: working with community groups to exchange information about abuse on the local level and investigating incidences of abuse in area hospitals. In Madison, Wisconsin, activists with the Near East Side Community Health Center collected information about sterilization in their community and aimed to persuade the city council to pass sterilization regulations.[42]

CESA in St. Louis focused the majority of its attention on dismantling the Program for International Education in Gynecology and Obstetrics (PIEGO), in which Washington University Medical School (located in St. Louis) participated. This program trained foreign doctors (primarily Latin American) in sterilization techniques. At the end of each four-to-six-week session held in St. Louis, PIEGO provided graduates with a $5,000 laparoscope to take back to their country of origin. PIEGO participants were not licensed to practice medicine in the United States; they could not operate on women while in America. Their training, therefore, consisted of observing surgeries performed by American doctors and practicing on rabbits. They did not operate on women until they returned home, which placed patients at risk, as the physicians who operated on them did not have experience sterilizing humans. CESA St. Louis accused the leaders of this program of using sterilization as a tool of population control in Latin American nations and called "for an end to this program and other population control measures used . . . to maintain social stability in the Third World and in this country."[43]

In California, the grassroots effort to end forced sterilization via the establishment of protective guidelines came from the Chicana community and radical white feminist groups like the Coalition for the Medical Rights of Women. Like poor black women, poor Chicanas also experienced the triple oppression of racism, sexism, and poverty. As a result, Chicana feminists advanced an inclusive philosophy of reproductive rights that championed women's right to determine the terms and conditions of their reproduction without interference and criticized white feminists for operating with racial blinders.[44]

Sterilization abuse became a unifying issue for the Chicana rights movement in the early 1970s, much like abortion was for white feminists in the late 1960s. Grassroots Chicana activism propelled *Madrigal v. Quilligan*, the lawsuit involving ten Chicanas forcibly sterilized in Los Angeles. Plaintiffs' attorneys Antonia Hernandez and Richard Nabarette worked for the Model Cities Center for Law and Justice, a local legal aid organization. They collaborated with the Comisión Femenil Mexicana Nacional, a Chicana organization dedicated to employment issues and reproductive rights. The Chicana Welfare Rights Organization and Chicana Service Action Center also created safe havens for victims to discuss their abuse.[45]

Chicanas' sterilization abuse activism extended beyond the courtroom and into local communities, where activists educated women about forced sterilization at local hospitals and taught them resistance tactics. Activists' efforts proved so successful that in the wake of the *Madrigal* suit, Dr. Edward James Quilligan, chairman of the Obstetrics and Gynecology Department at the University of Southern California, Los Angeles County Medical Center (USC L.A. County Hospital), remarked to journalist Claudia Dreifus, "The thing that's bothered me most is how the adverse publicity has affected our patients. . . . They come here in great fear, feeling that we're going to grab them and sterilize them."[46]

In 1975, the Coalition for the Medical Rights of Women coordinated the efforts of local feminist, legal, consumer, and medical groups and petitioned the California Department of Health to develop and implement guidelines to prevent sterilization abuse. White feminists who adopted the reproductive rights philosophy articulated by women of color were the majority in this organization. The coalition coordinated a larger ad hoc committee—which included the Berkeley-Oakland Women's Union, CESA San Francisco, the Mexican-American Legal Defense and Education Fund, the Women's Litigation Union (a San Francisco neighborhood legal assistance foundation), and the Bay Area

Committee Against Forced Sterilization—to plead in favor of the guidelines.[47] Like CESA, the ad hoc committee was a multicultural group.

Working with sterilization abuse activists, the California Department of Health formally proposed a series of guidelines in the spring of 1976 that established a fourteen-day waiting period between the time of consent and surgery, mandated that sterilization patients be at least eighteen years old, standardized the informed consent process for all public and private hospitals in the state, devised mandatory informed consent documents and educational booklets, and ordered that patients interested in sterilization receive complete information regarding the risks and benefits of surgery as well as about alternative methods of contraception before consenting to surgery. In addition, the Coalition for the Medical Rights of Women joined with the attorneys in the *Madrigal* case to develop a "patient's information booklet" for the department to disseminate to ensure that patients received all information about sterilization, as well as their reproductive rights, before making the decision about whether to undergo sterilization. Activists' demand that the guidelines govern all sterilizations exemplifies the local nature of sterilization abuse activism. Not a single plaintiff in *Madrigal v. Quilligan*, the most famous case of abuse in California, received welfare at the time of her surgery. *Madrigal* plaintiffs' experiences taught activists that all poor women, not just those covered by Medicaid, were vulnerable to forced sterilization. In April 1976, California's Health Facilities Advisory Board voted to recommend approval of the proposed regulations, and in the fall of 1976 and again in February 1977 the Department of Health held public hearings on the matter.[48]

Chicana feminists prepared for the hearings by soliciting oral and written testimony from victims of sterilization abuse, relatives and friends of victims, community organizations familiar with discrimination in public institutions, and health workers concerned with patients' rights. The Sterilization Abuse and Informed Consent Rights Research, Education, and Organizing Project of the Coalition for the Medical Rights of Women conducted workshops to prepare witnesses to testify and offered to translate testimonies for victims who did not speak fluent English. It also offered witnesses the option of having a representative read their statement at the hearings.[49]

As in New York, a coalition of sterilization abuse activists dominated by feminists with broad definitions of reproductive freedom rallied community support for the guidelines, and physicians—this time represented by the California Medical Association (CMA)—fervently opposed the proposed policy on the grounds that it interfered with the doctor-patient relationship and violated women's right to voluntary sterilization. The California Hospital Association,

Zero Population Growth (ZPG), and California NOW joined the CMA protest. Although NOW New York had broken with the national organization and supported the sterilization guidelines, California NOW chose to stand with the national organization and oppose any policy that restricted women's access to surgery. California NOW argued that the guidelines degraded women. ZPG used the same argument. More concerned with population control than reproductive rights, ZPG did not want to see its investment in Operation Lawsuit undone by state regulations.[50]

Again, as in New York, some California physicians opposed the guidelines because they believed the rules interfered with doctors' ability to sterilize "unfit" women during labor and delivery. They operated according to an outdated model of medical authority that presumed that their decision-making abilities were stronger than their patients' and resented the interference of the state in their ability to practice medicine. One local doctor told the *Medical Tribune* that he feared "many of these patients will conceive" in the interim between consent and surgery. And who exactly were "these patients"? "I'm not talking about private patients," the doctor explained. "But here we have a large population of illegal aliens from Mexico. If we don't get them while they're here—while the getting is good—we're in trouble."[51] This physician was convinced that Mexican women could not control their reproduction in a socially responsible manner (for fourteen days!) and therefore this duty fell to him, the physician. Unfortunately for him and other guidelines opponents, the California Department of Health ignored their protests and in May 1977 adopted the proposed regulations, the most comprehensive sterilization guidelines to date.

Following the lead of physicians in New York, the CMA immediately moved to prevent the state from implementing the policy by filing for a preliminary injunction against the guidelines. The court denied this motion, and the guidelines went into effect on December 1, 1977. Unwilling to concede, the CMA took its case to trial. In *California Medical Association v. Lackner* (the suit named Jerome A. Lackner, director of the California Department of Health, as the primary defendant), the CMA accused the California Department of Health of exceeding its regulatory powers. It argued that the authority to establish informed consent requirements for sterilization lay with the legislature.[52]

As CESA did in New York, the Coalition for the Medical Rights of Women and Comisión Femenil intervened in the lawsuit on behalf of the Department of Health in October 1977. Lawyers from the Women's Litigation Unit of the San Francisco Neighborhood Assistance, Public Advocacy, and Equal Rights Advocates represented the coalition in the suit. On April 24, 1978, the trial court ruled against the physicians on all counts but one: it added conditions to the prohibition of sterilization of individuals under eighteen. In this way, the court liberalized the guidelines to permit the sterilization of minors if they were married, over fifteen and emancipated, or in the armed services.[53]

The CMA appealed the decision, but a California appeals court affirmed the lower court's ruling on September 30, 1981, holding that the Department of Health possessed the legal authority to promulgate the guidelines. The court also rejected the CMA's claim that the guidelines were not "reasonably" necessary because patients sterilized without their informed consent could recover damages for their injuries. The appellate court's dismissal of this claim echoed a similar ruling handed down by Judge Gessell in *Relf v. Weinberger*, in which the judge rejected HEW's motion for dismissal on the grounds that sterilization abuse had to occur before plaintiffs could contest the new federal policy. In *California Medical Association v. Lackner*, the California court held that "CMA advances the extraordinary thesis that the hospital regulations are not 'reasonably necessary' because a patient sterilized without his or her informed consent can recover damages for negligence." It continued, "the merit of the principle by which recovery for an injury is exalted over prevention of an injury wholly escapes us."[54] Both courts agreed that prevention of abuse was far more important than the ability to recover damages after abuse had occurred.

While the trial court ruling constituted a clear victory for sterilization abuse activists, the appellate court ruling offered a victory in principle only because by the time the case was decided, new federal sterilization guidelines had been enacted. In 1978, HEW published new sterilization guidelines and ordered California to revise its policy accordingly, warning that failure to comply would result in nonreimbursement for Medicaid sterilizations. The logic behind HEW's request is questionable, however, for with one exception (the waiting period), California's guidelines were more comprehensive than the federal guidelines. Adopting HEW's policy would actually weaken California's regulations, as the federal guidelines applied only to publicly funded surgeries, whereas the state guidelines applied to all surgeries.[55]

Twice, California Department of Health officials requested that HEW allow the state to continue to operate according to its own guidelines, but HEW refused these requests and threatened to withhold federal funds if the state failed to comply with the new federal regulations. In early January 1980, Beverlee Myers, director of the California Department of Health, conceded and brought the state into compliance with the new federal regulations. When she rescinded the guidelines as applied to private patients, Myers promised to wage an educational campaign to prevent sterilization abuse of poor women not receiving welfare. The Coalition to Defend Reproductive Rights testified against this decision at a public hearing in June 1980, arguing that "everyone needs protection from sterilization abuse. Private pay patients are no less vulnerable than MediCal recipients," as the *Madrigal* case had shown.[56] Other activists responded to Myers's promise by declaring the educational campaign to be "NO substitute for material restrictions on abusive providers."[57] The Coalition for the Medical Rights of Women testified that the change in state guidelines would allow "the conditions to be re-created in California under which thousands of women and men were robbed of their ability to bear children."[58] Their protests failed. When the federal regulations went into effect in 1981, California bore the distinction of being the only state to have to weaken its guidelines to accommodate new federal policy.

Feminists and the Federal Guidelines

The victory in New York City combined with the defeat of the Nadler bill in the state legislature convinced CESA that combating sterilization abuse on a national level would be more expedient than addressing the issue community by community. Activists began to coordinate their efforts with those of other local sterilization groups across the country, especially in the Northeast, where sterilization abuse groups in Philadelphia, Hartford, western Massachusetts, Boston, and New York met in May 1978 to formally establish a regional network on the eastern seaboard. This informal network of local activists shared organizational tools (pamphlets, booklets, slide show presentations, and so forth) and kept each other updated about local struggles through newsletters. They also collaborated to pressure HEW to issue stricter national guidelines, which it did in December 1977. Unable to satisfy the judge in *Relf v. Weinberger* with HEW's first set of revised guidelines, Secretary of HEW Joseph Califano withdrew them (with the consent of the plaintiffs) and began the rule-making process anew.[59]

The debate over federal guidelines generally mirrored the conflicts in New York and California and pitted sterilization abuse activists against physicians, Planned Parenthood, the AVS, NOW, and NARAL. The 1978 sterilization guidelines became another contest in which feminists competed to have their respective reproductive rights agenda translated into public policy. Modeled on the New York law, the proposed federal guidelines replaced the seventy-two-hour waiting period with a thirty-day wait, continued the moratorium on sterilization of individuals under twenty-one years old, and authorized the sterilization of individuals over twenty-one residing in a penal or mental institution with the approval of both a special review committee and court order. The policy also strengthened informed consent requirements by mandating that sterilization candidates be counseled in their primary language and that counselors inform patients of all of the known risks and benefits of surgery, as well as alternative methods of temporary contraception, before eliciting their consent. In addition, it banned the federal funding of nonmedically indicated hysterectomies, or hysterectomies performed primarily for contraceptive reasons, and put forth two proposals for the sterilization of persons mentally incompetent to consent. Under the first policy, the department would continue its current moratorium. Under the second, the department would authorize the sterilization of mentally incompetent persons provided that the individual in question could offer her or his informed consent and then only after both a court and a special review committee formally approved.[60]

HEW conducted public hearings on the proposed regulations in Washington, D.C., and then sent representatives to conduct ten regional hearings in the Kansas City, Denver, San Francisco, Seattle, Boston, New York, Dallas, Philadelphia, Chicago, and Atlanta areas. Grassroots sterilization activists mobilized their constituents, and liberal feminists sent their leaders to testify at these meetings. HEW omitted one important site when convening these hearings: Native American reservations. Testifying at the Boston hearings, a representative of the Native American Solidarity Committee deemed this a "gross omission," and also drew attention to the fact that HEW failed to notify Native American organizations about the hearings. This failure was indeed glaring given that between 1970 and 1976, Indian Health Service (IHS) hospitals and affiliates sterilized between 25 and 42 percent of all Native American women of childbearing age.[61]

Liberal feminists and antisterilization abuse activists agreed on a few points. In their testimonies, both condemned the practice of forced sterilization and commended HEW for taking action to combat abuse. Both groups urged HEW to adopt stricter enforcement and monitoring mechanisms and proposed that the department punish abusive providers by refusing to reimburse them for sterilizations covered with federal funds. With the exception of NOW, representatives of both groups of feminists participated in the first national sterilization abuse conference sponsored by the Interreligious Foundation for Community Organization. Roughly eighty activists traveled to Washington, D.C., in September 1977 (two months before Califano published his new guidelines) to share their knowledge and devise strategies to end forced sterilization through educational campaigns, research, and legislation.[62]

Yet here the similarities between feminists ended, for when the groups weighed women's right to be free from coercion against their right to reproductive health services, they produced different results. Antisterilization abuse activists held that women's right to be free from coercion trumped women's right to have unrestricted access to reproductive health services and insisted that all women abrogate whatever race and class privileges they possessed in order to protect those women most vulnerable to abuse. "We are aware that the 30 day waiting period and the 21 year age minimum will create undue hardships for some persons," the Boston Women's Health Book Collective testified at a regional hearing. "However," it continued, "such difficulties must be considered in the context of an urgent need to protect a far greater number from unjustifiable and inappropriate sterilization."[63]

NOW and NARAL disagreed. NARAL refused to endorse regulations that imposed restrictions on women's immediate access to sterilization. The abortion rights group never explicitly said that women's right to reproductive health services trumped that of women's right to be free of coercion, but in its testimony to HEW, it did "respectfully submit that a more just balance could have been achieved to protect against abuses resulting from coercion while protecting against abuses resulting in denial of sterilization services for individuals who voluntarily request them."[64] NOW and NARAL denounced the "paternalistic" waiting period and age minimum on the grounds that these proposed policies denied women their "right to reproductive choice." "Restrictive sterilization policies—even when drafted to protect individuals against abuses—can result in even greater abuses if appropriate medical care is delayed," NARAL testified at the Washington hearings.[65] Speaking on behalf of the organization, Executive Director Karen Mulhauser asserted that the waiting period and age minimum penalized poor women for their poverty by denying them equal access to reproductive health services. Further, evidence suggested the physicians ignored the existing seventy-two-hour waiting period. How would imposing a longer waiting period remedy this problem, NARAL wondered. "It would be far more appropriate," Mulhauser suggested, "to more rigorously enforce a more lenient policy and penalize instead the practitioners—not the women."[66] As with the New York and California policies, liberal feminists' self-interest—fear of having the right to sterilization on demand removed and fear of the loss of abortion rights—led them to oppose the waiting period and age minimum in the proposed policy.

In its resolution on sterilization, NOW sought to increase patient education and to make "sterilization abuse a criminal offense with stringent, enforced punishments for abusing physicians and institutions."[67] Antisterilization abuse activists also strove to implement a stronger method of enforcing guidelines, but did not believe this to be sufficient to deter abuse. To prove this point, they pointed to a 1975 survey of hospital sterilization practices undertaken by the ACLU Reproductive Freedom Project, which found that few hospitals across the country complied with the 1974 sterilization guidelines. Only three of fifty-one hospitals that responded to the survey fully complied with the 1974 guidelines.

Elissa Kraus, the author of the study, concluded, "HEW has taken no action to enforce the regulations other than distribution of the regulations to participating programs and projects." The results of her study "indicate that in the absence of any enforcement effort by HEW, the sterilization guidelines are being widely ignored, if not deliberately evaded."[68] A 1975 study by Ralph Nader's Health Research Group (HRG) yielded similar conclusions: 33 percent of the hospitals surveyed remained ignorant of the interim guidelines existence, and HRG investigators found that 76 percent of these hospitals violated one or more of the regulations.[69]

NOW presented the most controversial objection to the guidelines by a liberal feminist organization in the summer of 1978 when its executive board adopted a formal statement (by a vote of twenty-four to one) against the proposed regulations, and its Human Rights and Minority Women's Task Forces also drafted antiguidelines statements. Significantly, neither task force consulted with NOW members before issuing its statement, and NOW's position angered many feminists within the organization and outside of it who supported the guidelines and who sought to protect poor women and women of color from forced sterilization. A NOW member who petitioned the executive board to support the guidelines described her failed attempt: "I couldn't believe the insensitivity and lack of understanding. . . . I hate to see the organization I have been in so long—since 1967–68—being so insensitive to the flow of the women's movement as a whole."[70]

Enraged at NOW's position, CARASA sent letters to 300 organizations informing them of the NOW executive board's decision to oppose the guidelines and outlining its own rationales in favor of the guidelines. CARASA's mailing prompted other feminists to send their own letters of protest, causing NOW to be "flooded with indignant letters from women's health groups all over the country." CESA and CARASA also invited NOW executives to travel to New York and observe the city's guidelines in practice, but according to CARASA, "the NOW leadership was too busy getting the ERA extension through Congress to come to New York."[71] NOW's rejection of CARASA's invitation illustrated the low priority that sterilization abuse assumed within the organization's national agenda.

NOW responded to internal and external criticisms by conducting a workshop on the guidelines at its next annual convention, but it appears that conference organizers used the opportunity to minimize resistance to its controversial position instead of actively listening to its members' concerns. At the last minute, organizers rescheduled the workshop from Saturday evening to early Sunday morning. CARASA interpreted this change as an attempt to make it so that "as few people as possible would hear about the opposition to the Board resolution." The minority women's workshop passed a counterresolution in favor of the proposed waiting period, but NOW executives prevented the distribution of this measure at the Sunday workshop. As a result, most NOW delegates remained unaware that women of color within NOW opposed the Minority Women's Task Force's position against the guidelines.[72]

Finally, just as in New York and California, physicians and family planners sided with NOW and NARAL. ACOG, the National Commission for Human Subjects, the AVS, and other physicians, family planners, and population controllers rejected the proposed waiting period and age minimum. The National Commission for the Protection of Human Subjects, the federal committee created by Congress in 1974 to guard the rights of participants in medical research, found both measures to be "more stringent than necessary" and warned that the implementation of the proposed regulations "may result in the denial of access to proper medical care." Without evidence indicating that the seventy-two-hour waiting period had proven insufficient to guard against abuse, the commission dismissed HEW's extended waiting period as arbitrary and invasive. "*The inescapable burden created by the need to protect against abuse should not be made to fall too heavily on the potentially abused*," it instructed.[73] Dr. Martin L. Stone, the president-elect of the ACOG and one of the six New York physicians to have filed a lawsuit against the HHC policy, called the waiting period a "classic case of legislative overkill."[74] And although the AVS expressed its support for the idea behind the guidelines, it submitted that "the 30-day waiting period may cause as much hardship as it is intended to prevent."[75]

The National Medical Association (NMA), a group that represented about 8,000 black physicians, proved one of only a few exceptions to this rule and voiced its support for the guidelines. "We are advocates of the population we serve," said Dr. Ezra Davidson, immediate past chairman of the group's obstetrics and gynecology section, "and we have a duty to speak out." The NMA endorsed a seventy-two-hour waiting period, but rejected antisterilization abuse activists' calls for a thirty-day wait, saying that longer interims between consent and sterilization constituted an "undue incursion on the patient-physician relationship."[76] Doctors affiliated with the HRG also testified in favor of the guidelines.[77]

On November 8, 1978, HEW published its final guidelines in the *Federal Register*, and despite the opposition of physicians, family planners, and liberal feminists, the formal policy differed little from the proposed regulations issued nearly a year earlier. Effective February 1979, the new policy upheld the prohibition of the sterilization of minors under twenty-one years of age and prolonged the existing moratorium on the sterilization of mentally incompetent persons.

It forbade the sterilization of any institutionalized individual, unless the person provided her or his informed consent, met the federal requirements for sterilization, and received the authorization of a review board and court, and it also prohibited the performance of hysterectomies for sterilization purposes. It replaced the seventy-two-hour waiting period with a thirty-day delay between the time of consent and surgery. Liberal and radical feminists had urged HEW to waive the waiting period for women undergoing emergency abdominal surgeries and premature deliveries, provided that seventy-two hours had elapsed between the time of consent and surgery, and HEW modified the final regulations accordingly. As it had under the interim guidelines, HEW threatened noncompliant doctors with nonreimbursement, and this time strengthened its monitoring mechanisms to include periodic audits, for which it ordered providers to keep patient records for at least three years and submit these records to HEW upon request. Finally, HEW ordered the new policy to be reevaluated in thirty-six months. The department (then operating as the Department of Health and Human Services [HHS]) conducted a formal review of the policy in 1982, but made no serious changes to the original regulations.[78]

Evaluating the Effectiveness of the Federal Guidelines

A significant reduction in reports of forced sterilization and in forced sterilization litigation suggests that the practice declined in the mid-to-late 1970s. It is impossible to tell, however, the extent to which this can be attributed to the guidelines or to the efforts of antisterilization abuse activists who began their public education and community awareness campaigns during the same years. Greater public awareness and the development of the 1974 interim guidelines likely reduced the incidence of flagrant abuses, as did changes to the standards of informed consent within the medical community.[79]

Yet even after the 1978 guidelines took effect, reports of physicians' and institutions' violation of the new guidelines continued to emerge. Most commonly, medical professionals failed to abide by the waiting period and the age minimum. Such violations of federal policy continued because of the absence of effective enforcement mechanisms in the new policy. A CESA study of New York hospitals found that 88 percent of the thirty-three hospitals surveyed complied with the thirty-day waiting period established by the 1978 guidelines. But although CESA documented an improvement in physicians' compliance since the development of local guidelines, it still reported gross noncompliance. Only 58 percent of the hospitals surveyed complied with the age minimum, and only 64 percent complied with the prohibition on obtaining consent during delivery or abortion.[80] A 1981 HRG study documented continued noncompliance with the new federal guidelines, despite the addition of a new audit and record-keeping system. This study reported that more than 13 percent of states attempted to submit for reimbursement for sterilizations performed on individuals under twenty-one years old and that twelve of the forty-five states surveyed submitted for Medicaid reimbursements for cases in which institutions violated the waiting period.[81] Government investigations drew similar conclusions. A 1981 HHS audit revealed nine states' violation of the federal guidelines. (HEW became HHS in 1980.) The audit found ample violations of the age minimum and waiting period and identified about $1 million of improper payments for surgeries that failed to meet federal standards. In one instance, Maine submitted ninety-one improperly prepared signed consent forms. In another, HHS auditors found evidence of sixty-six women sterilized in North Carolina without their informed consent.[82]

Physicians themselves confessed to intentionally violating the guidelines. For example, a professor of obstetrics and gynecology told HRG investigators, "I know several doctors who have *good reasons* to use other policies."[83] Dr. David M. Priver wrote a letter to the editor of the *Medical Tribune* in which he argued that the sterilization of minors, mentally incompetent persons, or women who had not complied with the thirty-day waiting period or other consent requirements was not illegal. Priver informed his colleagues that while the government would not reimburse them for these surgeries, doctors risked no other penalties for their noncompliance. He then encouraged his peers to operate when they deemed it "appropriate," regardless of the regulations. Priver boldly declared that if he received a request for sterilization from a woman who did not meet federal qualifications, "I certainly would comply, even without pay, as I have done in the past."[84] Dr. William Scragg, chairman of obstetrics and gynecology at Texas Tech University in El Paso, openly violated the guidelines, so much so that the *Washington Star* published an article about him in 1980. He explained his actions as follows: "You take a lady 35 years old who has seven kids. She can't come to the clinic. She has no transportation. Her husband has left her, and she hasn't been able to come in for a 30-day waiting period. So she comes in during labor and says, 'Doctor, please tie my tubes.' And the government says we can't—or at least we can't and get paid for it. But we do it anyway. Sometimes we don't tell the government and sometimes the government bounces it back."[85]

In 1980, the *Washington Star* undertook a two-month investigation of sterilization in Maryland and found that the state "is one of the country's most flagrant violators of the federal regulations."[86] It found incidence of violations in hospitals across the state, especially violations of the age minimum. For example, the chairman of obstetrics and gynecology at Prince George's General Hospital in

Cheverly was unaware of the federal policy prohibiting sterilization of individuals under twenty-one years old, and, as a result, his hospital performed sterilizations on minors. Greater Baltimore Medical Center, a private hospital, performed the most sterilizations of any hospital in the state in 1978. It also failed to comply with the federal age minimum. Its chairman of gynecology, Dr. Everett Diggs, explained, "Some of our 19-year-olds in the black community have three or four children. We don't have a policy that says you can't do it at any age." The chairman of obstetrics and gynecology at Sinai Hospital, a private hospital in Baltimore, also rejected the federal age minimum, stating, "We think there are 19- and 20-year-olds who are capable of making that decision [to be sterilized]." He continued, "If we think it's right, we'll take the loss (and forego Medicaid payments for the operation). If there's any resistance by the state or the feds, we'll do what's right morally and not be bound by economics."[87] Clearly, the threat of nonreimbursement did not scare physicians into compliance.

A spokeswoman for HEW recognized this serious limitation. "We realized there's a problem," she admitted. "But . . . all we can do is disallow the costs. We don't have the authority to penalize the states, other than taking the money back."[88] The threat of nonpayment did not provide sufficient leverage to deter abuse because the penalty rarely affected offending physicians directly. The majority of federal sterilizations occurred in teaching hospitals, where interns and residents performed the procedures. Unlike private physicians paid on a fee-for-service basis, these physicians received a salary. As such, the threat of nonreimbursement did not endanger their livelihood, and no evidence suggests that hospitals punished physicians who violated the guidelines.[89] In this context, physicians could continue to abide by their own sterilization agendas instead of federal policy, secure that they would not be reprimanded for their actions. Because HEW rejected the suggestion of NOW and NARAL that violators be subject to criminal offense, doctors who chose not to comply with the guidelines faced no real penalty for their actions. Without an effective enforcement mechanism, the guidelines could not prevent physicians from sterilizing "unfit" patients.

Cognizant of these serious limitations, some activists sought to create their own grassroots monitoring programs. CESA in New York was the most successful. It began to survey New York City hospitals' compliance with PL37 in 1978. After the new federal guidelines went into effect in early 1979, the National Women's Health Network joined with CARASA, CESA, Healthright, the New York Civil Liberties Union, and the Center for Constitutional Rights to establish a similar project that monitored New York hospitals' compliance with the federal policy. With a $15,000 grant from a New York foundation, these groups developed an instruction manual for local watchdog and consumer groups, with an emphasis on organizations in New York.[90] Feminists' monitoring of local programs, however, was limited both because of their lack of resources and because of new threats to abortion rights that drew their attention away from forced sterilization.

Abortion Once Again Overshadows Sterilization Abuse

HEW's publication of its revised sterilization regulations in November 1978 signaled the end of the guidelines debates, and many local antisterilization abuse groups and coalitions disbanded soon after the 1978 guidelines took effect. Their central objective had been met (although not necessarily to their satisfaction): protective policies had been implemented at the federal level. At this time, most feminists—even those committed to a broad reproductive rights movement—turned their attention to new threats to abortion, chief among them the Hyde Amendment.

Congress passed the Hyde Amendment (named for its sponsor, Henry Hyde, a Republican representative from Illinois) in 1976. This rider to an appropriations bill denied Medicaid reimbursement for abortion unless pregnancy endangered the recipient's life or the recipient was the victim of rape or incest. Abortion rights activists filed cases claiming that the law discriminated against poor women by funding childbirth but not abortion. Three such cases made their way to the Supreme Court, which ruled against them each time.[91] The Hyde Amendment effectively granted women with financial resources more reproductive autonomy than women receiving state assistance.

Abortion rights activists faced similar threats in the late 1970s and early 1980s. Pro-life congresspersons worked to call a constitutional convention with the sole purpose of introducing an amendment that banned the procedure. Pro-life state legislators introduced bills that criminalized abortion, created spousal and parental consent requirements, and established mandatory waiting periods, all designed to dissuade women from seeking abortion. And on the grassroots level, pro-life activists had begun to picket abortion clinics and to take to the streets to demand that *Roe* be overturned.

Both groups of feminists linked the Hyde Amendment to sterilization abuse in their testimonies regarding the 1978 guidelines, but predictably, did so in different ways. NOW and NARAL argued that the guidelines restricted women's reproductive choice by denying some women the right to sterilization on demand and that in the context of the Hyde Amendment, this constituted a severe restriction of the reproductive rights of poor women receiving government assistance. "Women who are affected by the discriminatory Hyde amendment against abortion funding would have their fertility problems further aggravated if the proposed sterilization regulations are adopted as they are now written," NARAL declared.[92] Antisterilization abuse activists in CARASA and other grassroots groups, however, argued that the ban on Medicaid funding created another form of sterilization abuse. The state refused to fund elective abortion but reimbursed Medicaid sterilization at 90 percent, activists revealed, and this created a coercive situation for poor women. The Hyde Amendment denied women on welfare access to abortion except under extreme circumstances. Knowing that they could not afford an abortion should they become pregnant unexpectedly, many women "chose" sterilization because it was the most effective method of contraception available to them. The Hyde Amendment forced women to "choose" sterilization by restricting their access to other forms of contraception and abortion; undergoing sterilization because of a discriminatory federal policy constituted coercion, sterilization abuse activists maintained.[93] In its book *Women Under Attack*, CARASA described "abortion cutbacks and sterilization abuse" as "two sides of a coin." "With the decision to fund sterilization and not abortion," it wrote, "the government has adopted a policy of *de facto* population control most directly affecting poor and minority people."[94] During their testimony on the guidelines in Boston, representatives from Low Income Planning Aid declared, "We know HEW's record. We've seen them accept the Hyde amendment. . . . If HEW is serious about ending sterilization abuse, it will initiate efforts to rescind that decision. Without such actions, efforts at new sterilization guidelines will prove a sham."[95] The California Committee to Defend Reproductive Rights provided evidence to support this claim when it publicized a study undertaken by a professor at Northeastern University that found "sterilization rates for women on welfare with three or more children are sixty-seven percent higher than for women not on welfare with the same number of children."[96]

Having achieved its goal of implementing sterilization guidelines, CESA disbanded in the late 1970s. Some members began to work with CARASA on its dual campaign to prevent forced sterilization and secure abortion rights. The Reproductive Rights National Network (R2N2) joined CARASA in its attempt to develop a new reproductive rights movement. Radical feminists established R2N2 in 1979 as an umbrella organization to coordinate the activities of radical health feminists across the nation. CARASA and R2N2 committed themselves to a range of women's health issues that included women's right to safe and affordable contraception, decent health care, quality child care, and adequate welfare benefits. They also promoted occupational safety and lesbian rights and opposed population control abroad.[97] CARASA and R2N2 saw abortion rights and sterilization abuse as fundamentally interconnected and placed this link at the center of their platforms. But as the guidelines debate concluded and the pro-life movement increased its threats, both groups dedicated the majority of their resources to defending women's right to abortion, which they perceived to be under the greatest threat. Activists continued to write about forced sterilization in their respective publications and to demand an end to sterilization abuse; however, operating with limited resources and dwindling membership, activists lacked the ability to wage two concurrent struggles. The shift toward abortion rights and away from sterilization abuse and other related issues was compounded by a new form of pro-life activism: clinic bombings and violence directed against clinic workers.

Despite activists' best efforts, CARASA and R2N2 lived short lives. The multitude of issues these organizations addressed attracted activists with divergent politics and interests, which generated considerable internal conflict. Debates surrounding the role of lesbianism in the new movement contributed in part to CARASA's decline, as did activists' fatigue and the group's homogenous membership. Despite efforts to recruit women of color to its ranks, CARASA remained a predominately white organization.[98]

CARASA's decline underscores a central feature of CESA's success: its single-issue focus. CESA constituted a racially and economically diverse group, and the organization endured and succeeded because activists shared both a philosophy of reproductive rights and a commitment to ending forced sterilization through the passage of government guidelines. This single-issue approach allowed the group to overcome individual and political differences and to remain focused on the goal at hand. CESA was not about feminist ideology or political dogma; it was about action, and it disbanded soon after it accomplished its goals.

Chapter 7

The Endurance of Neo-eugenics

In 1978—the same year the Department of Health, Education, and Welfare (HEW) implemented federal sterilization guidelines—the American Cyanamid Company established a fetal protection policy at its Willow Island, West Virginia, chemical plant that prohibited fertile women from working in departments (seven of nine) that exposed workers to lead. The company employed thirty women, eight of whom held jobs that involved lead exposure. Plant managers informed these eight white women that unless they consented to sterilization, they would either lose their jobs or be transferred to lower-paying positions with less seniority and no chance for advancement. Company insurance covered sterilization, and American Cyanamid promised to grant sick leave to workers who chose this option. Two of the women refused surgery and were transferred to the janitorial department, one woman already sterilized kept her current position, and the five remaining women "chose" sterilization in order to retain their jobs. American Cyanamid was the principal employer in Willow Island. The women had few employment options outside of the plant, and almost no opportunities to earn as much as they did in the pigments department, where they worked. "They don't have to hold a hammer to your head—all they have to do is tell you that it's the only way you can keep your job," one woman who "chose" sterilization explained.[1] In a cruel twist of fate, American Cyanamid closed the pigments department just a few months after establishing the new policy and transferred the newly sterilized women to the lesser-paying jobs they had undergone surgery to avoid. American Cyanamid's policy was not unique. In the late 1970s and early 1980s, companies like General Motors, Allied Chemicals, St. Joe's Minerals, Olin, and B. F. Goodrich adopted similar policies that banned all women of childbearing potential (defined by General Motors as fertile women between the ages of fifteen and fifty) from jobs that involved toxic chemicals, with the exception of those women surgically sterilized.[2]

American reproductive policy has historically rested on a central tenet: women cannot be trusted to govern their bodies "responsibly." Through bans on birth control, the criminalization of abortion, and the passage of eugenic sterilization laws, policy makers (lawmakers and judges) sought to substitute their politics and social goals for women's own and to reproduce citizens and a society that reflected the values and power of the dominant group, mainly white middle-class men. The notion that women could not be trusted to govern their reproduction dates back to the beginning of the Republic, when women lacked basic citizenship rights and were seen as incapable of equality solely on the basis of their sex. This distrust of women shifted over time, but never fully ended, even with the legalization of birth control and abortion in the 1960s and 1970s. *Roe v. Wade*, for example, requires that the decision to terminate a pregnancy must be made by a woman *and her doctor* rather than a woman alone.[3] Contemporary restrictions on abortion like mandatory waiting periods and parental consent laws function to deprive women (and girls) of the fundamental right to make independent decisions about their bodies and their reproduction. Forced sterilization and the age/parity policies operated in the same manner. They replaced women's self-determination with the will and the politics of physicians, social workers, and hospital administrators.

American Cyanamid's policy substituted women's self-determination with the company's own paternalism. The company banned fertile women from working in departments that exposed workers to toxic chemicals in order to protect itself against potential litigation. In doing so, it privileged its bottom line above women's reproductive rights, which by 1978 had been firmly established by the Supreme Court. Significantly, American Cyanamid did not establish similar policies for men, even though research had determined that toxic chemicals could alter sperm and cause congenital abnormalities and infertility in both sexes. In fact, a year before the American Cyanamid policy took effect, exposure to the pesticide DBCP had rendered ten male workers sterile at Occidental Chemical Co. in Lathrop, California.[4]

Fetal protection policies merged pro-life rhetoric with neo-eugenic ideas to argue that women working in factories could not be trusted to make "responsible" decisions about their bodies and their families. They also challenged women's recent movement into high-paying manufacturing jobs previously reserved for men. As such, they functioned as institutional resistance to the gains made by second-wave feminism. Companies created fetal protection policies only in heavy industries in which women had just begun to break down the gender barriers. Employers did not establish fetal protection policies in "female" industries, even though women working in fields like nursing were also routinely exposed to anesthetic gases shown to affect fertility negatively.[5] This distinction reflects the malleability of ideas about reproductive fitness and exemplifies yet another way in which those with social power used an unjust sterilization policy to resist women's challenges for social, economic, and political equality.

At their core, eugenic and neo-eugenic ideas were premised upon controlling women's reproduction in order to engineer a society that reproduced white middle-class values and bodies. Eugenicists active in the first half of the century did not trust native-born middle-class white women to bear as many children as eugenicists deemed necessary to protect their own privileged status, so they intervened and substituted their own political agendas for women's self-determination through fitter family and better baby contests and cries of "race suicide." Eugenicists distrusted poor "feebleminded" women even more, and forcibly sterilized thousands of "unfit" poor immigrant and white women in the name of racial betterment. In the post–World War II era, new anxieties about the expanding welfare system, racial equality, and overpopulation, combined with fears of Communist attempts to sabotage American society, caused standards of reproductive fitness to shift. In the immediate postwar years, industry and government pushed young white women back to the home and idealized their roles as wives and mothers, claiming women's conformity constituted a defense against Communist infiltration. Medical policy reinforced this ideology by implementing pronatalist policies like age/parity rules and abortion boards designed to promote white women's reproduction by barring them from accessing sterilization and abortion. Significantly, these policies were applied more stringently in white northern communities than in southern states with large black populations.

At the same time that they promoted "fit" women's reproduction, neo-eugenicists identified a new population of "unfit" women: poor women of color who gained access to federal services after civil rights activists successfully expanded the boundaries of American citizenship to include people of color. Having abandoned biological determinism for an environmental approach, neo-eugenicists targeted poor women, predominately women of color, whom they charged with exploiting the welfare system for their own profit, using the system to reproduce a culture of dependence, and nurturing children who would "inevitably" grow up to be criminals and unwed parents. The stereotypes of the "welfare queen" and "pregnant pilgrim" cast poor black and Mexican women as "dangerous" threats to white middle-class families who were forced to divert their hard-earned resources from their own "deserving" households in order to finance the illegitimate families of "undeserving" poor women.[6]

Citizens, policy makers, physicians, and other experts who endorsed neo-eugenic ideas of reproductive fitness shared a common belief that women who received state aid did not possess the right to govern their own reproduction. In their minds, this "privilege" resided with the government and the taxpayers who financed the welfare system. Simply put, poor women had no right to bear children whom they could not support. From its inception, the welfare system institutionalized this assumption by conditioning the receipt of stipends on recipients' submission to government regulation of their private relationships and family lives.[7] The Supreme Court struck down especially intrusive policies in the late 1960s, but the neo-eugenic notion that taxpayers held a direct investment in, and thus the right to determine, the reproductive choices of welfare recipients continued to gain favor. The rapid spread of coercive sterilization from the South throughout the rest of the nation attests to the strength of this trend.

In the late 1950s and early 1960s, southern physicians seized upon sterilization as a weapon to combat racial equality and reduce the expanding welfare system. They practiced "Mississippi appendectomies" and exploited existing eugenics statutes to sterilize poor black women who bore children out of wedlock. Physicians, nurses, and hospital administrators across the country adopted this strategy a few years later, aided by the abolition of legal segregation and creation of federal family planning. The legitimization of permanent contraception played a critical role in nurturing new forms of forced sterilization that developed through federal family planning programs because the rising rates of voluntary sterilization offered a "cover" for physicians who engaged in coercive practices. Such doctors routinely forced women to "consent" to unwanted surgery in order to shield themselves from allegations of abuse. The case of the ten Chicanas sterilized in Los Angeles epitomizes the genius of this strategy. In *Madrigal v. Quilligan*, Judge Jesse Curtis ruled that the consent forms some of the women signed under duress or under the influence of heavy pain medication were "unequivocal on their face" and absolved the defendant physicians of any wrongdoing.[8]

Even though they valued "fit" women's reproduction to a far greater extent than they did "unfit" women's reproduction, adherents to neo-eugenics continued to distrust "fit" women to reproduce according to their politics, as evidenced by age/parity policies like the 120 rule. But like their predecessors, whose birth rates continued to fall despite eugenicists' best efforts to stimulate them, "fit" women resisted in the 1970s, charging that age/parity restrictions violated their fundamental rights. Although they did not identify themselves as feminists, the women who challenged hospital policies, formally and informally, drew upon contemporary feminist notions of reproductive self-determination that had filtered into the mainstream. "Fit" women began to demand access to contraceptive sterilization after medical concerns about the safety of the Pill developed in the mid-to-late 1960s. They benefited from the efforts of the Association for Voluntary Sterilization (AVS), a former eugenics group that undertook an aggressive campaign to persuade physicians, family planners, politicians, and citizens in general of the social benefits of voluntary sterilization for contraceptive purposes in the 1950s and 1960s.

The shift from biological to environmental determinism in the 1930s provided the intellectual basis for the AVS's transition from a eugenics to a neo-eugenics organization in the 1950s. In the postwar years, the AVS began to promote voluntary sterilization as a solution to the social problems of poverty, overpopulation, and single motherhood. Its extensive media campaign brought the benefits of contraceptive sterilization to the attention of physicians, family planners, and the general public, and women seeking access to the surgery drew upon this publicity and the benefits of sterilization that the AVS touted when petitioning their physicians and hospitals for access to the elusive surgery. In the early 1970s, white women across class teamed with the AVS, the American Civil Liberties Union (ACLU), and Zero Population Growth (ZPG) to contest restrictive hospital policies that prohibited them from accessing their desired contraception. Their campaign, Operation Lawsuit, proved largely successful and culminated in victory in a landmark suit, *Hathaway v. Worcester City Hospital* (1973), which compelled hospitals across the country to rescind their age/parity rules and granted women access to contraceptive sterilization.

Operation Lawsuit's victories, however, created precedents that stymied sterilization abuse victims' efforts to seek recognition and reparations for the violations they endured. In *Griswold v. Connecticut, Roe v. Wade,* and *Hathaway v. Worcester City Hospital*, the courts adopted white women's conceptualization of reproductive rights. Reflective of white women's racial privilege—and for middle-class women, their socioeconomic status—these definitions of reproductive rights focused primarily on granting women access to reproductive health services on demand. But this narrow construction of rights left poor women and women of color vulnerable to sterilization abuse, as evidenced by the continuation of forced sterilization in the years following these landmark decisions. In the mid-1970s, victims of forced sterilization filed lawsuits in defense of their fundamental right to be free from coercion and asked the courts to expand women's right to reproductive privacy and self-determination to include this demand. But with one exception (*Relf v. Weinberger*), the courts rejected their claims. As a result, *Griswold, Roe,* and *Hathaway* made reproductive freedom a privilege of women who could afford reproductive health services and white women whose skin color protected them from medical racism. Anti-sterilization abuse activists had to fight for the establishment of local, state, and federal sterilization guidelines because the existing policies failed to protect the fundamental rights of poor women and women of color. The limitations of the guidelines shaped the reproductive experiences of vulnerable populations in the 1990s and today.

In the early 1990s, lawmakers, judges, and welfare workers began to promote Norplant as the newest solution to black urban poverty. The Food and Drug Administration (FDA) approved the contraceptive implant, developed by the Population Council, in December 1990. Norplant involves the surgical insertion of six matchstick-size silicone capsules filled with levonorgestral, a type of progestin found in some birth control pills, into a woman's upper arm. It is a type of long-term contraception; the implants protect against pregnancy for five years and cannot be removed without surgery. Legal scholar Dorothy Roberts characterizes the drug as "temporary sterilization."[9] Ninety-nine percent effective, Norplant offers users the benefits of the Pill without the daily hassles and routine medical care associated with oral contraceptives. Unfortunately, like the Pill, it also involves long-term side effects, not all of which were known in December 1990. Norplant has been linked to breast cancer, cervical cancer, and osteoporosis, and women who used Norplant, like those who used the Pill, complained about negative side effects including nausea, mood swings, headaches, and stomach pain. Norplant users have also reported infection, itching, soreness, and scabbing at the insertion site.[10]

Two days after the FDA approved the drug, Donald Kimelman of the *Philadelphia Inquirer* published an editorial that proposed offering welfare recipients financial incentives to use Norplant. "The main reason more poor black children are living in poverty," Kimelman wrote, "is that people having the most children are the ones least capable of supporting them."[11] His proposal reiterated two central neo-eugenic principles: first, poor black women are less capable mothers than white women with economic resources, and second, the government has a right to regulate the fertility of dependent women. Washington, D.C., mayor and supporter of Norplant incentives Marion Barry reiterated this second principle when he stated: "You can have as many babies as you want, but when you start asking the government to take care of them, the government now ought to have some control over you."[12] A black man, Barry's statement demonstrates that neo-eugenic sentiments were not always confined to whites.[13] In his mind, poor women across race relinquished their reproductive autonomy when they accepted government aid.

The *Philadelphia Inquirer* editorial set off a national controversy that reawakened earlier accusations of genocide and coercion. David Frankel, director of Population Sciences at the Rockefeller Foundation, rebuffed these concerns in a letter to the editor of the *Washington Post*. "Despite the infantile reaction of some black staffers," he maintained, " . . . birth control incentives would not be genocide. Such incentives would be a humane inducement to social responsibility."[14] But incentives were inherently coercive; they were explicitly intended to exploit poor women's financial desperation. Offering poor women anywhere from between $100 and $500 to accept Norplant and calling it a choice is an attempt to conceal the coercive intent of the proposed incentives. A real choice would have entailed offering poor women unconditional access to all available methods of contraception *and* respecting their decision not to employ birth control at all. The practice of offering women only a few reproductive options and insisting that they possessed full reproductive autonomy was not new. As the Committee for Abortion Rights and Against Sterilization Abuse (CARASA) pointed out in the late 1970s, women on welfare received government support for sterilization and childbirth, but not abortion. If a woman on welfare chose sterilization to avoid an unwanted pregnancy that she could not afford to terminate, was she expressing her reproductive rights or making a decision based upon the limited rights she possessed?

As they had in the 1950s and 1960s with punitive sterilization bills, state legislators in the 1990s introduced proposals that would pay welfare recipients to accept Norplant in order to limit poor women's reproduction and state welfare expenses. In the first legislative term following the FDA approval of the implant (1991–1992), policy makers in thirteen state legislatures introduced twenty Norplant-related bills, amendments, and welfare proposals. Legislators in Mississippi and South Carolina tried to pass bills that would have required welfare recipients to accept Norplant in order to receive benefits. In Kansas, State Representative Kerry Patrick introduced a bill that would pay welfare recipients an initial $500 to accept Norplant and an additional $50 each year the implants remained in their arms. Advancing ideas that dated back to the turn of the twentieth century, Patrick declared that he designed his bill to "save the taxpayers millions of their hard-earned dollars."[15] Eugenicists employed this same rationale to lobby for selective sterilization bills in the years between 1910 and 1930, and neo-eugenic legislators in the 1960s used it again to support punitive sterilization legislation. Determined to limit the "costly" reproduction of poor women whom he believed forfeited their right to reproductive self-determination when they accepted government assistance, Patrick went so far as to include a measure that would force women to return a portion of the original $500 if they removed the device before the five years concluded. In Louisiana, State Representative David Duke proposed a similar bill that would pay welfare recipients in his state $100 a year to use Norplant. This former Ku Klux Klan leader's motives were transparent. For their part, conservative North Carolina policy makers tried to link Norplant to their pro-life agenda by introducing a measure that would force welfare recipients who underwent abortion to accept the implant. Here, the insertion of the long-term contraceptive would be used to punish women who terminated unwanted pregnancies. None of these bills passed, but failure did not prevent legislators from proposing similar measures over the next several sessions. The Norplant debate also inspired a small revival in sterilization proposals. In 1993, legislators in Oklahoma introduced bills that would pay welfare recipients between $2,000 and $5,000 to undergo sterilization.[16]

In the 1990s, some judges required convicted women to use Norplant. On January 2, 1991, one month after the FDA approved the implant, Judge Howard Broadman sentenced Darlene Johnson to three years on Norplant. The black woman from California had been convicted of child abuse, and Broadman granted her request for probation on the condition that she accept the contraceptive device. The judge acknowledged that his sentence violated California law, but he did not apologize for his offense. In 1984, the California Court of Appeals had ruled that courts could not condition probation on contraceptive use because such sentences violated the right to privacy. Broadman intentionally violated the appeals court ruling and went on national television to justify his decision using both neo-eugenic and pro-life language. In a *60 Minutes* interview, Broadman explained that his responsibility as a judge was to "balance conflicting constitutional rights," and in Johnson's case, he "found that there were the constitutional rights of the children, the born children and her unconceived children." "I balanced their rights against her rights, and they won," Broadman stubbornly proclaimed.[17] Johnson's case bears a striking similarity to the 1966 case of Nancy Hernandez, who was sentenced to sterilization for occupying a room that contained marijuana. The judges in both cases characterized the defendants as "unfit" mothers and administered sentences unrelated to the crime for which the women had been convicted. Both judges exploited their government-sanctioned authority to inscribe their own social policy upon women's bodies. Neither apologized for his actions.

Similar practices continue today. In May 2004, a judge in upstate New York prohibited a woman from getting pregnant until she could prove to the court that she could care for her existing children. This woman had four children, three of whom shared the same father and were born addicted to cocaine. All four children had been placed in foster care. Family Court Judge Marilyn L. O'Connor decided that "the generosity and kindness of society have been abused enough," and that "she [the mother] should not get pregnant again soon, if ever." O'Connor ruled that neither the mother nor the father of the three drug-addicted children could have any more children until they regained custody of and demonstrated their ability to care for their existing children. She insisted that "the court is not directing what steps the mother take in order not to get pregnant or what steps the father should take in order not to get any woman pregnant"; that is, she did not order one or both of them to undergo sterilization or order the wife to use Norplant or Depo-Provera. Nevertheless, the judge forbade this couple from reproducing on the grounds that their "irresponsible" reproduction contributed to the state welfare budget, which she described as "a shockingly large number." O'Connor's ruling was not novel. Judges in two other states had issued similar decisions against "dead-beat dads."[18]

The most recent neo-eugenic practice to emerge has been to offer drug-addicted women cash in exchange for sterilization and long-term contraception like the IUD, Norplant, or Depo-Provera. In 1997, Barbara Harris, an adoptive mother of four children born to a drug-addicted woman, founded Children Requiring a Caring Kommunity (CRACK) in Anaheim, California. CRACK pays drug addicts (both users and those in recovery) $200 to undergo sterilization or accept long-term contraception. Harris's concern for drug-addicted babies motivated her to establish the program, which has "assisted" 2,242 women and twenty-seven men between its inception in 1997 and 2007.[19] But like the Norplant bills that offered women cash incentives in exchange for their acceptance of the long-term contraceptive, CRACK's use of financial incentives constitutes another form of coercion. CRACK preys upon the economic vulnerability of women addicted to drugs and those recovering from drug addiction. As one mother of three children who was recovering from her addiction to speed stated, "I'm not going to lie. . . . I need the money right now."[20] CRACK advertises through the justice system, among other places, and sometimes incarcerated women convicted of drug offenses consent to the exchange before they receive treatment for their addiction. CRACK also advertises in drug rehab centers, where it targets poor, emotionally and financially vulnerable women struggling to reconstruct their lives and families. As of November 2007, CRACK operated forty-two chapters in twenty-seven states and the District of Columbia. Also by this time the reward for sterilization or Norplant (which was pulled from the market in 2002 but is still being offered on the CRACK Web site) had increased to $300. Women who chose Depo-Provera or an IUD were offered $75 for every three months they use these contraceptives, up to $300.[21]

Although CRACK denies such intentions, it clearly operates according to neo-eugenic principles. "If you can not trust someone with their reproductive choices, how can you trust them with a child?" CRACK's Web site (which used to be www.cashforbirthcontrol.com) read in 2004.[22] This statement reiterates the neo-eugenic argument for coercive sterilization: poor women cannot be trusted to control their reproduction "responsibly." This rationale holds that the state, or in this instance a group of private citizens, possesses the right to interfere in one of the most personal decisions an individual can make (whether to bear a child) if it determines that interference is in the best interest of society precisely because the women in question have "demonstrated" their lack of reproductive fitness through their poverty, illegitimacy, and/or criminality. Medicaid and state insurance programs finance many of CRACK's sterilizations, signaling government endorsement of the coercive quid pro quo "cash for birth control."

This link to eugenics was not lost on critics. Lynn Paltrow, executive director of National Advocates for Pregnant Women, insisted, "It's hard not to think that some of the people who support this just think it's a good way to get those they don't like to stop reproducing,"[23] Dr. Van Dunn, chief medical officer at the New York City Health and Hospitals Corporation (which passed the first set of local sterilization guidelines in 1975), refused to allow the hospitals his organization oversaw to participate with CRACK because he believed that "reproductive choice should always be an option, and people shouldn't be paid."[24] The National Association for the Advancement of Colored People (NAACP) and the ACLU have also declared their opposition to the program. But CRACK's Web site is filled with letters of support from people recovering from addiction, lawmakers, and parents who adopted children born from women with addictions, demonstrating the continuity of neo-eugenic ideas. "I wish a program like this would have been available while I was addicted. Then I wouldn't have so many children," said a woman in recovery with seven children. A foster parent added, "It is immoral to have a baby that no one can care for. We're adopting number 7 from a mom who has had 12."[25] Sympathy and support for Harris's mission have also been visible in the dozens of articles published about CRACK in newspapers across the country over the last ten years.[26]

For the past century, women have struggled to resist social engineering practices designed to control their reproduction and undermine their fundamental rights to access reproductive health services and to be free from coercion. White middle-class women, those deemed "fit" to reproduce, succeeded in overturning medical policies designed to encourage their reproduction and gained access to sterilization on demand, but the legal precedents they set established standards of reproductive freedom that failed to protect women of color and poor women from coercion, as evidenced by Norplant incentives and the CRACK program. Antisterilization abuse activists understood that the eradication of forced sterilization depended upon the elimination of the structural forces that drove neo-eugenics, namely racism and poverty. These forces continue to remain in place today. Until the structures that reinforce and reproduce social and economic inequalities are abolished, negative neo-eugenics will continue to permeate American culture and shape American social and medical policy, depriving poor women and women of color of their fundamental right to reproductive self-determination.

Notes

Introduction

1. Charles F. Westoff and Elise F. Jones, "Contraception and Sterilization in the United States, 1965–1975," *Family Planning Perspectives* 9 (1977): 156, 157.
2. Phillip Reilly, *The Surgical Solution: A History of Involuntary Sterilization in the United States* (Baltimore: Johns Hopkins University Press, 1991), 97.
3. Ibid., 137–138.
4. Allison C. Carey, "Gender and Compulsory Sterilization Programs in America," *Journal of Historical Sociology* 11 (March 1998): 81.
5. Vivian Cadden, "A Very Private Decision," *Good Housekeeping* 174 (May 1972), 148; Report of Consultation for Florence Caffarelli, Association for Voluntary Sterilization (AVS) Records, University of Minnesota Social Welfare History Archives, Minneapolis, box 111, folder Caffarelli (hereafter cited as Records-AVS); *Caffarelli v. Peekskill Community Hospital*, Affidavit, Florence Caffarelli, 2, Records-AVS, box 111, folder Caffarelli.
6. *Caffarelli v. Peekskill Community Hospital*, Plaintiff's Memorandum of Law in Support of Motion for Preliminary Injunction, 2, Records-AVS, box 111, folder Caffarelli.
7. Jane A. Lawrence, "Indian Health Service: Sterilization of Native American Women, 1960s–1970s" (M.A. thesis, Oklahoma State University, 1999).
8. *Madrigal v. Quilligan*, No. CV 75–2057-JWC, Plaintiffs' Finding of Fact and Conclusions of Law: Elena Orozco, 11, 12, 13, 14, Carlos Velez-Ibanez Sterilization Papers, University of California, Los Angeles, Chicano Studies Research Center Library and Special Collections, Los Angeles, box embargoed, folder [ca. November 1974] (hereafter cited as Records-UCLA); *Madrigal v. Quilligan*, No. CV 75–2057-JWC, Opinion, 19, Records-UCLA, box embargoed, folder [ca. 1978] transcript of judge's opinion on case.

Chapter 1 — From Eugenics to Neo-eugenics

1. Wendy Kline, *Building a Better Race: Gender, Sexuality, and Eugenics from the Turn of the Century to the Baby Boom* (Berkeley: University of California Press, 2001), 143–155; Alexandra Minna Stern, *Eugenic Nation: Faults and Frontiers of Better Breeding in Modern America* (Berkeley: University of California Press, 2005), 4–5, chap. 5; Reilly, *Surgical Solution*, 128; William H. Tucker, *The Funding of Scientific Racism: Wickliffe Draper and the Pioneer Fund* (Urbana: University of Illinois Press, 2002).
2. "One-Fifth of U.S. Couples—More Than 7 Million—Rely on Contraceptive Sterilization; Procedures Doubled in 4 Years," *Family Planning Perspectives* 7 (1975): 113; Westoff and Jones, "Contraception and Sterilization," 156, 157.
3. Some historians challenge the validity of the terms "positive eugenics" and "negative eugenics." Stern, *Eugenic Nation*, 154–155; Martin Pernick, "Taking Better Baby Contests Seriously," *Journal of Public Health* 92 (May 2002): 707–708.
4. Reilly, *Surgical Solution*, 2; Daniel J. Kevles, *In the Name of Eugenics: Genetics and the Use of Human Heredity* (New York: Knopf, 1985), 4, 12, 18–19, 46–48, 70–71.

5. Frank Dikotter, "Race Culture: Recent Perspectives on the History of Eugenics," *American Historical Review* 103 (April 1998): 467–468.

6. Reilly, *Surgical Solution*, 42–43; Diane Paul, *Controlling Human Heredity: 1865 to the Present* (Atlantic Highlands, N.J.: Humanities Press, 1995), 10–11; Kevles, *In the Name of Eugenics*, chaps. 3 and 4.

7. Sean Dennis Cashman, *America Ascendant: From Theodore Roosevelt to FDR in the Century of American Power, 1901–1945* (New York: New York University Press, 1998), 88–89.

8. Sara M. Evans, *Born for Liberty: A History of Women in America* (New York: Free Press, 1997), chap. 7; Kathy Peiss, *Cheap Amusements: Working Women and Leisure in Turn-of-the-Century New York* (Philadelphia: Temple University Press, 1986).

9. Kline, *Building a Better Race*, 20, 24–25; Kevles, *In the Name of Eugenics*, 107, 131; Miroslava Chavez-Garcia, "Intelligence Testing at Whittier State School, 1890–1920," *Pacific Historical Review* 76 (May 2007): 193–228; Stern, *Eugenic Nation*, 86–99.

10. Theodore Roosevelt, "Race Decadence," *Outlook*, April 8, 1911, quoted in Andrea Tone, ed., *Controlling Reproduction: An American History* (Wilmington, Del.: Scholarly Resources, 1997), 159–162; Kline, *Building a Better Race*, 11–12.

11. Kline, *Building a Better Race*, 19–20; Peiss, *Cheap Amusements*.

12. California bears responsibility for 2,558 of the 3,233 total eugenic sterilizations performed between 1907 and 1921. Reilly, *Surgical Solution*, 40, 45, 49.

13. Reilly, *Surgical Solution*, 11–15, 25–26, 30–40, 49; Kline, *Building a Better Race*, 32–60; Kevles, *In the Name of Eugenics*, 92–95.

14. Reilly, *Surgical Solution*, 52–55; Kevles, *In the Name of Eugenics*, 109–110.

15. Nine state legislatures actually passed bills, but two governors exercised their vetoes, so only seven bills became law. Reilly, *Surgical Solution*, 84.

16. Ibid., 68, 86.

17. *Buck v. Bell*, 274 U.S. 200 (1927).

18. Reilly, *Surgical Solution*, 87.

19. Stephan Jay Gould, "Carrie Buck's Daughter," *Natural History* (July 1984): 16.

20. Reilly, *Surgical Solution*, 97.

21. Stephen Kuhl, *The Nazi Connection: Eugenics, American Racism, and German National Socialism* (New York: Oxford University Press, 1994); Reilly, *Surgical Solution*, 106–110.

22. Carey, "Gender and Compulsory Sterilization Programs," 76, 80–83, 84.

23. Ibid., 76, 90–91; Reilly, *Surgical Solution*, 98; Kevles, *In the Name of Eugenics*, 167; William Ray Vanessendelft, "A History of the Association for Voluntary Sterilization, 1935–1964" (Ph.D. diss., University of Minnesota, 1978), 83.

24. Carey, "Gender and Compulsory Sterilization Programs," 81–82, 86–88.

25. Ibid., 93–94; Reilly, *Surgical Solution*, 34.

26. Historians who argue that the eugenics movement was in decline by the 1930s include Reilly, *Surgical Solution*; Carl Degler, *In Search of Human Nature: The Decline and Revival of Darwinism in American Social Thought* (New York: Oxford University Press, 1991); and Hamilton Cravens, *The Triumph of Evolution: The Heredity-Environment Controversy, 1900–1941* (Baltimore: Johns Hopkins University Press, 1988). Edward J. Larson argues that while mainstream eugenics fell from favor by the mid-1930s in other regions, southern institutions and individuals continued to practice eugenics throughout the decade. Edward J. Larson, *Sex, Race, and Science: Eugenics in the Deep South* (Baltimore: Johns Hopkins University Press, 1995), 119–120. Daniel J. Kevles makes the slightly more nuanced argument

that mainstream eugenics was discredited in the 1930s and that it was replaced by a "reform eugenics" movement that recognized the intersection between heredity and nature. Kevles, *In the Name of Eugenics*, 164–175. Diane B. Paul proposes a similar chronology in *Controlling Human Heredity: 1865 to the Present* (Atlantic Highlands, N.J.: Humanities Press, 1995). Kline and Stern argue for continuity through the 1950s. Kline, *Building a Better Race*, 6, 124–126; Stern, *Eugenic Nation*, 9–10.

27. Kline, *Building a Better Race*, 98, 99, 100–101, 104–105, 125; Stern, *Eugenic Nation*, chap. 5.

28. *Skinner v. Oklahoma*, 316 U.S. 535 (1942); Reilly, *Surgical Solution*, 130; Gayle Binion, "Reproductive Freedom and the Constitution: The Limits on Choice," *Berkeley Women's Law Journal* 4 (1988): 24.

29. Reilly, *Surgical Solution*, 128.

30. Kline, *Building a Better Race*, 100–101, 124–126; Michael B. Katz, *The Undeserving Poor: From the War on Poverty to the War on Welfare* (New York: Pantheon Books, 1989), 17–23, 29–35; Mimi Abramovitz, *Regulating the Lives of Women: Social Welfare Policy from Colonial Times to the Present* (Boston: South End Press, 1998), 321; Ellen Reese, *Backlash against Welfare Mothers: Past and Present* (Berkeley: University of California Press, 2005), 40, 48–49, 54–57.

31. Kline, *Building a Better Race*, chap. 1; Kevles, *In the Name of Eugenics*, 74–75; Carey, "Gender and Compulsory Sterilization Programs," 81; Stern, *Eugenic Nation*, chap. 2, 92–99, 188–192.

32. Stern, *Eugenic Nation*, 5.

33. Reilly, *Surgical Solution*, 94–95; Alan F. Guttmacher, "Facts and Arguments: Sterilization . . ." *Nation*, April 6, 1964, 346; Eugene D. Fleming, "Our Sterilization Scandal," *Cosmopolitan* 147 (July 1959), 58, 59.

34. "One-Fifth of U.S. Couples," 113; "Series B 5–10. Birth Rate—Total and Fertility Rate for Women 15–44 Years Old, by Race: 1800–1997," in *Datapedia of the United States 1790–2005, America Year by Year*, 2nd ed., ed. George Thomas Kurian (Lanham, Md.: Bernan, 2001), 42.

35. San Gabriel Valley Chapter, Zero Population Growth (ZPG), "Report on Operation Lawsuit, Chapter Program," July 13, 1971, 3–5, Records-AVS, box 91, folder Operation Lawsuit; C. Hastings to C. T. Faneuff, Sub: Operation Lawsuit—Status, March 20, 1973, 1–6, Records-AVS, box 91, folder Operation Lawsuit; "Sterilization Lawsuits Compiled by the Association for Voluntary Sterilization, Inc.," December 20, 1974, Records-AVS, box 91, folder Operation Lawsuit; Judy Kutulas, *The American Civil Liberties Union and the Meaning of Modern Liberalism, 1930–1960* (Chapel Hill: University of North Carolina Press, 2006), 212–214.

36. Larry L. Bumpass and Harriet B. Presser, "Contraceptive Sterilization in the U.S.: 1965 and 1970," *Demography* 9, no. 4 (November 1972): 533.

37. "Editorial: Voluntary Sterilization," *American Journal of Public Health* 63 (July 1973): 573, Records-AVS, box 91, folder ACOG, AMA, APHA, AHA; American Public Health Association, "APHA Recommends Program Guide for Voluntary Sterilization," Records-AVS, box 91, folder ACOG, AMA, APHA, AHA; H. Curtis Wood Jr., "The Changing Trend in Voluntary Sterilization," *Contemporary Ob/Gyn* 1 (April 1973): 32.

38. Rickie Solinger, "'A Complete Disaster': Abortion and the Politics of Hospital Abortion Committees, 1950–1970," in *Women and Health in America*, 2nd ed., ed. Judith Waltzer Leavitt (Madison: University of Wisconsin Press, 1999), 659–680;

Kristin Luker, *Abortion and the Politics of Motherhood* (Berkeley: University of California Press, 1984), 56–57.

39. H. Pystowsky and N. J. Eastman, "Puerperal Tubal Sterilization: Report of 1,830 Cases," *Journal of the American Medical Association* 158 (June 11, 1955): 463–467; P. L. Garrison and C. J. Gamble, "Sexual Effects of Vasectomy," *Journal of the American Medical Association* 144 (September 23, 1950): 293–295; T. N. Evans, "Simplified Method for Sterilization of the Female," *American Journal of Obstetrics and Gynecology* 66 (Autumn 1953): 393–395; Jerome A. Weinbaum, M.D., and Carl T. Javert, M.D., "Sterilization at the New York Hospital Over a Twenty Year Period, 1932–1952," *Western Journal of Surgery, Obstetrics and Gynecology* 62 (February 1954): 95–100; Theron H. Funk, M.D., F.A.C.S., Frank Weyrens, M.D., and Paul Pollinger, M.D., "The Modern Trend of Sterilization," *Medical Records and Annals* 46 (March 1952): 891–893.

40. Weinbaum and Javert, "Sterilization at the New York Hospital," 96.

41. Funk, Weyrens, and Pollinger, "Modern Trend of Sterilization," 891.

42. Lyle Bachman, M.D., "Tubal Sterilization in the Human Female," *Hawaii Medical Journal* 13 (March–April 1954): 265.

43. Goodrich C. Schauffler, M.D., "Tell Me Doctor . . .," *Ladies' Home Journal* 76 (1959), 22.

44. Bachman, "Tubal Sterilization," 265–266.

45. Reilly, *Surgical Solution*, 94–95.

46. Molly-Ladd Taylor, "Saving Babies and Sterilizing Mothers: Eugenics and Welfare Policies in the Interwar United States," *Social Politics* 4 (Spring 1997): 147; Johanna Schoen, *Choice and Coercion: Birth Control, Sterilization, and Abortion in Public Health and Welfare* (Chapel Hill: University of North Carolina Press, 2005), 5; James Ridgeway, "Birth Control by Surgery," *New Republic* 151 (November 14, 1964), 9; H. Curtis Wood Jr., "A Prescription for the Alleviation of Welfare Abuses and Illegitimacy," *Henry Ford Hospital Medical Bulletin* 12 (March 1964): 80; "Experts Outline Views on Voluntary Vasectomy," *Medical World News*, April 26, 1963, 83–84, 86, Population Council Records, Rockefeller Archive Center, Sleepy Hollow, N.Y., box 91, folder 1719 (hereafter cited as Records–Population Council); Fred P. Graham, "New Fight Grows on Sterilization," *New York Times*, April 4, 1965.

47. Weinbaum and Javert, "Sterilization at the New York Hospital," 97.

48. Fleming, "Our Sterilization Scandal," 58.

49. "Experts Outline Views on Voluntary Vasectomy," 84. His advice was repeated in Jim E. Davis and Jaroslav F. Hulka, "Elective Vasectomy by American Urologists in 1967," *Fertility and Sterility* 21 (August 1970): 618.

50. Vanessendelft, "History of the Association for Voluntary Sterilization," chap. 3; Sterilization League of New Jersey, "Platform of the Sterilization League of New Jersey," Adopted November 20, 1937, Records-AVS, box 42, folder Human Betterment Program Development (since 1948).

51. H. Curtis Wood Jr., M.D., Read at the April 19th 1979 Membership Meeting of the Association for Voluntary Sterilization, Records-AVS, box 110, folder minutes 1979, 1.

52. Vanessendelft, "History of the Association for Voluntary Sterilization," 72–73, 75; Wood, Read at the April 19th 1979 Membership Meeting of the Association for Voluntary Sterilization, 1.

53. Kline, *Building a Better Race*, 98–101; Reilly, *Surgical Solution*, 95; Julius Paul, "Population 'Quality' and 'Fitness for Parenthood' in the Light of State Eugenic Sterilization Experience, 1907–1966," *Population Studies* 21 (November 1967): 297.

54. Vanessendelft, "History of the Association for Voluntary Sterilization," 104, 107, 109, 112.

55. Ibid., 109–112.

56. Ibid., 111; Human Betterment Association for Voluntary Sterilization (HBAVS), "Family Planning Program in Eastern Kentucky," n.d., Records-AVS, box 57, folder Hartman Plan-KY.

57. H. Curtis Wood Jr. to Dear Friend, October 31, 1949, Records-AVS, box 42, folder Human Betterment Program Development (since 1948); Birthright, Inc., "Sterilization for Human Betterment: A Presentation," Records-AVS, box 42, folder Human Betterment Program Development (since 1948); AVS, "A Statement of Purpose and Program: To Make Known the Benefits of Voluntary Sterilization and the Solution of Family and Population Problems," 2, 3, Records–Population Council, box 98, folder 1812; HBAVS, "To Protect the Retarded Adolescent," 11, Seeley G. Mudd Manuscript Library, Princeton University, Princeton, N.J., box 1973, folder 16 (hereafter cited as Records-ACLU); Hugh Moore to Dear Friend, October 1966, Records-ACLU, box 1973, folder 16; Vanessendelft, "History of the Association for Voluntary Sterilization," 81, 82, 110–111; "The Association for Voluntary Sterilization, Inc. Cordially Invites You to Attend the First National Conference on Public Welfare, Voluntary Sterilization, and the Public Health," Thursday, October 7, 1965, Afternoon Program Guide, Records–Population Council, box 98, folder 1812; AVS, List of Committee Members, Records-AVS, box 47, folder AVS resolutions; "General Draper, Population Control Expert, Takes Role in International Conference on Voluntary Sterilization," For Release, Sunday, March 22, 1964, Records-AVS, box 92, Gen. Draper; Hugh Moore to Dear Friend, November 1966, Records–Population Council Organizational Files, box 98, folder 1812; Donald T. Critchlow, *Intended Consequences: Birth Control, Abortion, and the Federal Government* (Oxford: Oxford University Press, 1999), 42–43.

58. Kuhl, *Nazi Connection*, 58–59, 66, 101. Wood's presidency extended from 1945 to 1961. Vanessendelft, "History of the Association for Voluntary Sterilization," 154.

59. Lisa McGirr, *Suburban Warriors: The Origins of the New American Right* (Princeton, N.J.: Princeton University Press, 2001), 75–79; Elaine Tyler May, *Homeward Bound: American Families in the Cold War Era* (New York: Basic Books, 1988); Birthright, "Sterilization for Human Betterment," 5–7; Vanessendelft, "History of the Association for Voluntary Sterilization," 107, 164.

60. Birthright, "Sterilization for Human Betterment," 1.

61. Vanessendelft, "History of the Association for Voluntary Sterilization," 108; Wood, "Prescription for the Alleviation of Welfare Abuses."

62. Birthright, "Sterilization for Human Betterment," 1, 3; H. Curtis Wood Jr. to Dear Friend, October 31, 1949; HBAVS, "To Protect the Retarded Adolescent"; Robert W. Laidlow, M.D., to All Concerned with Helping the Mentally Handicapped, n.d., Records-AVS, box 47, folder retarded memorandum.

63. HBAVS, "To Protect the Retarded Adolescent," 1.

64. Ibid., 4, 5.

65. Kline, *Building a Better Race*, 64, 66, 77; Elizabeth Siegel Watkins, *On the Pill: A Social History of Oral Contraceptives, 1950–1970* (Baltimore: Johns Hopkins University Press, 1998), 12–13, 33, 39–40.

66. C. Lee Buxton, "The Doctor's Responsibility in Population Control," *Northwest Medicine* 65 (1966): 113–114.

67. Luke T. Lee and Richard K. Gardiner, "Law and Family Planning," *Studies in Family Planning* 2 (April 1971): 81.

68. Wood, "Prescription for the Alleviation of Welfare Abuses," 76.
69. Buxton, "Doctor's Responsibility in Population Control," 114, 115.
70. Wood, "Prescription for the Alleviation of Welfare Abuses."
71. Critchlow, *Intended Consequences*, 13–24; Hugh Moore to Dear Friend, November 1966.
72. See, for example, Paul Ehrlich, *The Population Bomb* (New York: Ballantine Books, 1968); Winfield Best, "The New Swing to Small Families," *Parents Magazine* 47 (November 1972), 64; Garrett Hardin, "Parenthood: Right or Privilege?" *Science* 169 (July 31, 1970): 425; Lawrence Lader, "A Platform on Population," 1970, NARAL records, Schlesinger Library, Cambridge, Mass., MC-313, folder population and environment (hereafter cited as Records-NARAL).
73. Critchlow, *Intended Consequences*, 135, 156.
74. Ibid., 56; George H. Gallup, ed., *The Gallup Poll: Public Opinion 1935–1971*, vol. 3, *1959–1971* (New York: Random House, 1972), 2299.
75. AVS, "Minutes, Executive Committee meeting," May 21, 1969, 1, Records-AVS, box 110, folder minutes 1967.
76. Vanessendelft, "History of the Association for Voluntary Sterilization," 170–171, 178–179; AVS, "Report of the Executive Committee," March 23, 1966, 3, Records-AVS, box 110, folder 1966 Board of Directors Mtgs; AVS, "Report of the Executive Director, Annual Meeting of the Association for Voluntary Sterilization," 3, Records-AVS, box 110, folder 1967 Board of Directors/Executive Committee; AVS, "Report of the Executive Director, Annual Meeting," March 22, 1967, 3, Records-AVS, box 110, folder minutes 1967; AVS, "Report of the Legal and Scientific Committee, Annual Meeting," March 22, 1967, 1–2, Records-AVS, box 110, folder minutes 1967; AVS, "Report of the Executive Director, presented at Annual Meeting," March 24, 1971, 12, Records-AVS, box 110, folder annual meeting minutes March 1971.
77. Vanessendelft, "History of the Association for Voluntary Sterilization," 157–159, 184–185.
78. AVS, "For Immediate Release: Catholic Physician John Rock, M.D., Developer of Birth Control 'Pill,' and Jack Lippes, M.D., Inventor of the 'Lippes Loop' Contraceptive Device, Jointly Endorse Voluntary Sterilization," Records-AVS, box 54, folder Rock, John M.D.; AVS, "Executive Committee Meeting Minutes," June 21, 1967, 1, Records-AVS, box 110, folder minutes 1967.
79. Draft of Hugh Moore Press Release, "Eminent Catholic Doctor, John Rock, Assails the Stand of the Catholic Hierarchy Against Voluntary Sterilization," June 2, 1967, Records-AVS, box 54, folder Rock, John M.D.
80. AVS, "For Immediate Release."
81. HBAVS, "The Physician and Sterilization," Records-ACLU, box 1973, folder 16; HBAVS, "Voluntary Sterilization: Questions and Answers," Records-ACLU, box 1973, folder 16; HBAVS, "The Lawyer Speaks on Contraceptive Sterilization: A Statement by Harriet F. Pilpel HBAVS' Legal Counsel," Records-ACLU, box 1973, folder 16; AVS, "A Statement of Purpose and Program: To Make Known the Benefits of Voluntary Sterilization in the Solution of Family and Population Problems," Records-ACLU, box 1973, folder 16; AVS, "AVS Progress Report," February 16, 1966, 1, Records-AVS, box 110, folder minutes 1966; AVS, "AVS Progress Report," June 15, 1966, 1, Records-AVS, box 110, folder minutes 1966.
82. See, for example, AVS, "AVS Progress Report," February 16, 1966, 1–2; AVS, "Executive Committee Minutes," May 18, 1966, 2, Records-AVS, box 110, folder minutes 1966;

AVS, "AVS Progress Report," July 20, 1966, 1, Records-AVS, box 110, folder minutes 1966; AVS, "TV and Radio Requests for AVS Speakers, Jan. to Mid-March, 1967," Records-AVS, box 110, folder minutes 1967; AVS, "Minutes, Annual Membership Meeting," March 22, 1967, 2, 4, Records-AVS, box 110, folder minutes 1967; AVS, "Report of the Executive Director, Annual Meeting," March 22, 1967, 1–2, Records-AVS, box 110, folder minutes 1967; Helen Edey, "Questions Parents Ask about Sterilization," *Parents Magazine* 46 (March 1971), 66–67, 90.

83. AVS, "AVS Progress Report," June 15, 1966, 2; Barbara Seaman, "The Dangers of Birth Control Operations," *Ladies' Home Journal* 84 (July 1967), 50.

84. Handwritten statistical reports of sterilization referrals organized by month for 1965–1970, Records-AVS, box 111, folder Service Department Statistical Reports, 1965–1970; "January 1970 Operations," Records-AVS, box 111, folder Service Department Statistical Reports, 1965–1970; "Press, Magazine Publicity Sweeps AVS Service Dept.: Over 11,000 Referrals Made in First 6 Months of 1971," *AVS, Inc. Bulletin* (Summer 1971): 4, Records-ACLU, box 1973, folder 16; John R. Rague, "AVS Progress Report," May 21, 1969–June 18, 1969, 2, Records-AVS, box 110, folder reports 1969; Michael Shane to Merrie Spaeth, Memorandum: Monthly Summary of Activities, February 8, 1978, 1, Records-AVS, box 112, MTS Chrons 1978–January.

85. Vanessendelft, "History of the Association for Voluntary Sterilization," 188–189.

86. Joanna Poletti to A.M., May 8, 1962, Records-AVS, box 65, folder Assistance Fund Loan, Paid by HBAA 1/10/62.

87. Evelyn E. Bryant, "AVS' Past Role as a Supplier of Patient Services Presented at the Board of Directors Meeting, River Club, New York City, March 24, 1976," 1, Records-AVS, box 49, folder Hartman Plan–KY 1964–1965.

88. Application of G.B., Received April 2, 1964, Records-AVS, box 58, folder Loan Pd by HBA 6/17/64, B. G. Broward Gen. Hospital, Kirkely, W.H., M.D.

89. Application for Mrs. M.L.A., submitted April 3, 1964, Records-AVS, box 58, folder Loan Pd by HBA 5/20/64 A., Mrs. J.H.

90. Application for Assistance in Securing a Sterilization Operation for Mr. M.B. of Barbourville, Kentucky, received January 24, 1963, Records-AVS, box 58, folder Loan Pd by HBA 2/19/63, B.M., Berea College Hospital, (Jones, H.C., M.D.).

91. Ava H. Parks to Association for Voluntary Sterilization, March 7, 1966, Records-AVS, box 58, folder Operation Loan Paid by AVS 7/66, B.M., Barnes Hosp.

92. For example, see Application for Mrs. M.L.A.; Application of D.M.A., received February 13, 1964, Records-AVS, box 58, folder loan H.D. Pd by HBA 3/19/64, A. Mr. D.M.; Application of R.A., received July 31, 1964, Records-AVS, box 58, folder loan pd by HBA 10/16/64, A. Mrs. R. (L).

93. Mrs. Carl B. Benson to Human Betterment Association of America, Inc., July 21, 1958, Records-AVS, box 58, folder French Fund Loan, A., Mrs. A. (A), Pd by HBAA 12/31/59.

94. Edna Estes, R.N. to Mrs. James Daugherty, May 22, 1959, Records-AVS, box 58, folder Assistance Loan Fund, A.H. Pd by HBAA 6–8-59.

95. A.P.B. to c/o Mr. Gram [*sic*] French, Human Betterment Association of America, Inc., July 24, 1959, Records-AVS, box 58, folder Assistance Loan Fund Pd by HBAA 8–10–59, B.A.P.

96. C.W.A. Application for Assistance in Securing a Sterilization Operation, February 22, 1965, Records-AVS, box 58, folder Operation No Loan 6/15/65, W.A.

97. "Mrs. P.D. Follow-up Questionnaire, January 6, 1964," Records-AVS, box 84, folder follow-up female 1965.

98. "AVS Cooperating Physicians Donate 2100 Voluntary Contraceptive Sterilization Operations to Help the Poor," *AVS, Inc. Bulletin* (Summer 1965): 1, Records-ACLU, box 1973, folder 16. The total number of sterilizations performed via AVS's sterilization loan fund for 1965 is not available; however, statistics for the months of October, November, and December of that year are. Twenty-seven surgeries were performed in October and December, and thirty-one surgeries were performed in November. A total of eighty-five surgeries were performed during the last three months of the year. Assuming this number is representative, I estimate that about 340 sterilizations were performed during 1965. "October 1965 cases closed (operations)," Records-AVS, box 111, folder Service Department Statistical Referrals, 1965–1970; "November 1965 cases closed (operations)," Records-AVS, box 111, folder Service Department Statistical Referrals, 1965–1970.

99. Evelyn Bryant, "Service Department Report," May 1966, 1–2, Records-AVS, box 111, folder Service Department Statistical Reports, 1965–1970; AVS, "Service Department Report," October 31, 1966, 1–2, Records-AVS, box 111, folder Service Department Statistical Reports, 1965–1970; "January 1968 Service Department Report," February 21, 1968, 1, Records-AVS, box 111, folder Service Department Statistical Reports, 1965–1970; AVS, "January 1968 Service Department Report," February 21, 1968, 1–2, Records-AVS, box 111, folder Service Department Statistical Reports, 1965–1970; "Annual Report," March 26, 1969, 10, Records-AVS, box 111, folder Service Department Statistical Reports, 1965–1970.

100. "Service Department Report–1971," *AVS, Inc. Bulletin* (Spring 1972): 4, Records-ACLU, box 1973, folder 16.

101. "Mrs. M.B.P. Follow-up Questionnaire, April 11, 1958," Records-AVS, box 84, folder follow-up female 1958.

102. "Mrs. E.S. Follow-up Questionnaire, October 6, 1961," Records-AVS, box 84, folder follow-up female 1958.

103. "Mr. H.P. Follow-up Questionnaire, September 8, 1958," Records-AVS, box 84, folder follow-up male 1958.

104. "Mrs. O.C. Follow-up Questionnaire, December 6, 1962," Records-AVS, box 84, folder follow-up female 1962.

105. "Mrs. L.C.G. Follow-up Questionnaire, March 6, 1965," Records-AVS, box 84, folder follow-up female 1965.

106. "Mrs. H.T. Follow-up Questionnaire, October 6, 1961," Records-AVS, box 84, folder follow-up female 1958.

107. Gerald Grant, "The Fauquier Hospital Sterilization Story," *Background Reports* (January 1973): 2.

108. Julius Paul, "The Return of Punitive Sterilization Proposals: Current Attacks on Illegitimacy and the AFDC Program," *Law and Society Review* 3 (August 1968): 99; Gregory Michael Dorr, "Segregation's Science: The American Eugenics Movement and Virginia, 1900–1980" (Ph.D. diss., University of Virginia, 2000), 8.

109. Grant, "Fauquier Hospital Sterilization Story," 2, 3; "Clinic Offers Aid by Sterilization," *New York Times*, September 9, 1962; "Washington Prelate Denounces Sterilization Clinic in Virginia," *New York Times*, September 10, 1962; "Sterilization: New Argument," *U.S. News and World Report*, September 24, 1962, 55.

110. Grant, "Fauquier Hospital Sterilization Story," 3.

111. Ibid., 4; "Washington Prelate Denounces Sterilization Clinic," 25.

112. Reilly, *Surgical Solution*, 118–122; Sharon Mara Leon, "Beyond Birth Control: Catholic Response to the Eugenics Movement in the United States, 1900–1950" (Ph.D. diss., University of Minnesota, 2004); "A Sterile Issue?" *Newsweek*, September 24, 1962, 88.

113. Grant, "Fauquier Hospital Sterilization Story," 6; "Sterile Issue?" 88. Orthodox Jews opposed sterilization; however, members of less traditional (Reformed, Reconstructionist, and Conservative) congregations tolerated the procedure.
114. Grant, "Fauquier Hospital Sterilization Story," 7.
115. Ibid.
116. "Sterile Issue?" 88.
117. "Clinic Offers Aid by Sterilization"; "Sterilization: New Argument," 55; David Binder, "Clinic Is Backed on Sterilization," *New York Times*, September 9, 1962.
118. "Sterilization: New Argument," 55.
119. Grant, "Fauquier Hospital Sterilization Story," 3.
120. "Clinic Offers Aid by Sterilization"; David Binder, "Virginians Calm on Sterilization," *New York Times*, September 13, 1962; Binder, "Clinic Is Backed on Sterilization," 31; "Sterilization: New Argument," 55; Grant, "Fauquier Hospital Sterilization Story," 8.
121. Bryant, "AVS' Past Role," 1; "$25,000 Gift Speeds Voluntary Sterilization Program in Appalachia to Control Poverty Bomb," June 19, 1964, 1, 4, Records-AVS, box 57, folder Hartman Plan–KY; "Hartman Plan–Kentucky Project," July 23, 1964, Records-AVS, box 57, folder Hartman Plan–KY; " "HBAVS War on Poverty," *HBAVS Bulletin* (Summer 1964): 2, Records-AVS, box 49, folder Hartman Plan–KY, 1964–1965.
122. Evelyn E. Bryant, "Memo to Mr. Higgins," October 24, 1966, Records-AVS, box 49, folder Hartman Plan–KY 1964–1965. A letter from Louise G. Hutchins, M.D., director of the Mountain Maternal Health League, to Jesse Hartman, dated July 8, 1965, indicates that 196 sterilizations had been performed. I have found no other evidence to indicate which figure is correct. Louise G. Hutchins, M.D., to Jesse Hartman, July 8, 1965, Records-AVS, box 49, folder Hartman Plan–KY 1964–1965.
123. "Among Ky. Poor $25,000 Fund Starts Sterilization Plan," *Boston Globe*, July 9, 1964, in *Human Betterment Association for Voluntary Sterilization Bulletin* (Summer 1964), Records-AVS, box 49, folder Hartman Plan–KY 1964–1965; Ruth Proskauer Smith to Dear Kentucky Friends, June 12, 1964, 1, Records-AVS, box 57, folder Hartman Plan–KY.
124. Ruth Proskauer Smith to Editor, Letter to the Editor, *New York Times*, April 30, 1964, Records-AVS, box 45, folder U.S. Office of the President.
125. "War on Poverty: To President Lyndon B. Johnson," *New York Times*, n.d., Records-AVS, box 45, folder U.S. Office of the President.
126. "$25,000 Gift," 1; John D. Morris, "Appalachia Plan Gathers Support," *New York Times*, April 30, 1964, Records-AVS, box 45, folder U.S. Office of the President.
127. "$25,000 Gift"; A. S. Holmes, M.D., Letter to the Editor of the *Cincinnati Enquirer*, August 12, 1964, Records-AVS, box 57, folder Hartman Plan-KY.
128. Abramovitz, *Regulating the Lives of Women*, 318–329; Lisa Levenstein, "The Gendered Roots of Modern Urban Poverty: Poor Women and Public Institutions in Post–World War II Philadelphia" (Ph.D. diss., University of Wisconsin–Madison, 2002), 252–258; Dorothy Roberts, *Killing the Black Body: Race, Reproduction and the Meaning of Liberty* (New York: Vintage Books, 1997), 92, 102–103; "Family Planning Program in Eastern Kentucky," 1, Records-AVS, box 57, folder Hartman Plan–KY.
129. "$25,000 Gift," 1, 3.
130. "Family Planning in Eastern Kentucky," 1.
131. "Report on Meeting to Inaugurate the Hartman Plan," June 11, 1964, 2, Records-AVS, box 57, folder Hartman Plan-KY; Ruth Proskauer Smith, "Memo Re: Hartman Plan for Voluntary Sterilization—Florida Project," October 26, 1964, Records-AVS, box 49, folder Hartman Plan Florida 1965; John R. Rague to Frank M. Craft, March 31, 1965, Records-AVS, box 49, folder Hartman Plan Florida 1965; Frank M. Craft

to John R. Rague, May 5, 1965, Records-AVS, box 49, folder Hartman Plan Florida 1965; "AVS Offers $25,000 'Challenge Grant' to Public Health and Welfare Units; Special Effort Made in Florida," *AVS, Inc. Bulletin* (Summer 1965): 5, Records-ACLU, box 1973, folder 16; Bryant, "AVS' Past Role," 2.

Chapter 2 — "Fit" Women and Reproductive Choice

1. Watkins, *On the Pill*, 34, 50–51; Andrea Tone, *Devices and Desires: A History of Contraceptives in America* (New York: Hill and Wang, 2001), 233, 240–241.
2. Tone, *Devices and Desires*, 270.
3. As quoted in ibid., 271.
4. Carole R. McCann, *Birth Control Politics in the United States, 1916–1945* (Ithaca, N.Y.: Cornell University Press, 1994), 134, 201.
5. Watkins, *On the Pill*, 70.
6. Ibid., 70–71.
7. Ibid., 89–91, 120–128.
8. Tone, *Devices and Desires*, 257.
9. Bumpass and Presser, "Contraceptive Sterilization," 534, 540, 542.
10. Beth Bailey, *Sex in the Heartland* (Cambridge, Mass.: Harvard University Press, 1999), 11–12.
11. Bumpass and Presser, "Contraceptive Sterilization," 532–534.
12. Ellen Graham, "Vasectomies Increase as Concern Over 'Pill,' Overpopulation Grows," *Wall Street Journal*, November 11, 1971.
13. Jane E. Brody, "Pregnancies Follow Birth Pill Publicity," *New York Times*, February 15, 1970; Jane E. Brody, "More Than 100,000 Persons a Year Are Reported Seeking Sterilization as Method of Contraception," *New York Times*, March 22, 1970.
14. Graham, "Vasectomies Increase"; ZPG-AVS-ACLU, "Should You Sue Your Hospital for the Sterilization Operation You Want?" Records-AVS, box 91, folder Operation Lawsuit; Hjalmar E. Carlson, M.D., "Vasectomy of Election," *Southern Medical Journal* 63 (July 1970): 767.
15. Carlson, "Vasectomy of Election," 766.
16. Robert E. Hackett, M.D., and Keith Waterhouse, M.D., "Vasectomy—Reviewed," *Journal of Obstetrics and Gynecology* 116 (1973): 442.
17. "Vasectomy Service," February 5, 1970, 1, Records-AVS, box 54, folder Sanger, Margaret Vasectomy Service.
18. Joan Rattner Heilman, "What Vasectomy Means to a Man and His Marriage," *Reader's Digest* 116 (April 1980), 33–36; Charlotte Muller, "The Cost of Contraceptive Sterilization," *Family Planning Perspectives* 6 (Winter 1974): 39; Alice Lake, "Sterilization: The Growing Alternative to the Pill," *Good Housekeeping*, 183 (February 1976), 204d; "The Facts about Voluntary Sterilization," 170 *Good Housekeeping* (June 1970), 155; Jane E. Brody, "Sterilization," *New York Times*, April 4, 1971; Judy Klemserud, "Sterilization Is an Answer for Many," *New York Times*, January 18, 1971; "Vasectomy: That Controversial Surgery," *Ebony* 34 (November 1978), 134. The cost of tubal ligation here refers to the surgery before the development of endoscopic techniques. Memo from Ruth Proskauer Smith to HBAVS Hartman Plan Committee for Kentucky Appalachia; Louise G. Hutchins, M.D., Chairman; Mary P. Fox, M.D.; A. M. Holmes, M.D.; William R. Kelsey Jr., M.D.; Elwood L. Woosley, M.D.; and William H. Suters Jr., July 21, 1964, 1, Records-AVS, box 49, folder Hartman Plan–KY 1964–1965; Ruth Proskauer Smith to Kentucky Friends, June 12, 1964, 1, Records-AVS, box 49, folder Hartman Plan–KY 1964–1965.

19. Leslie Aldridge Westoff, "Sterilization," *New York Times Magazine*, September 29, 1974, 31.

20. Lake, "Sterilization," 73, 203, 204d.

21. "L.A. Application for Referral for a Sterilization Operation," November 26, 1969, Records-AVS, box 65, folder Operation No Loan, 2/16/70, A., L.J.

22. "R.A. Application for Referral for a Sterilization Operation," February 10, 1970, Records-AVS, box 65, folder Operation No Loan, 4/18/70, A., G.W.

23. AVS, "Service Department Report," November 20, 1968, Records-AVS, box 111, folder Service Department Statistical Reports, 1965–1970.

24. Lake, "Sterilization," 73.

25. Follow-up survey, Mr. J.H.W., August 23, 1965, Records-AVS, box 84, folder follow-up male rec 1965.

26. Follow-up from Mr. W.B., January 1966, Records-AVS, box 84, folder follow-up males 1966.

27. Follow-up from Mr. C.E.G., July 1970, Records-AVS, box 84, folder [July 1970].

28. "At 22, My Husband Chose Sterilization," *Good Housekeeping* 172 (January 1971), 39, 41, 42, 44.

29. See, for example, "Facts about Voluntary Sterilization," 155; David R. Zimmerman, "Medicine Today," *Ladies' Home Journal* 90 (March 1970), 26, 127; "One Man's Answer to Overpopulation," *Life*, March 6, 1970, 42–47; Evan McLeon Wylie, "Sterilization: Now First for Birth Control," *Reader's Digest* 109 (November 1976), 150–152.

30. Westoff and Jones, "Contraception and Sterilization," 155; Tone, *Devices and Desires*, 279.

31. Lake, "Sterilization," 203.

32. Westoff and Jones, "Contraception and Sterilization," 155.

33. "F.A. Application for Assistance in Securing a Sterilization Operation," September 28, 1962, Records-AVS, box 65, folder Operation No Loan, A. F. A.

34. "J.C. AVS Follow-Up Survey," July 23, 1970, Records-AVS, box 84, folder [July 1970].

35. Klemesrud, "Sterilization Is an Answer for Many," 24.

36. "One Man's Answer to Overpopulation," 42–47.

37. Critchlow, *Intended Consequences*, 150.

38. Melva Weber, "When Men Take Over Birth Control Are Women Glad or Sorry?" *Vogue* 159 (February 1972), 195; Larry L. Bumpass, "The Risk of Unwanted Birth: The Changing Context of Contraceptive Sterilization in the U.S.," *Population Studies* 41 (November 1987): 348; Claudia Dreifus, "Sterilization: The Not-So-Simple Facts," *Right Now* 104 (October 1976): 47–48.

39. Harriet B. Presser and Larry L. Bumpass, "The Acceptability of Contraceptive Sterilization among U.S. Couples: 1970," *Family Practice Perspectives* 1, no. 4 (October 1972): 20.

40. Ibid., 19, 20.

41. Lake, "Sterilization," 204d.

42. Ibid., 204.

43. Ibid., 204d.

44. Critchlow, *Intended Consequences*, 156–157; "Childless—and Unfettered," *U.S. News and World Report*, October 4, 1976, 59–60.

45. "Make Love, Not Babies," *Newsweek*, June 15, 1970, 111.

46. Lake, "Sterilization," 204d.

47. Ms. D.C. to Whom It May Concern, May 24, 1974, Records-AVS, box 112, folder correspondence cases 1974.

48. Ellen Peck, *The Baby Trap: A Devastating Attack on the Motherhood Myth* (New York: Bernard Geis, 1971), 73, 140–144, 160–163.

49. Based upon a review of letters from Americans to AVS from the 1950s through the 1970s. See, for example, Ms. S.W. to People, November 12, 1974, Records-AVS, box 112, folder correspondence other 1974; Ms. K.K. to AVS, November 12, 1974, Records-AVS, box 112, folder correspondence other 1974; Mrs. S.W.C. to AVS, November 18, 1974, Records-AVS, box 112, folder correspondence cases 1974; Mr. S.L.S. to Sir, June 19, 1974, Records-AVS, box 112, folder correspondence cases 1974; Evelyn E. Bryant to Mrs. Charles Westoff, May 1, 1974, Records-AVS, box 112, folder correspondence other 1974; Ms. G.S. to Madame or Sir, September 8, 1974, Records-AVS, box 112, folder correspondence cases 1974; Mrs. L.P. to Sirs, December 12, 1974, Records-AVS, Supp. II, box 3, folder correspondence cases 1974.

50. Mrs. P.W. to AVS, July 11, 1974, 1, Records-AVS, box 112, folder correspondence cases 1974; Evelyn E. Bryant to Mrs. P.B., July 16, 1974, Records-AVS, box 112, folder correspondence cases 1974.

51. Evelyn E. Bryant to Mrs. P.B., July 16, 1974.

52. David Wolfers and Helen Wolfers, "Vasectomania," *Family Planning Perspectives* 5 (Autumn 1973): 196–199; Gallup, *Gallup Poll*, 2000; "80% of Americans Favor V.S. New Study Shows," *Association for Voluntary Sterilization Inc.* (Spring 1972): 3, Records-ACLU, box 1973, folder 16; Peter M. Layde, David Fleming, Joel R. Greenspan, Jack C. Smith, and Howard W. Ory, "Demographic Trends of Tubal Sterilization in the United States, 1970–1975," *American Journal of Public Health* 70 (August 1980): 809; Ronald R. Rindfuss and Futing Liao, "Medical and Contraceptive Reasons for Sterilization in the United States," *Studies in Family Planning* 19 (November–December 1988): 370–380.

53. Aquiles J. Sobrero to John R. Rague, November 6, 1970, 1, Records-AVS, box 54, folder Sanger, Margaret Vasectomy Services; "AVS Progress Report," October 20, 1971–November 17, 1971, November 15, 1971, 6, Records-ACLU, box 1973, folder 16.

54. "Vasectomy Clinics Burgeon to Meet National Demand," *AVS, Inc. Bulletin* (Summer 1971): 3, Records-ACLU, box 1973, folder 16.

55. "Midwest Population Center," Records-AVS, box 46, folder Midwest Population Center.

56. Simone M. Caron, *Who Chooses? American Reproductive History since 1830* (Gainesville: University Press of Florida, 2008), 218–219.

57. Ernest Dunbar, "For Men Only: Foolproof Birth Control," *Look*, March 9, 1971, 45.

58. John Rague to Mildred Mayers Re: MIDWEST POPULATION CENTER LOAN GUARANTY AGREEMENTS, March 18, 1971, Records-AVS, box 46, folder Midwest Population Center; Midwest Population Center, "Vasectomy Clinic to Open in Chicago," For Release: February 16, 1971, 3, Records-AVS, box 46, folder Midwest Population Center; Rev. Canon Don C. Shaw to Chicago Area Physician, January 6, 1971, Records-AVS, box 46, folder Midwest Population Center. This was not the first time *Playboy* and Hugh Hefner contributed to efforts designed to increase Americans' access to reproductive health services. In 1966, Hefner lent his support to Illinois Citizens for the Medical Control of Abortion, and *Playboy* printed materials for the group. Caron, *Who Chooses?* 193.

59. Midwest Population Center, "Vasectomy Clinic to Open in Chicago," For Release: February 16, 1971, 2.

60. Dunbar, "For Men Only," 47, 48.

61. Hackett and Waterhouse, "Vasectomy—Reviewed," 442.

62. "One-Fifth of U.S. Couples," 113; Charles F. Westoff, "The Modernization of U.S. Contraceptive Practice," *Family Practice Perspectives* 4, no. 3 (July 1972): 10–11; Davis and Hulka, "Elective Vasectomy by American Urologists," 618.

63. Presser and Bumpass, "Acceptability of Contraceptive Sterilization," 19.

64. Westoff, "Modernization of Contraceptive Practice," 11; Presser and Bumpass, "Acceptability of Contraceptive Sterilization," 19; Jennifer A. Nelson, "From Abortion Rights to Reproductive Freedom: Feminism, Nationalism, and the Politics of Identity" (Ph.D. diss., Rutgers University, 1999), 113–154; "Vasectomy: That Controversial Surgery," 134; "Family Size and the Black American," *Population Bulletin* 30, no. 4 (1975); Reilly, *Surgical Solution*, 28–29; Jennifer Nelson, *Women of Color and the Reproductive Rights Movement* (New York: New York University Press, 2003), 104–107; Caron, *Who Chooses?* 168–177; *Pittsburgh Press*, February 24, 1969, quoted in Caron, *Who Chooses?* 173.

65. Memorandum to Members of AVS Boards, Committees & Other Correspondents from Betty Gonzales, Public Relations Director Re: Medicaid Reimbursement for Voluntary Sterilization, Records-AVS, box 86, folder Medicaid Survey General, 1968–1974; Albert J. Richter to Evelyn E. Bryant, May 23, 1973, Records-AVS, box 86, folder Medicaid Survey General, 1968–1974; AVS to Medicaid Administrators, August 17, 1972, Records-AVS, box 86, folder Medicaid Survey General, 1968–1974; AVS to Blue Cross and Blue Shield administrators who do not pay for voluntary sterilization for socioeconomic reasons, August 1972, Records-AVS, box 86, folder Medicaid Survey General, 1968–1974; Jim E. Davis, Ph.D., "Considerations Relevant to the Inclusion of Voluntary Sterilization in Health Insurance Coverage, 1968," Records-AVS, box 86, folder Medicaid Survey General, 1968–1974; Inter-Office Memorandum from Donald H. Higgins to John R. Rague Re: Letter from Paul Douglas, Attorney in Vermont, Re: Non-Coverage of A.V.S. Operation by Blue Cross–Blue Shield, March 16, 1972, Records-AVS, box 86, folder Blue Cross Blue Shield Surveys (Alabama–Mississippi) 1968–1972; C. Hastings to J. R. Rague Sub: Michigan BLUE SHIELD, June 23, 1972, Records-AVS, box 86, folder Blue Cross Blue Shield Surveys (Alabama–Mississippi) 1968–1972; AVS, "Blue Cross, Blue Shield Insurance Companies in Most States Pay for Voluntary Sterilization, New AVS Survey Reveals: Federal/State Medicaid Program Also Pays for Operations in 34 States and the District of Columbia," 1, Records-AVS, box 86, folder Medicaid Survey General, 1968–1974.

66. Caron, *Who Chooses?* 154–155; Critchlow, *Intended Consequences*, 82.

67. Louis J. Lefkowitz to Honorable George K. Wyman, August 21, 1967, Records-AVS, box 90, folder Blumenthal–Goodwin Bills (NYS); "State Medical Handbook, Policies and Standards for Physician Services, Family Planning Policy," August 31, 1967, 1–2, Records-AVS, box 90, folder Blumenthal–Goodwin Bills (NYS).

68. John R. Rague to Harriet F. Pilpel, Re: AVS, March 18, 1971, Records-AVS, box 90, folder Blumenthal–Goodwin Bills (NYS).

69. Sherry Davis to Association for Voluntary Sterilization, July 26, 1973, Re: Information on doctors in East Tennessee (or closest area) who will perform sterilization surgery on women without unnecessary hassle about husband's permission, Records-AVS, box 112, folder Correspondence Agencies 1973; Evelyn E. Bryant to Sherry Davis, August 9, 1973, Records-AVS, box 112, folder Correspondence Agencies 1973.

70. AVS, "Blue Cross, Blue Shield Insurance Companies in Most States Pay for Voluntary Sterilization," 3; AVS, "Blue Cross–Blue Shield and Medicaid Insurance for Voluntary

Sterilization," January 3, 1972, Records-AVS, box 86, folder Medicaid Survey General, 1968–1974; AVS, "Blue Cross–Blue Shield and Medicaid Insurance for Voluntary Sterilization," June 4, 1973, Records-AVS, box 86, folder Blue Cross Blue Shield Surveys (Alabama–Mississippi) 1968–1972. Arizona and Alaska were the two states without Medicaid programs. Memorandum from Evelyn E. Bryant to John R. Rague, September 17, 1971, Records-AVS, box 86, folder Medicaid Survey General, 1968–1974. Three of the four remaining carriers covered female sterilization for medical reasons only. Charlotte F. Muller, "Insurance Coverage of Abortion, Contraception, and Sterilization Services," *Family Planning Perspectives* 10 (March–April 1978): 73.

71. Hackett and Waterhouse, "Vasectomy–Reviewed," 440.

72. A. Marsh Poulson Jr., "Analysis of Female Sterilization Techniques," *Obstetrics and Gynecology* 42 (July 1973): 131–135.

73. Jaroslav F. Hulka, M.D., *Complications of Laparoscopy* (New York: Year Book Medical Publishers, 1981), 7; J. Wortman, "Female Sterilization by Mini-Laparotomy," *Population Reports* Series C, no. 4 (November 1974): C-53; "Voluntary Sterilization Becoming More Popular as Method of Birth Control," *Population Chronicle* 5 (1971): 8.

74. Critchlow, *Intended Consequences*, 73, 78; Caron, *Who Chooses?* 160.

75. Muller, "Cost of Contraceptive Sterilization," 39–40; "Safety and Effectiveness of Tubal Ligation via Laparotomy and Laparoscopic Sterilization with Cautery Are Debated," *Family Planning Perspectives* 6 (November–December 1975): 275; "Georgia Sterilization Costs Range from $120–$513," *Family Planning Perspectives* 4 (July–August 1975): 153; "Contraceptive Tubal Sterilization Rate Increases More Than Twice during the Period 1970–1976," *Family Planning Perspectives* 11 (July–August 1979): 254; Margaret F. McCann and Lynda Painter Cole, "Laparoscopy and Minilaparoscopy: Two Major Advances in Female Sterilization," *Studies in Family Planning* 11 (April 1980): 119–127.

76. "Sterilization Method for Women Reported That's Simple, Cheap," *Wall Street Journal*, March 28, 1972; Bruce Thompson and R. Clifford Wheeless, "Outpatient Sterilization by Laparoscopy: A Report of 666 Patients," *Obstetrics and Gynecology* 38 (December 1971): 912–915.

77. Thompson and Wheeless, "Outpatient Sterilization by Laparoscopy," 912, 915.

78. Jane E. Brody, "Sterilization: For Women, an Easier Way," *New York Times*, March 24, 1976.

79. Cedric W. Porter Jr. and Jaroslav F. Hulka, "Female Sterilization in Current Clinical Practice," *Family Perspectives* 6 (1974): 33–34.

80. "Minilap Reduces Sterilization Risk: More Suitable for Outpatient Procedures than Laparoscopic Technique," *Family Planning Perspectives* 9 (1977): 85–86; Arthur J. Horowitz, Letter to the Editor, *Journal of the American Medical Association* 223 (March 12, 1973): 1286–1287; J. F. Hulka, Letter to the Editor, *Journal of the American Medical Association* 223 (March 12, 1973): 1287; Marguerite K. Shepard, "Review: Female Contraceptive Sterilization," *Obstetrical and Gynecological Survey* 29 (November 1974): 745; American College of Obstetrics and Gynecology, "Guidelines for Gynecologic Laparoscopy," May 1973, Records-AVS, box 91, folder ACOG, AMA, APHA, AHA.

81. "The Growing Use of Sterilization for Birth Control," *Good Housekeeping* 176 (May 1973), 196–197; Lake, "Sterilization"; Evan McLeod Wylie, "Sterilization: Now First for Birth Control," *Reader's Digest* 109 (November 1976), 150–152; W. M. Wolfe, "Questions about Sterilization," *Redbook* 136 (March 1971), 22, 24, 28, 31; "A Simple New Kind

of Sterilization for Women," *Good Housekeeping* 180 (June 1975), 157; Julia Kagan, "Sterilization Techniques," *Right Now* 106 (October 1978): 69.

82. Elaine Randell, "On Being 29 and Having a Tubal Ligation," *Mademoiselle* 82 (May 1976), 14.

83. Ibid.; "A Simple New Kind of Sterilization for Women," 157.

84. "Growing Use of Sterilization for Birth Control," 196–197; "Sterilization Techniques," 69; Dreifus, "Sterilization"; "Facts about Voluntary Sterilization," 155.

85. "Contraceptive Tubal Sterilization Rate Increases," 253.

Chapter 3 — Sterilizing "Unfit" Women

1. Carlos G. Velez-I, "Se Me Acabo La Cancion: An Ethnography of Non-Consenting Sterilizations among Mexican Women in Los Angeles," in *Mexican Women in the United States: Struggles Past and Present*, ed. Magdalena Mora and Adelaida R. Del Castillo (Los Angeles: Chicano Studies Research Center Publications, University of California, Los Angeles, 1980), 79–82; Janet Karsten Larson, "And Then There Were None," *Christian Century*, January 26, 1977, 61.

2. Kay Mills, *This Little Light of Mine: The Life of Fannie Lou Hamer* (New York: Plume Books, 1993), 22.

3. Bernard Rosenfeld, M.D., Sidney M. Wolfe, M.D., and Robert E. McGarrah Jr., *A Health Research Group Study on Surgical Sterilization: Present Abuses and Proposed Regulations* (Washington, D.C.: Health Research Group, 1973); Ted Bogue and Daniel W. Sigelman, *Sterilization Report Number 3: Continuing Violations of Federal Sterilization Guidelines by Teaching Hospitals in 1979* (Washington, D.C.: Health Research Group, 1979); Daniel W. Sigelman, *Health Research Group Study Number 4 on Sterilization Abuse of the Nation's Poor under Medicaid and Other Federal Programs* (Washington, D.C.: Health Research Group, 1981); Elissa Krauss, *Hospital Survey on Sterilization Policies* (New York: American Civil Liberties Union, 1975), 1570.

4. Larson, *Sex, Race, and Science*, 153–154; Carey, "Gender and Compulsory Sterilization Programs," 99.

5. Linda Gordon, *Pitied but Not Entitled: Single Mothers and the History of Welfare, 1890–1935* (New York: Free Press, 1994), 293–303.

6. Abramovitz, *Regulating the Lives of Women*, 319, 320, 321.

7. Ibid., 334.

8. Ibid., 335.

9. Gallup, *Gallup Poll*, 1919–1920.

10. "The Welfare Backlash," *America* 115 (November 26, 1966): 680–681.

11. Lisa Levenstein, "From Innocent Children to Unwanted Migrants and Unwed Moms: Two Chapters in Public Discourse on Welfare in the United States, 1960–1961," *Journal of Women's History* 11 (Winter 2000): 12, 15–16.

12. Rickie Solinger, *Wake Up Little Susie: Single Pregnancy and Race before* Roe v. Wade (New York: Routledge, 2000), 49–53; Abramovitz, *Regulating the Lives of Women*, 325–326; Gordon, *Pitied but Not Entitled*, 298; Levenstein, "From Innocent Children to Unwanted Migrants," 12.

13. Solinger, *Wake Up Little Susie*, 42; Gordon, *Pitied but Not Entitled*, 43–46, 51–52.

14. Cravens, *Triumph of Evolution*, 158.

15. National rates of illegitimacy tripled between 1940 and 1957, during which time the number of illegitimate births increased by 125 percent. Black women tended to bear more children out of wedlock than white women did, but the illegitimacy rate of

white women rose faster than that of blacks during these years. Solinger, *Wake Up Little Susie*, 13.

16. Daniel Patrick Moynihan, *The Negro Family: A Case for National Action* (Westport, Conn.: Greenwood Press, 1981).

17. Paul, "Return of Punitive Sterilization Proposals," 84–85.

18. Mississippi Legislature, "House Bill No. 479: An Act to Discourage Immorality of Unmarried Females by Providing for Sterilization of the Unwed Mothers Under Conditions of this Act; and for Related Purposes," Regular Session 1958, Records-AVS, box 90, folder Mississippi State Board of Trustees of Mental Institutions.

19. Paul, "Return of Punitive Sterilization Proposals," 83, 87, 90, 91, 92.

20. Ibid.; Roberts, *Killing the Black Body*, 94; Solinger, *Wake Up Little Susie*, 57–58; Kutulas, *American Civil Liberties Union*, 212.

21. ACLU, "Minutes Board of Directors February 5–6, 1972," 2, Records-ACLU, box 25, folder 5.

22. "Is the Quality of U.S. Population Declining? Interview with a Nobel Prize-Winning Scientist," *U.S. News and World Report*, November 22, 1965, 68–71, William Shockley Papers, Series II, Stanford University Department of Special Collections, Stanford, Calif., box A13, folder FSM Master Set 1–18 (hereafter cited as Shockley Papers).

23. "NAS Again Says No to Shockley," *Science* 168 (May 8, 1970): 685.

24. Dwight J. Ingle, "Racial Differences and the Future," *Science* 146 (October 16, 1964): 378, quoted in William H. Tucker, *The Science and Politics of Racial Research* (Urbana: University of Illinois Press, 1994), 182.

25. Richard J. Herrnstein and Charles Murray, *The Bell Curve: Intelligence and Class Structure in American Life* (New York: Free Press, 1994).

26. Arthur R. Jensen, "How Much Can We Boost IQ and Scholastic Achievement?" *Harvard Educational Review* 33 (February 1969): 1–123.

27. William Shockley, "Academy Ruling Unjust: Resolution Proposed Again," October 17, 1972, 2, Shockley Papers, box A13, folder FSM Master Set 1–18.

28. "'FREED' Eugenic Research Board Established," *Berkeley Daily Gazette*, March 30, 1970.

29. Tucker, *Science and Politics of Racial Research*, 193.

30. Joel N. Shurkin, *Broken Genius: The Rise and Fall of William Shockley* (London: Macmillan, 2006), 221; Tucker, *Science and Politics of Racial Research*, 190–191, 194.

31. Dwight J. Ingle, *I Want to See the Elephant* (New York: Vantage, 1963), quoted in Tucker, *Science and Politics of Racial Research*, 182–183.

32. William Shockley, Letter to the Editor, *Palo Alto Times*, December 28, 1967.

33. William Shockley, "The Voluntary Sterilization Bonus Plan—An Answer to Population Pollution?" paper written for a meeting of the Lake Merritt Breakfast Club in Oakland, Calif., June 14, 1973, Shockley Papers, box A13, folder FSM Master Set 1–18; "Shockley's Eugenic 'Bonus' Plan," *San Francisco Chronicle*, May 28, 1970; Karen Klinger, "New Shockley Genetic Proposal," *San Jose Mercury*, June 15, 1973, Shockley Papers, box A13, folder FSM Master Set 1–18; "Bounty Hunters for Sterilization," *San Jose News*, June 15, 1973, Shockley Papers, box A13, folder FSM Master Set 1–18; Harold V. Streeter, "Shockley Argues Case for Sterilization Bonuses," *San Francisco Examiner*, August 24, 1974, Shockley Papers, box A13, folder noncomposed letters.

34. Shurkin, *Broken Genius*, 218, 238–239; Tucker, *Science and Politics of Racial Research*, 206; Committee Against Racism, "Demonstrate Against Shockley's Racist Lies, N.Y.U., Tuesday, April 9, 1:30 P.M., Washington Square South," Shockley Papers, box A13, white envelope; "No 'Freedom' to Advocate Genocide: Stop Nazi

Shockley at NYU," Shockley Papers, box A13, white envelope; "Recent Events at NYU and Yale, Future Schedule, Intentions for FREED Activities," April 22, 1974, Shockley Papers, box A13, folder FSM Master Set 1–18; "Race Geneticist Shouted Down at Georgia U.," *Washington Star-News*, March 6, 1974, Shockley Papers, box A13, folder FSM Master Set 1–18.

35. Mallory Nagle to Prof. Wm. Shockley, December 12, 1973, FREED Records, Department of Special Collections, Stanford University Library, Stanford, Calif., box 4, folder 27 Dec 73 1–1222 (hereafter cited as Records-FREED).

36. Joseph C. Miller to Dr. William Shockley, February 2, 1973, Records-FREED, box 4, folder 27 Dec 73 1–1222.

37. Mrs. N. Richard Seligh to Dr. William Shockley, February 19, 1974, Records-FREED, box 4, folder FREED income January 4–October 18, 1974, 123–300.

38. Vincil Penny Crowe to Professor Shockley, August 30, 1974, Records-FREED, box 4, folder FREED income January 4–October 18, 1974, 123–300.

39. Mike Culbert, "Shockley Fires New Pattern of Torpedoes," *Berkeley Daily Gazette*, December 2, 1970.

40. William H. Chafe, *The Unfinished Journey: America since World War II*, 3rd ed. (New York: Oxford University Press, 1995), 112.

41. Stephanie Coontz, *The Way We Never Were: American Families and the Nostalgia Trap* (New York: Basic Books, 1992), 76–77, 80–81; Lizabeth Cohen, *A Consumers' Republic: The Politics of Mass Consumption in the Postwar America* (New York: Vintage Books, 2004), 190–191.

42. May, *Homeward Bound*, chap. 1, 16–36, 94.

43. Elena R. Gutiérrez, "Policing 'Pregnant Pilgrims': Situating the Sterilization Abuse of Mexican-Origin Women in Los Angeles County," in *Women, Health, and Nation: Canada and the United States since 1945*, ed. Georgina Feldberg, Molly Ladd-Taylor, Alison Li, and Kathryn McPherson (Montreal: McGill-Queen's University Press, 2003), 390–391.

44. Letters from Don T. Wilson to John Tanton, September 24, 1972, and April 7, 1973, quoted in Elena R. Gutiérrez, "The Racial Politics of Reproduction: The Social Construction of Mexican-Origin Women's Fertility" (Ph.D. diss., University of Michigan, 1999), 159.

45. "Aliens Reportedly Get $100 Million in Welfare," *Los Angeles Times*, January 27, 1973.

46. McGirr, *Suburban Warriors*, 154–155.

47. Gutiérrez, "Racial Politics of Reproduction," chap. 3, 115, 116.

48. Ibid., 150, 172.

49. Letter from Elaine Stansfield, director of ZPG-LA, to Phyllis Eisen, October 20, 1978, quoted in Gutiérrez, "Racial Politics of Reproduction," 178.

50. Paul, "Return of Punitive Sterilization Proposals," 81.

51. "The Difficulties of Getting Sterilized," *Time*, November 13, 1964, 88; Paul, "Return of Punitive Sterilization Proposals," 79.

52. "Jail or Sterilization?" *Time*, June 3, 1966, 46.

53. Ibid.; "Cruel and Unusual?" *Newsweek*, June 13, 1966, 46.

54. Peter Bart, "Sterilization or Jail Order Is Reversed on Coast," *New York Times*, June 9, 1966.

55. Paul, "Return of Punitive Sterilization Proposals," 79; Wm. F. Buckley Jr., "Sterilize That Woman!" *National Review* 18 (July 12, 1966), 666.

56. Bart, "Sterilization or Jail Order Is Reversed on Coast," 77.

57. "Judge Gives View of Sterilization," *New York Times*, May 25, 1966.

58. Bart, "Sterilization or Jail Order Is Reversed on Coast," 77.

59. Buckley, "Sterilize That Woman!" 666.

60. Ibid.

61. "Woman on Coast Chooses Jail Over Sterilization," *New York Times*, May 24, 1966.

62. Schoen, *Choice and Coercion*, 108.

63. Molly-Ladd Taylor, "Saving Babies and Sterilizing Mothers: Eugenics and Welfare Policies in the Interwar United States," *Social Politics* 4 (Spring 1997): 147; Schoen, *Choice and Coercion*, 5.

64. Schoen, *Choice and Coercion*, 112–124.

65. Reproductive Freedom Project, "Legal Docket," March 22, 1979, 53, Records-ACLU, box 387, folder 10.

66. Schoen, *Choice and Coercion*, 121–124; *Cox v. Stanton*, 529 F.2d 47 (4th Cir. 1975); *Cox v. Stanton*, 381 F. Supp. 349 (D.N.C. 1974); Edward Hudson, "Suit Seeks to Void Sterilization Law," *New York Times*, July 13, 1973.

67. *Cox v. Stanton*, 381 F. Supp. 349 (D.N.C. 1974); "Forced Sterilization in North Carolina," *ACLU News*, 1973, NARAL Records Vertical Files (microfiche) 82-M217, Schlesinger Library, Radcliffe Institute for Advanced Study, Harvard University, Cambridge, Mass. (hereafter cited as Records-NARAL Vertical Files); *Nial Ruth Cox, Plaintiff v. A. M. Stanton M.D. et al.*, "Complaint: Preliminary Statement," Records-NARAL Vertical Files; "Forced Sterilization in North Carolina," *ACLU News*, 1973, 3, Records-NARAL Vertical Files.

68. *Cox v. Stanton*, 381 F. Supp. 349 (D.N.C. 1974); *Cox v. Stanton*, 529 F.2d 47 (4th Cir. 1975); Congress, Senate, Committee on Labor and Public Welfare, *Quality of Health Care–Human Experimentation, 1973*, 93rd Cong., 1st sess., July 10, 1973, 1585–1586; Hudson, "Suit Seeks to Void Sterilization Law," 43; Jack Slater, "Sterilization: Newest Threat to the Poor," *Ebony* 28 (October 1973), 150–151; *Cox v. Stanton*, 381 F. Supp. 349 (D.N.C. 1974).

69. Psychological tests taken after Trent learned of her sterilization showed her to be of normal intelligence. ACLU, Reproductive Freedom Project, *Annual Report* (New York: American Civil Liberties Union, 1982), 24, Records-ACLU, box 1924, folder 3.

70. "ACLU News, For Immediate Release, January 21, 1974," American Civil Liberties Union Papers, Records-ACLU, box 1924, folder 3.

71. *Walker v. Pierce*, 560 F.2d 609 (4th Cir. 1977), and *Madrigal v. Quilligan*, as discussed in Gutierrez, "Policing 'Pregnant Pilgrims,'" 392–393; Virginia Espino, "'Woman Sterilized As Gives Birth': Forced Sterilization and Chicana Resistance in the 1970s," in *Las obreras: Chicana Politics of Work and Family*, ed. Vicki Ruíz (Los Angeles: Chicano Studies Research Center Publications, University of California, Los Angeles, 2000), 76; Velez-I, "Se Me Acabo La Cancion," 85–87.

72. Critchlow, *Intended Consequences*, 78–80.

73. Ibid., 72.

74. Family Planning Services and Population Research Act of 1970, Public Law 91–572, 1504 (1970); Critchlow, *Intended Consequences*, 91.

75. Family Planning Services and Population Research Act of 1970.

76. *Relf v. Weinberger*, 372 F. Supp. 1196 (D.D.C. 1974); "Sterilization Guidelines: 22 Months on the Shelf," *Medical World News*, November 9, 1973, 53–61.

77. The policy also prohibited the use of federal funds to advertise family planning. Office of Economic Opportunity, "Policy Regarding Family Planning Activities Under Community Action Programs," March 12, 1965, Records–Population Council Organizational Files, box 116, folder 2133; Sargent Shriver, "Statement of the

U.S. Office of Economic Opportunity, on Family Planning Programs," November 15, 1966, Records-ACLU, box 1144, folder 1; OEO, "Policy Regarding Family Planning Activities Under Community Action Programs," 1; Center for Family Planning Program Development (Planned Parenthood–World Population) and the National Center for Family Planning Services, *Family Planning, Contraception, and Voluntary Sterilization: An Analysis of Laws and Polices in the United States, Each State and Jurisdiction (as of September, 1971)* (Rockville, Md.: U.S. Department of Health, Education, and Welfare, Public Health Service, Health Services Administration, Bureau of Community Health Services, 1974), 27.

78. *OEO Instruction 6130–1*, May 18, 1971, in Congress, Senate, Committee on Labor and Public Welfare, *Quality of Health Care*, 1505–1506.

79. The survey found that 78 percent of respondents wanted to add sterilization services for women, and 81 percent wanted to add sterilization services for men. "Sterilization Guidelines," 54.

80. Letter from George Contis, M.D., to All OEO Community Agency Directors, June 28, 1971, in Congress, Senate, Committee on Labor and Public Welfare, *Quality of Health Care*, 1506, emphasis added.

81. Letter from George Contis, M.D., to All OEO Community Action Directors, November 5, 1971, in Congress, Senate, Committee on Labor and Public Welfare, *Quality of Health Care*, 1507.

82. *OEO Instruction 6130–2, Voluntary Sterilization Services*, in Congress, Senate, Committee on Labor and Public Welfare, *Quality of Health Care*, 1518–1520.

83. Congress, Senate, Committee on Labor and Public Welfare, *Quality of Health Care*, 1578.

84. Ibid., 1518–1536, 1576–1579; Stephen Trombley, *The Right to Reproduce: A History of Coercive Sterilization* (London: Weidenfeld and Nicolson, 1988), 183; Thomas M. Shapiro, *Population Control Politics: Women, Sterilization, and Reproductive Choice* (Philadelphia: Temple University Press, 1985), 115. Cooper's role in the printing of the guidelines remains contested. *A Medical World News* article insisted that Cooper signed the order to print the guidelines but that he could not later account for his signature. But an OEO Office of Program Audit of July 19, 1973, reported that Cooper did not know who authorized the printing and believed the printing to have been premature. "Sterilization Guidelines," 55, 57, 61; OEO Office of Program Audit, July 19, 1973, in Congress, Senate, Committee on Labor and Public Welfare, *Quality of Health Care*, 1573, 1578.

85. "Sterilization Guidelines," 53–61; Congress, Senate, Committee on Labor and Public Welfare, *Quality of Health Care*, 1503, 1509–1513, 1552, 1553–1556, 1572–1584; Bill Kovach, "Guidelines Found on Sterilization," *New York Times*, July 7, 1973; Shapiro, *Population Control Politics*, 115.

86. Congress, Senate, Committee on Labor and Public Welfare, *Quality of Health Care*, 1555–1556; "Sterilization Guidelines," 54.

87. Jeannie I. Rosoff, "Sterilization: The Montgomery Case—and Its Aftermath," *Hastings Center Report* 3 (September 1973): 6.

88. "Sterilization Guidelines," 54.

89. "A Well-Meaning Act," *Newsweek*, July 16, 1973, 31; Slater, "Sterilization," 150.

90. Congress, Senate, Committee on Labor and Public Welfare, *Quality of Health Care*, 1947; Trombley, *Right to Reproduce*, 181.

91. Congress, Senate, Committee on Labor and Public Welfare, *Quality of Health Care*, 1496; Carol Levine, "Depo-Provera and Contraceptive Risk: A Case Study of Values in Conflict," *Hastings Center Report* 9 (October 1979): 8–11; Roberts, *Killing the Black Body*, 93.

92. Congress, Senate, Committee on Labor and Public Welfare, *Quality of Health Care*, 1502; "Well-Meaning Act," 31.

93. B. Drummond Ayres Jr., "Racism, Ethics and Rights at Issue in Sterilization Case," *New York Times*, July 2, 1973.

94. Congress, Senate, Committee on Labor and Public Welfare, *Quality of Health Care*, 1503; Bill Kovach, "Sterilization Consent Not Given, Father Tells Kennedy Panel," *New York Times*, July 11, 1973.

95. Congress, Senate, Committee on Labor and Public Welfare, *Quality of Health Care*, 1502.

96. W. Shockley, "The Relf Tragedy: Berserk Humanism or Benevolent Genocide?" September 18, 1973, 3, Shockley Papers, box A13, folder FSM Master Set 1–18; Congress, Senate, Committee on Labor and Public Welfare, *Quality of Health Care*, 1552. Mary Alice Relf was mentally challenged, which most likely contributed to her inability to comprehend the consequences of her surgery. There is no definitive evidence that her sister was also mentally challenged.

97. Ayres, "Racism, Ethics, and Rights at Issue"; Kovach, "Sterilization Consent Not Given."

98. Ayres, "Racism, Ethics, and Rights at Issue."

99. Congress, Senate, Committee on Labor and Public Welfare, *Quality of Health Care*, 1570.

100. Rosenfeld, Wolfe, and McGarrah, *Health Research Group Study*, 2.

101. Harry Ring, "Doctor Exposes Forced Sterilization," *Militant*, September 5, 1975, 26.

102. Claudia Dreifus, "Sterilizing the Poor," in *Seizing Our Bodies: The Politics of Women's Health*, ed. Claudia Dreifus (New York: Vintage, 1977), 115.

103. Robert Kistler, "Women Pushed into Sterilization, Doctor Charges," *Los Angeles Times*, December 2, 1974.

104. Dreifus, "Sterilizing the Poor," 115.

105. Elena Orozco, quoted in the trial transcript of *Madrigal v. Quilligan*, in Gutiérrez, "Policing 'Pregnant Pilgrims,'" 387.

106. Affidavit of V.A., 2, Records-UCLA.

107. "PF#344–39–01," Ricardo Cruz Católicos por La Raza Papers, California Ethnic and Multicultural Archives, University of California, Santa Barbara, box 15, folder 3 (hereafter cited as Records-UCSB).

108. "PF#347–34–55," Records-UCSB, box 15, folder 3; "PF#321–49–45," Records-UCSB, box 15, folder 3; "PF#349–66–30," Records-UCSB, box 15, folder 3; "Hospital No. 346–40–39," Records-UCSB, box 15, folder 3; "PF#254–22–90," Records-UCSB, box 15, folder 3.

109. "PF#254–22–90," Records-UCSB, box 15, folder 3.

110. Dreifus, "Sterilizing the Poor," 110.

111. Maria Gomez Affidavit, Records-UCLA, box sterilization papers embargoed, folder [ca. January 1975]; "Gomez, Maria. PF#332–75–85," Records-UCLA, box sterilization papers embargoed, folder [ca. January 1975].

112. Maria Hernandez, "L.A. Women Protest Forced Sterilizations," *Militant*, December 20, 1974, 17.

113. Rosenfeld, Wolfe, and McGarrah, *Health Research Group Study*, 3–9.

114. "Exhibit A," Ricardo Cruz Católicos por La Raza Papers, Records-UCSB, box 15, folder 3.

115. "PF#348–93–26," Records-UCSB, box 15, folder 3; "PF#259–6–46," Records-UCSB, box 15, folder 3; "PF#347–34–55," Records-UCSB, box 15, folder 3; "PF#318–37–72,"

Records-UCSB, box 15, folder 3; "PF#320–83–59," Records-UCSB, box 15, folder 3; "PF#122–21–08," Records-UCSB, box 15, folder 3; "PF#349–66–30," Records-UCSB, box 15, folder 3; "PF#349–80–90," Records-UCSB, box 15, folder 3; "PF#254–22–90," Records-UCSB, box 15, folder 3; "PF#318–29–71," Records-UCSB, box 15, folder 3; "PF#249–88–25," Records-UCSB, box 15, folder 3; "PF#349–08–14," Records-UCSB, box 15, folder 3; "PF#342–88–91," Records-UCSB, box 15, folder 3; "PF#344–39–01," Records-UCSB, box 15, folder 3; "PF#331–26–06," Records-UCSB, box 15, folder 3; "PF#307–64–71," Records-UCSB, box 15, folder 3.

116. "PF#259–6–46," Records-UCSB, box 15, folder 3.
117. "PF#348–93–26," Records-UCSB, box 15, folder 3.
118. "PF#305–05–12," Records-UCSB, box 15, folder 3.
119. "PF#351–29–80," Records-UCSB, box 15, folder 3; "PF#245–61–38," Records-UCSB, box 15, folder 3; "PF#249–88–25," Records-UCSB, box 15, folder 3.
120. "PF#305–05–12," Records-UCSB, box 15, folder 3.
121. "PF#334–01–03," Records-UCSB, box 15, folder 3.
122. "PF#331–26–06," Records-UCSB, box 15, folder 3.
123. Ibid.
124. David Rothman, *Strangers at the Bedside: A History of How Law and Bioethics Transformed Medical Decision Making* (New York: Basic Books, 1991), 145–147.
125. Ring, "Doctor Exposes Forced Sterilization," 26.
126. Kistler, "Women Pushed into Sterilization," 26.
127. Dreifus, "Sterilizing the Poor," 113.
128. Ibid.
129. Rosenfeld, Wolfe, and McGarrah, *Health Research Group Study*, 11; Adele Clark, "Subtle Forms of Sterilization Abuse: A Reproductive Rights Analysis," in *Test-Tube Women: What Future for Motherhood*, ed. Rita Arditti et al. (London: Pandora Press, 1984), 193.
130. Rosenfeld, Wolfe, and McGarrah, *Health Research Group Study*, 3, 4, 11.
131. Kisler, "Women Pushed into Sterilization," 26.
132. Lawrence, "Indian Health Service," 1–2, 80.
133. "Shortage of Doctors and Money Poses Serious Indian Health Treat: Nixon Impounds Funds 4 of Last 5 Years," *Liberation News Service* (July 6, 1974), quoted in Sally J. Torpy, "Endangered Species: Native American Women's Struggle for their Reproductive Rights and Racial Identity, 1970s–1990s" (M.A. thesis, University of Nebraska at Omaha, 1998), 49, 62–63.
134. Torpy, "Endangered Species," 46, 51; "Growing Fight against Sterilization of Native Women," *Akwesasne Notes* 11 (Late Winter 1979): 29.
135. "Killing Our Future: Sterilization and Experiments," *Akwesasne Notes* (Early Spring 1977): 4.
136. "Oklahoma: Sterilization of Native Women Charged to I.H.S.," *Akwesasne Notes* 6 (Early Winter 1974): 6.
137. Joan Burnes, "Shocking Sterilization Statistics Surface," *Indian County Today*, August 22, 1994, 8; Torpy, "Endangered Species," 1, 40; Lawrence, "Indian Health Service," 400.
138. [Letter Report Concerning Activities of the Indian Health Service to U.S. Senator James G. Abourezk,] (Washington, D.C.: Government Accounting Office, 1975), 18–26.
139. "Sterilization of Young Native Women Alleged at Indian Hospital—48 Operations in July, 1974 Alone," *Akwesasne Notes* (Early Summer 1974): 22; "Killing Our Future,"

4–6; "Growing Fight against Sterilization of Native Women," 29; "An Interview with Barbara Moore, On Sterilization," *Akwesasne Notes* (Spring 1979): 11–12; Richard Bevilacqua, "Sterilization by Appendectomy," *Boston Herald*, February 23, 1978, Women's Education Center Inc. Records, Northeastern University, Boston, M47, box 13, folder 443 (hereafter cited as Records-WEC); Dee Fairbanks, "Our Children Are Our Wealth," *Akwesasne News*, Records-WEC, M47, box 13, folder 444; Richard M. Harley, "Indian Women Plan to Sue U.S. in Sterilization Case," *Christian Science Monitor*, May 27, 1977; Mark Miller, Judith Miller, and Chris Szechenyi, "Native American Peoples on the Trail of Tears Once More," *America* 139 (December 9, 1978): 422–425; Lawrence, "Indian Health Service," chap. 5; [Letter Report Concerning Activities of the Indian Health Service to U.S. Senator James G. Abourezk], 21–26.

140. "Growing Fight against Sterilization of Native Women," 29.

141. Ibid.

142. Torpy, "Endangered Species," 45.

143. Larson, "And Then There Were None," 61.

144. "Killing Our Future," 4.

145. Patricia A. Moore, "Indian Woman's Suit Starts," *National Catholic Reporter* 15 (January 19, 1979): n.p.; "Native American Woman Challenges Forced Sterilization, Removal of Children," *Liberation News Service* 704 (May 31, 1975): 5.

146. "Native American Woman Challenges Forced Sterilization," 5; Torpy, "Endangered Species," 38; Jean Horan, "Condition: Socio-economic—Treatment; Sterilization," *off our backs* 6 (January 31, 1977), 6.

147. Horan, "Condition," 5, 6; "Native American Woman Challenges Forced Sterilization," 5.

148. Horan, "Condition," 6.

149. "Native American Woman Challenges Forced Sterilization," 5.

150. Bruce E. Johansen, "Forced Sterilizations: Sterilization of Native American Woman Reviewed by Omaha Master's Student," *Ratville Times*, www.ratical.org/ratville/sterilize.html, accessed June 18, 2008.

151. Rothman, *Strangers at the Bedside*, 128–133.

152. Kisler, "Women Pushed into Sterilization," 26.

153. Paul Starr, *The Social Transformation of American Medicine: The Rise of a Sovereign Profession and the Making of a Vast Industry* (New York: Basic Books, 1982), 5, 14; Kisler, "Women Pushed into Sterilization," 26.

154. Dreifus, "Sterilizing the Poor," 106.

Chapter 4 — "Fit" Women Fight Back

1. *Yohn v. Riverview Hospital*, Civil Action No. 1820–71, Verified Complaint, filed December 6, 1971, 4, Records-AVS, box 111, folder Mrs. Anne Yohn v. Riverview and St. Barnabas Hospitals.

2. "Sterilization Subject of Sex Suit," in *Liberties Report: Civil Liberties Union of New Jersey*, December 1971, Records-AVS, box 111, folder Mrs. Anne Yohn v. Riverview and St. Barnabas Hospitals; *Yohn v. Riverview Hospital*, Civil Action No. 1820–71, Verified Complaint, filed December 6, 1971, 4–5.

3. *Yohn v. Riverview Hospital*, Civil Action No. 1820–71, Verified Complaint, filed December 6, 1971, 5. This administrator died before the Yohns filed their suit.

4. Ibid., 6–8.

5. Mary P. Ryan, *Mysteries of Sex: Tracing Men and Women through American History* (Chapel Hill: University of North Carolina Press, 2006), 264.

6. *Yohn v. Riverview Hospital*, Civil Action No. 1820–71, Stipulation of Dismissal, May 1972, Records-AVS, box 111, folder Mrs. Anne Yohn v. Riverview and St. Barnabas Hospitals; Golden Johnson, Esq., to Jeremiah S. Gutman, Esq., Re: *Yohn v. Riverside Hospital, et al.*, September 15, 1972, Records-AVS, box 111, folder Mrs. Anne Yohn v. Riverview and St. Barnabas Hospitals. The hospital is Riverview Hospital, but this memo refers to it as Riverside. As the memo is attached to a court document that lists the hospital as Riverview, I assume this is an error on the part of the author. Doris Fulman, "Sterilization Case Attorney Cites U.S. Court Decision," *Red Bank, New Jersey Register*, December 31, 1971, Records-AVS, box 111, folder Mrs. Anne Yohn v. Riverview and St. Barnabas Hospitals.

7. See, for example, *Hathaway v. Worcester City Hospital*, 475 F.2d 701 (1st Cir. 1973); *McCabe v. Nassau County Medical Center*, 453 F.2d 698 (2nd Cir. 1971); *Ponter v. Ponter*, 125 N.J. Super. 50, 342 A2d 572 (N.J. Super. 1975).

8. Wendy Kline found a similar phenomenon in her research on *Our Bodies, Ourselves*. Wendy Kline, " 'Please Include This in Your Book': Readers Respond to *Our Bodies, Ourselves*," *Bulletin of the History of Medicine* 79 (Spring 2005): 81–110.

9. "80% of Americans Favor V.S."

10. John J. Meister to the Director of San Gabriel Community Hospital, June 29, 1971, 1–2, Records-AVS, box 91, folder Operation Lawsuit; Wood, "Changing Trend in Voluntary Sterilization," 32.

11. "A Compendium of Policies of Legal Actions Pertinent to Female Sterilization," July 1971, in San Gabriel Valley Chapter, ZPG, "Report on Operation Lawsuit," 1–5, July 13, 1971, Records-AVS, box 91, folder Operation Lawsuit; "Hospital Policy Listings: Female Sterilization, Tubal Ligation," 1–3, in San Gabriel Valley Chapter, ZPG, "Report on Operation Lawsuit."

12. "Editorial: Voluntary Sterilization," 573; American Public Health Association, "APHA Recommends Program Guide for Voluntary Sterilization."

13. "Population and the American Future, The Report of the Commission on Population Growth and the American Future, 1972, Excerpts from Chapter 11: Human Reproduction," Records-AVS, box 91, folder ACOG, AMA, APHA, AHA.

14. Anthony J. Ferraro to Jeremiah S. Gutman, Esq., June 16, 1971, Records-AVS, box 111, folder Lawsuits Caffarelli.

15. *Florence E. Caffarelli v. Peekskill Community Hospital*, Plaintiff's Memorandum of Law in Support of Motion for a Preliminary Injunction, 19, Records-AVS, box 111, folder Lawsuits Caffarelli; Kay Etzler, "Sterilization Denial Brings Suit," *Mount Kisco, N.Y., Patent Trader*, April 19, 1971, 2, Records-AVS, box 111, folder Caffarelli.

16. "Editorial: Voluntary Sterilization," 573.

17. AVS, "Operation Lawsuit," 2, Records-AVS, box 91, folder Operation Lawsuit.

18. John de J. Pemberton Jr. to John R. Rague, July 21, 1966, Records-ACLU, box 2023, folder 10.

19. A proposed resolution calling on federal agencies and government-sponsored organizations to provide access to contraceptive services, information, and facilities (including voluntary sterilization and abortion) circulated at the ACLU's biennial conference in 1970, but the board of directors did not approve this resolution until September 29, 1973. Edward J. Ennis to ACLU Affiliates, March 10, 1971, Records-AVS, box 47, folder Ennis, Edward J; "American Civil Liberties Union Board of Directors Meeting, September 29–30, 1973," 3–6, Records-ACLU, box 26, folder 6.

20. Reproductive Freedom Project, ACLU Foundation, *Women's Legal Guide to Reproductive Rights* (New York: Reproductive Freedom Project American Civil

Liberties Foundation, 1981), Records-ACLU, box 1134, folder 1; "Reproductive Freedom Project Proposal 1980," Records-ACLU, box 382, folder 21; ACLU, "The ACLU's Campaign for Choice: The Right of a Woman to Control Her Own Body," Records-ACLU, box 1898, folder 5.

21. "ACLU's Campaign for Choice."

22. Ibid., 1.

23. ACLU, "Liberal Abortion Policies Campaign," August 1973, 3, Joan Dunlop Papers, Rockefeller Archive Center, Sleepy Hollow, N.Y., box 2, no folder (hereafter cited as Dunlop Papers).

24. AVS, "Operation Lawsuit," 2.

25. Memo from C. Hastings to C.T. Faneuff, January 3, 1973, 1–2, Records-AVS, box 91, folder Operation Lawsuit.

26. Evelyn E. Bryant to Senator Anthony C. Beilenson, January 10, 1974, Records-AVS, box 91, folder Operation Lawsuit; Anthony C. Beilenson to Mr. W.D. Schroeder, January 15, 1974, Records-AVS, box 91, folder Operation Lawsuit.

27. San Gabriel Valley Chapter, ZPG, "Report on Operation Lawsuit, Chapter Program," July 13, 1971, 1, Records-AVS, box 91, folder Operation Lawsuit; John J. Meister to Director, San Gabriel Community Hospital, June 29, 1971, Records-AVS, box 91, folder Operation Lawsuit.

28. San Gabriel Valley Chapter, ZPG, "Report on Operation Lawsuit, Chapter Program," 2.

29. See, for example, AVS, "Operation Lawsuit," 2.

30. Memo from Courtland Hastings to Evelyn Bryant and carbon copied to Ira Lubell and Betty Gonzales, December 10, 1973, Records-AVS, Supp. II, box 2, folder Operation Lawsuit.

31. James A. Sweet, "Differentials in the Rate of Fertility Decline," *Family Planning Perspective* 6 (Spring 1974): 104–105.

32. "One-Fifth of U.S. Couples," 113.

33. Center for Disease Control, *Surgical Sterilization Surveillance: Tubal Sterilization, Summary 1970–1975* (Washington, D.C.: U.S. Department of Health, Education, and Welfare, 1979), 12.

34. AVS, "Operation Lawsuit," 3.

35. San Gabriel Valley Chapter, ZPG, "Report on Operation Lawsuit, Chapter Program," 5.

36. "Sterilization Lawsuits Compiled by the Association for Voluntary Sterilization, Inc.," December 20, 1974, Records-AVS, box 91, folder Operation Lawsuit.

37. *Stein v. Northern Westchester Hospital*, Affidavit Janet S. Stein, 3, Records-AVS, box 111, folder Janet S. Stein v. Northern Westchester Hospital, Mt. Kisco, N.Y., CONCLUDED.

38. "Woman Sues Mt. Kisco Hospital After Being Denied Sterilization," *New York Times*, May 12, 1970; *Stein v. Northern Westchester Hospital*, Affidavit Janet S. Stein, 4.

39. *Stein v. Northern Westchester Hospital*, Amended Complaint, 6, Records-AVS, box 111, folder Janet S. Stein v. Northern Westchester Hospital, Mt. Kisco, N.Y., CONCLUDED; "Woman Sues Mt. Kisco Hospital," 49. Abortion boards frequently used a quota system to limit the number of therapeutic procedures they performed. Luker, *Abortion and the Politics of Motherhood*, 57.

40. Deirdre Carmody, "Hospital Shifts on Sterilizations," *New York Times*, July 4, 1970.

41. *Stein v. Northern Westchester Hospital*, Stipulation Index No. 70 Civ. 1904, October 29, 1973, Records-AVS, box 91, folder Operation Lawsuit; "For Immediate Release: Hospital Pays $2,000 Damages to Woman to Whom Sterilization Was Delayed"

(draft), November 21, 1973, Records-AVS, box 91, folder Operation Lawsuit; Jeremiah S. Gutman to Association for Voluntary Sterilization, November 21, 1973, Records-AVS, box 91, folder Operation Lawsuit; Jeremiah S. Gutman to Harold B. Berel, Esq., October 25, 1973, Records-AVS, box 91, folder Operation Lawsuit.

42. *McCabe v. Nassau County Medical Center.*

43. Ibid.

44. Ibid.

45. *Stein v. Northern Westchester Hospital*, Amended Complaint, 8; *Caffarelli v. Peekskill Community Hospital*, Affidavit Florence E. Caffarelli, 2, Records-AVS, box 111, folder Lawsuits Caffarelli.

46. *McCabe v. Nassau County Medical Center.*

47. Cadden, "Very Private Decision," 85.

48. Ibid.

49. Ibid., 148; Walter P. Gage, M.D., "Report of Consultation," Records-AVS, box 91, folder Caffarelli.

50. Cadden, "Very Private Decision," 148.

51. Ibid.

52. Ibid., 85; *Caffarelli v. Peekskill Community Hospital*, Plaintiff's Memorandum of Law in Support of Motion for a Preliminary Injunction, 2, 15–16, 19, 23–24; "The Policy Needs Review," *Mount Kisco, N.Y., Patent Trader*, August 21, 1971, Records-AVS, box 111, folder Caffarelli.

53. *Stein v. Northern Westchester Hospital*, Affidavit Janet S. Stein, 6.

54. Cadden, "Very Private Decision," 148.

55. Ibid., 85, 148; Etzler, "Sterilization Denial Brings Suit," 2.

56. AVS, "Mother of Ten Children Sues Fordham Hospital and the City of New York to Obtain Sterilization Operation Refused Her; Asks $250,000 Damages," For Immediate Release, February 9, 1971, 3, Records-AVS, box 91, folder Operation Lawsuit.

57. Mrs. F.B. to Gentlemen, November 18, 1971, Records-AVS, box 91, folder Operation Lawsuit.

58. *Stein v. Northern Westchester Hospital*, Affidavit Janet S. Stein, 3.

59. Ellen Goodman, "A Suit for Sterilization," *Boston Globe*, July 8, 1973, Records-AVS, box 91, folder Operation Lawsuit.

60. Eltzer, "Sterilization Denial Brings Suit," 1.

61. Donald H. Higgins to John R. Rague, Re: Latest on Caffarelli Case (Peekskill Community Hospital), September 27, 1971, 1, Records-AVS, box 111, folder Lawsuits Caffarelli; *Caffarelli v. Peekskill Community Hospital*, Judgment and Order, January 4, 1972, 1–2, Records-AVS, box 111, folder Caffarelli; Cadden, "Very Private Decision," 150.

62. *Caffarelli v. Peekskill Community Hospital, Yohn v. Riverview and St. Barnabas Hospitals, Ivesaj v. Fordham Hospital* in Memo from C. Hastings to C. T. Fareuff, Sub: Operation Lawsuit–Status, March 20, 1973, 2, Records-AVS, box 91, folder Operation Lawsuit; *Hathaway v. Worcester City Hospital; McCabe v. Nassau County Medical Center*; Mrs. F.B. to Gentleman.

63. John R. Rague to Women's Liberation Leader, May 15, 1970, Records-AVS, box 91, folder Operation Lawsuit; Untitled list of women's organizations, n.d., Records-AVS, box 55, folder Women's Liberation list—1970; Memo from Donald H. Higgins to John R. Rague Re National Conference on Voluntary Sterilization and Women's Rights, September 24, 1971, Records-AVS, box 49, folder First National Conference on Sterilization and Women's Rights; John R. Rague to Joseph E. Davis, M.D., September 27, 1971, Records-AVS, box 49, folder First National Conference on

Sterilization and Women's Rights; "Minutes—Executive Committee Meeting," November 17, 1971, Records-AVS, box 110, folder Minutes 1971.

64. "Landmark Ruling by 2nd Circuit Federal Court of Appeals Makes Hospital Liable for Proven Damages in Arbitrary Refusal of Sterilization Operations for Women Demanding Them," December 23, 1971, 2, Records-AVS, box 111, folder LS/NY *McCabe v. Nassau County.*

65. Ibid.

66. *Hathaway v. Worcester City Hospital.*

67. Goodman, "Suit for Sterilization."

68. Ibid.; *Hathaway v. Worcester City Hospital.*

69. Goodman, "Suit for Sterilization"; *Hathaway v. Worcester City Hospital.*

70. Goodman, "Suit for Sterilization."

71. Ibid.

72. The hospital also rejected petitions for vasectomy submitted by seven physicians. Goodman, "Suit for Sterilization"; Memo from Carol Petrick to Shirley L. Radl, Subj: Progress of Operation Lawsuit, 4, Records-AVS, box 91, folder Operation Lawsuit.

73. Goodman, "Suit for Sterilization."

74. Ibid.

75. Ibid.

76. Nancy Cott, *Public Vows: A History of Marriage and the Nation* (Cambridge, Mass.: Harvard University Press, 2000), 11.

77. Goodman, "Suit for Sterilization."

78. *Doe v. Bolton*, 410 U.S. 179 (1973); Women's Rights Project, ACLU, "Spousal Consent for Voluntary Sterilization," n.d., Dunlop Papers, box 2, no folder; *Hathaway v. Worcester City Hospital.*

79. *Hathaway v. Worcester City Hospital.*

80. *Coe v. Gerstein*, 376 F. Supp (D. Fl. 1973); *Jones v. Smith*, 278 So.2d 339 (Fl. App. 1973); *Planned Parenthood v. Danforth*, 428 U.S. 54 (1976); *Doe v. Doe*, 314 N.E.2d 128 (1974).

81. *Coe v. Gerstein.*

82. *Jones v. Smith.*

83. Women's Right Project, ACLU, "Spousal Consent for Voluntary Sterilization," 12; *Pound v. Pound*, 42 USLW 2456 (Ill. Cir. Ct., January 31, 1974); *Doe v. Doe*, 365 Mass. 556 (1974).

84. *Planned Parenthood v. Danforth.*

85. *Bellotti v. Baird*, 443 U.S. 622 (1979).

86. Quoted in Women's Right Project, ACLU, "Spousal Consent for Voluntary Sterilization," 4.

87. Women's Right Project, ACLU, "Spousal Consent for Voluntary Sterilization," 6–8.

88. *Ponter v. Ponter.*

89. "Woman Takes Hospital to Court for Denying Her Sterilization," *Glouster Times*, November 14, 1972, Records-AVS, box 91, folder Operation Lawsuit.

90. Thomas Wright, "Wayward Husband Can't Be Found, Refuses to Sterilize Mother of Seven," *Forward Times*, Houston, August 2, 1975, n.p., Records-AVS, box 91, folder Operation Lawsuit.

91. Ibid.

92. Ibid.

93. Ibid.

94. *Murray v. VanDevander*, 522 P.2d 302 (OK CIV APP. 1974).

95. Ibid.; J. G. Zimmerly, "Consent to Sterilization: Are We Creating New Problems?" *Journal of Legal Medicine* 3 (February 1975): 2.

96. Affidavit of Elona Gilbert, Records-AVS, box 91, folder ACLU Reproductive Freedom docket.

97. "Judge Sidesteps in Vasectomy Case," *Newsday*, December 20, 1974, Records-AVS, box 91, folder ACLU Reproductive Freedom Project.

98. Ibid.

99. Jeremiah S. Gutman, "Can Hospitals Constitutionally Refuse to Permit Abortions and Sterilizations?" *Family Planning/Population Reporter* 2 (December 1973): 146.

100. Ibid.

101. Ibid., 146–148.

102. "Reaction to the Church Amendment: A Typical Letter," *Association for Voluntary Sterilization* (Summer 1973): 3, Records-AVS, box 91, folder Operation Lawsuit.

103. "American Medical Doctors Attacked by U.S. Senate in 92–1 Vote: Senator Frank Church Spearheads Catholic Hierarchy's Assault on U.S. Supreme Court Voluntary Abortion and Voluntary Sterilization Decisions," For Release May 1, 1973, 2, Records-ACLU, box 1147, folder 1.

104. *Greco v. Orange Memorial Hospital Corporation*, 43 U.S. 1000 (1975), cert denied; *Greco v. Orange Memorial Hospital Corporation*, 513 F.2d 873 (5th Cir. 1975); *Greco v. Orange Memorial Hospital Corporation*, 374 F. Supp. 227 (1974).

105. A few women unaffiliated with Operation Lawsuit filed their own claims against Catholic hospitals. See, for example, Joe Frein, "S.J. Woman's Suit Asks Sterilization," n.p., June 2, 1973, Records-AVS, box 91, folder Operation Lawsuit. The name of the San Jose newspaper that published this article was not listed on the document.

106. *Ham v. Holy Rosary Hospital*, 529 P2d 361 (1974).

107. Ibid.

108. Mrs. F.B. to Gentlemen.

109. *Padin v. Fordham Hospital*, 392 F. Supp. 447 (1975).

110. Ibid.

111. *Chrisman v. St. Josephs of the Peace*, 506 F.2d 308 (9th Cir. 1974); *Taylor v. St. Vincent's Hospital*, 523 F.2d 75 (9th Cir. 1975); *Watkins v. Mercy Medical Center*, 520 F.2d 894 (9th Cir. 1975).

Chapter 5 — "Unfit" Women Fight Too

1. Nadine Brozan, "The Volatile Issue of Sterilization Abuse," *New York Times*, December 2, 1977.

2. Ibid.

3. Ibid.

4. Nelson, "From Abortion Rights to Reproductive Freedom," 94.

5. This group of lawsuits does not include *Stump v. Sparkman* because this case falls outside the bounds of my study. This book examines surgeries performed on "healthy" women, defined as having no disabilities. *Stump v. Sparkman* involved the sterilization of a white fifteen-year-old Indiana girl whose mother deemed her "somewhat retarded," and expressed concern about her daughter's sexual behavior. In 1971, a circuit court judge authorized this girl's sterilization without a hearing and without appointing a guardian *ad litem* for her. The daughter was subsequently sterilized without her knowledge: she believed she had an appendectomy. She later learned the truth about her surgery, which led her and her husband to file suit against the judge who authorized it. *Stump v. Sparkman* (which went all the way to the Supreme Court and concluded with a ruling in the judge's favor) was about judicial immunity, not sterilization policy or sterilization trends. *Stump v. Sparkman*, 435 U.S. 349 (1978); *Stump v. Sparkman*, 552 F.2d 172 (1977).

6. The race of plaintiffs in *Harris v. Karem* is not listed on the ACLU Reproductive Freedom Docket.

7. Http://www.splcenter.org/center/about.jsp, accessed June 27, 2008.

8. *White v. Druid City Hospital*, as described in Lourdes Soto, ed., *Legal Docket, American Civil Liberties Union Foundation, Reproductive Freedom Project* (New York: American Civil Liberties Union, 1983), 156, Records-ACLU, box 388, folder 14.

9. *Johnson v. City of New York* 10784/77 (N.Y. Sup. Ct., Kings Cty., filed 1977), in Soto, *Legal Docket*, 70; "On the Count Docket," *New York Times*, December 9, 1977.

10. Soto, *Legal Docket*, 70.

11. Arizona did not participate in the federal Medicaid program. In Arizona, each individual county could establish its own policy. Soto, *Legal Docket*, 39. The ACLU dockets do not list these plaintiffs' race(s).

12. *Cox v. Stanton*, 381 F. Supp. 349 (D.N.C. 1974); *Cox v. Stanton*, 529 F.2d 47 (4th Cir. 1975); *Cox v. Stanton*, Complaint: Preliminary Statement, Records-NARAL Vertical Files.

13. Http://www.law.cornell.edu/uscode/42/1983.html, accessed June 30, 2008; *Walker v. Pierce*, 560 F.2d 609 (4th Cir. 1977); *Cox v. Stanton*, 381 F. Supp. 349 (D.N.C. 1974).

14. *Relf v. Weinberger*, 372 F. Supp. 1196 (D.D.C. 1974).

15. James Howard Jones, *Bad Blood: The Tuskegee Syphilis Experiment*, rev. ed. (New York: Free Press, 1993); Rothman, *Strangers at the Bedside*, 183; Susan Lederer, "The Tuskegee Syphilis Study in the Context of American Medical Research," in *Tuskegee's Truths: Rethinking the Tuskegee Syphilis Study*, ed. Susan Reverby (Chapel Hill: University of North Carolina Press, 2000), 266–275; Vanessa Northington Gamble, "Under the Shadow of Tuskegee: African Americans and Health Care," in Reverby, *Tuskegee's Truths*, 431–456.

16. Vernon E. Jordan Jr., "Sterilization: A Scandal," *Peabody Times*, July 20, 1973, Records-AVS, box 91, folder Alabama compulsory sterilization of mentally retarded girls.

17. Carmen Fields, "Blacks Major Victims of Medical Experiments," *Boston Globe*, July 17, 1973, Records-AVS, box 91, folder compulsory sterilization of mentally retarded girls.

18. Sharla M. Fett, *Working Cures: Healing, Health, and Power on Southern Slave Plantations* (Chapel Hill: University of North Carolina Press, 2002), 151–152.

19. Susan E. Lederer, *Subjected to Science: Human Experimentation in America before the Second World War* (Baltimore: Johns Hopkins University Press, 1995), xv.

20. Ibid., 13–14, 20–23, 25, 119, 126–127.

21. Ibid., 106.

22. Ibid., 110–111, 113.

23. Rothman, *Strangers at the Bedside*, 74–75.

24. Ibid., 78–81; Lederer, *Subjected to Science*, 140–141; Tone, *Devices and Desires*, 221.

25. Rothman, *Strangers at the Bedside*, 80–81.

26. Jones, *Bad Blood*, 213.

27. Elizabeth Siegel Watkins, *The Estrogen Elixir: A History of Hormone Replacement Therapy in America* (Baltimore: Johns Hopkins University Press, 2007), 26: Rothman, *Strangers at the Bedside*, 185.

28. Sandra Morgen, *Into Our Own Hands: The Women's Health Movement in the United States, 1969–1990* (New Brunswick, N.J.: Rutgers University Press, 2002); Sheryl Burt Ruzek, *The Women's Health Movement: Feminist Alternatives to Medical Control* (New York: Praeger, 1978); Kline, "'Please Include This in Your Book.'"

29. Rothman, *Strangers at the Bedside*, 146.

30. Ibid.

31. Trombley, *Right to Reproduce*, 190.
32. *Walker v. Pierce*, 560 F.2d 609 (4th Cir. 1977); Nancy Hicks, "Sterilization of Black Mother of 3 Stirs Aiken, S.C.," *New York Times*, August 1, 1973; Trombley, *Right to Reproduce*, 189, 190.
33. Trombley, *Right to Reproduce*, 189; Scott Derks, "Sorta Dampens Your Spirits," *Nation*, September 16, 1978, 675; Linda Jenness, "Black Women Fight Sterilization," *Militant*, August 15, 1975, 12; Hicks, "Sterilization of Black Mother," 27.
34. *Walker v. Pierce*, 560 F.2d 609 (4th Cir. 1977).
35. Hicks, "Sterilization of Black Mother," 27; Roberts, *Killing the Black Body*, 92.
36. *Walker v. Pierce*, 560 F.2d 609 (4th Cir. 1977).
37. Ibid.
38. Ibid.
39. Hicks, "Sterilization of Black Mother," 27.
40. "Two Join Suit Seeking Limits on Sterilization," *Washington Star News*, August 14, 1973, Records-AVS, box 91, folder Alabama compulsory sterilization of mentally retarded girls.
41. Http://dictionary.law.com/default2.asp?selected=1332&bold=｜｜｜｜, accessed June 27, 2008; http://www.businessdictionary.com/definition/nominal-damages.html, accessed June 27, 2008.
42. Reproductive Freedom Project, ACLU Foundation, "Legal Docket, August 13, 1978," 91, Records-ACLU, box 387, folder 4; *Walker v. Pierce*, 560 F.2d 609 (4th Cir. 1977); *Walker v. Pierce*, 434 U.S. 1075 (1978), cert. denied.
43. *Walker v. Pierce*, 560 F.2d 609 (4th Cir. 1977).
44. Ibid.
45. Ibid.
46. Ibid.
47. Ibid.
48. Ibid.
49. Trombley, *Right to Reproduce*, 189–191.
50. Antonia Hernandez, "Chicanas and the Issue of Involuntary Sterilization: Reforms Needed to Protect Informed Consent," *Chicano Law Review* 3, no. 3 (1976): 9.
51. *Madrigal v. Quilligan*, No. CV 75–2057-EAC, Vol. 1, Deposition of Edward James Quilligan, 37–39, Records-UCLA, box embargoed, folder transcript of defendant's statement D. M.V.Q.
52. Ibid., 13–14; *Madrigal v. Quilligan*, No. CV 715–2057-EC, Finding of Fact and Conclusions of Law, 9–21, Records-UCLA, box 4, folder 27.
53. *Madrigal v. Quilligan*, No. CV 74–2057-JWC, Reporter's Transcript of Proceedings, Tuesday, May 30, 1978, 12, Records-UCLA, box 7, folder 1.
54. Gutiérrez, "Policing 'Pregnant Pilgrims,'" 391; Espino, "Women Sterilized as Gives Birth," 75.
55. Joseph J. Levin to Charles Nabarette, October 9, 1972, Re: California Sterilization Cases, Records-UCSB, box 15, folder 4; *Madrigal v. Quilligan*, No. CV 75–2057-EC, Findings of Fact and Conclusions of Law, 1, Records-UCLA, box 4, folder 27.
56. *Madrigal v. Quilligan*, No. CV 94–2057-JWC, Reporter's Transcript of Proceedings, Wednesday, June 7, 1978, and Thursday, June 8, 1978, 789–790, Records-UCLA, box 2, folder 7.
57. *Madrigal v. Quilligan*, No. CV 74–2057-JWC, Reporter's Transcript of Proceedings, Tuesday, May 30, 1978, 27–29, Records-UCLA, box 7, folder 1; Velez-I, "Se Me Acabo La Cancion," 85–86.

58. *Madrigal v. Quilligan*, No. CV 74-2057-JWC, Reporter's Transcript of Proceedings, Wednesday, June 7, 1978, and Thursday, June 8, 1978, 796–797.

59. "Deposition of Dr. Karen Benker," 58–59, quoted in Gutiérrez, "Racial Politics of Reproduction," 205.

60. *Madrigal v. Quilligan*, No. CV 74-2057-JWC, Reporter's Transcript of Proceedings, Wednesday, June 7, 1978, and Thursday, June 8, 1978, 823–825, 827, emphasis added; Velez-I, "Se Me Acabo La Cancion," 85.

61. Hernandez, "Chicanas and the Issue of Involuntary Sterilization," 5–9.

62. *Madrigal v. Quilligan*, No. CV 74-2057-JWC, Reporter's Transcript of Proceedings, Wednesday, June 7, 1978, and Thursday, June 8, 1978, 841-A, 852.

63. Ibid., 841-B, 843.

64. Ibid., 856–858.

65. Affidavit of Delia Gonzales, September 17, 1974, Records-UCLA, box embargoed, folder September 17, 1974, notarized statement of sterilization.

66. Karen E. Benker, "Statement on Sterilization Abuse," 3, quoted in Gutiérrez, "Racial Politics of Reproduction," 201.

67. Velez-I, "Se Me Acabo La Cancion," 211.

68. Ibid., 79.

69. Ibid., 81.

70. Ibid.

71. Terry A. Kupers, "10 Lose Their Fertility—and Their Case," *Los Angeles Times*, September 28, 1978, Records-UCLA, box 5, folder 16; *Madrigal v. Quilligan*, No. CV 74–2057-JWC, Reporter's Transcript of Proceedings, Friday, June 9, 1973, 1083–1134, Records-UCLA, box 20, folder 1.

72. Velez-I, "Se Me Acabo La Cancion," 81.

73. Dreifus, "Sterilizing the Poor," 109.

74. Ibid., 107.

75. *Madrigal v. Quilligan*, No. CV 75–2057-EAC, Order Dismissing Action as against Defendants E. J. Quilligan, M.D., and Roger K. Freeman, M.D., Records-UCLA, box embargoed, folder [ca. May 1978]; *Madrigal v. Quilligan*, No. CV 75–2057-JWC, Opinion, 2, Records-UCLA, box embargoed, folder [ca. May 1978].

76. *Madrigal v. Quilligan*, No. CV 75–2057-JWC, Opinion, 3, Records-UCLA, box embargoed, folder [ca. May 1978].

77. *Madrigal v. Quilligan*, No. CV 75–2057-JWC, Opinion, 11, Records-UCLA, box embargoed, folder [ca. May 1978].

78. Ibid., 19.

79. *Madrigal v. Quilligan*, No. CV 75–2057-JWC, Opinion, 19, Records-UCLA, box embargoed, folder [ca. 1978] transcript of judge's opinion on case.

80. Congress, Senate, Committee on Labor and Public Welfare, *Quality of Health Care*, 1607–1610.

81. Bill Kovach, "14 Organizations Urge the Government to Stop Providing Funds for Sterilization of Minors," *New York Times*, July 10, 1973.

82. Premilla Nadasen, "Expanding the Boundaries of the Women's Movement: Black Feminism and the Struggle for Welfare Rights," *Feminist Studies* (Summer 2002): 277. Nadasen estimates that remainder of the membership was 10 percent white, 5 percent Latina, and a few Native Americans.

83. Ibid., 274, 295.

84. Ibid., 279; Deborah Gray White, *Too Heavy a Load: Black Women in Defense of Themselves, 1884–1994* (New York: W. W. Norton, 1999), 228.

85. Anne M. Valk, " 'Mother Power': The Movement for Welfare Rights in Washington D.C., 1966–1972," *Journal of Women's History* 11 (January 2000): 34.

86. Nadasen, "Expanding the Boundaries," 283.

87. Doris Bland, quoted in *NOW News*, February 2, 1968, quoted in White, *Too Heavy a Load*, 237.

88. Association for Voluntary Sterilization Inc., National Welfare and Rights Organization Inc., "Joint Statement Against Forced Sterilization," July 18, 1973, Records-AVS, box 91, folder Alabama compulsory sterilization of retarded girls.

89. John R. Rague to Brenda Fasteau, May 26, 1972, Records-AVS, box 47, folder American Civil Liberties Union Correspondence, 1965–1972.

90. Congress, House, Subcommittee on Public Health and the Environment of the Committee on Interstate and Foreign Commerce, *Biomedical Research Ethics and the Protection of Human Subjects*, 93rd Cong., 1st sess., September 27, 1973, 93.

91. Bill Kovach, "H.E.W. Head Curbs Sterilization Aid," *New York Times*, July 6, 1973.

92. May, *Barren in the Promised Land*, 121; Lee, *For Freedom's Sake*, 80.

93. Nadasen, "Expanding the Boundaries," 273.

94. Nelson, "From Abortion Rights to Reproductive Freedom," 88–112; White, *Too Heavy a Load*, 216–223; Tracye A. Matthews, " 'No One Ever Asks What a Man's Role in the Revolution Is': Gender Politics and Leadership in the Black Panther Party, 1966–71," in *Sisters in the Struggle: African American Women in the Civil-Rights–Black Power Movement*, ed. Bettye Collier-Thomas and V. P. Franklin (New York: New York University Press, 2001), 237–238.

95. Combahee River Collective, "A Black Feminist Statement," in *Words of Fire: An Anthology of African-American Feminist Thought*, ed. Beverly Guy-Sheftall (New York: New Press, 1995), 234.

96. Toni Cade Bambara, "The Pill: Genocide or Liberation?" in *The Black Woman: An Anthology*, ed. Toni Cade Bambara (New York: Mentor, 1970), 166.

97. Nelson, *Women of Color*, 77–79.

98. "Third World Sisters," *Militant*, July 30, 1971, 21, quoted in Nelson, "From Abortion Rights to Reproductive Freedom," 75.

99. Frances Beale, "Double Jeopardy: To Be Black and Female," in Cade Bambara, *Black Woman: An Anthology*, 97.

100. Nelson, *Women of Color*, 97, 100.

101. Ibid., 108.

102. Ibid., 107.

103. Ibid., 109.

104. 38 FR 20930, *Sterilization Guidelines: Departmental Policy*, August 3, 1973; 39 FR 4730, *Sterilization Restrictions*, February 6, 1974; *Relf v. Weinberger*, 372 F. Supp. 1196 (D.D.C. 1974).

105. *Relf v. Weinberger*, 372 F. Supp. 1196 (D.D.C. 1974); Trombley, *Right to Reproduce*, 182.

106. "Two Join Suit Seeking Limits on Sterilization"; *Relf v. Weinberger*, 372 F. Supp. 1196 (D.D.C. 1974).

107. *Relf v. Weinberger*, 372 F. Supp. 1196 (D.D.C. 1974).

108. Ibid.

109. Ibid.

110. Ibid.

111. Ibid.; Rosenfeld, Wolfe, and McGarrah, *Health Research Group Study*.

112. Congress, Senate, *Quality of Health Care—Human Experimentation*, 1515.

113. Ibid., 1511.
114. Nelson, "From Abortion Rights to Reproductive Freedom," 16–17; *Relf v. Weinberger*, 372 F. Supp. 1196 (D.D.C. 1974).
115. *Relf v. Weinberger*, 372 F. Supp. 1196 (D.D.C. 1974).
116. Ibid.
117. *Relf v. Mathews*, 403 F. Supp. 1235 (D.D.C. 1975).
118. Ibid.; *Relf v. Weinberger*, 184 U.S. App. D.C. 147 (D.C. Cir. 1977).

Chapter 6 — Irreconcilable Conflicts

1. CESA, "Structure of Health Care Institutions," n.d., 4, National Women's Health Network (NWHN), Washington, D.C., box 2, folder sterilization abuse 1974–1977 (hereafter cited as Records-NWHN); Shapiro, *Population Control Politics*, 143; Nelson, *Women of Color*, 140.
2. NWHN, "Sterilization Abuse: What It Is and How It Can Be Controlled," 30–31, Records-NWHN, box 2, no folder; CESA, "Structure of Health Care Institutions," 5; Shapiro, *Population Control Politics*, 144.
3. NWHN, "Sterilization Abuse," 30; Shapiro, *Population Control Politics*, 150; Nelson, *Women of Color*, 141; CESA, "Sterilization: What You Need to Know before Making a Decision," 2, Records-WEC, box 13, folder 444.
4. Nelson, *Women of Color*, 141; Shapiro, *Population Control Politics*, 143.
5. CESA, "Statement of Purpose," Records-WEC, box 10, folder 324.
6. Nelson, *Women of Color*, 141–142.
7. NWHN, "Sterilization Abuse," 25–26; Shapiro, *Population Control Politics*, 138; Nelson, *Women of Color*, 142.
8. NWHN, "Sterilization Abuse," 3.
9. Ibid., 5; Advisory Committee on Sterilization, "Why Sterilization Guidelines Are Needed," 5, Records-NWHN, box 2, folder sterilization abuse, 1974–1977.
10. Advisory Committee on Sterilization, "Why Sterilization Guidelines Are Needed," 6–7.
11. NWHN, "Sterilization Abuse," 27; R2N2, "The Need for Regulations, DRAFT," 5, Records-NWHN, box 2, folder sterilization abuse 1974–1977.
12. Shapiro, *Population Control Politics*, 140; R2N2, "Need for Regulations," 4.
13. NWHN, "Sterilization Abuse," 27, 28; New York City Health and Hospitals Corporation, "Guidelines for Female Elective Sterilization," Effective November 1, 1975, Records-ACLU, box 1147, folder 10; Shapiro, *Population Control Politics*, 140.
14. "Suit Challenges Curbs on Sterilization of Women," *New York Times*, January 11, 1976; NWHN, "Sterilization Abuse," 28.
15. "Suit Challenges Curb on Sterilization of Women," 22; Maritza Arrastia, "A Suit against the People," *Claridad*, January 18, 1976, reprinted by the Committee to End Sterilization Abuse, Records-NWHN, box 2, folder sterilization abuse 1974–1977; NWHN, "Sterilization Abuse," 28; Helen Rodriguez-Trias, *Women and the Health Care System: Sterilization Abuse: Two Lectures* (New York: Barnard College, 1970), 21–22; Irwin H. Kaiser, "Against Sterilization Policy Here," *New York Times*, January 12, 1976; "Suit Challenges Curbs on Sterilization of Women," 22; John Elliot, "New York Law Found Failing to Protect Rights of Patient," *Medical Tribune*, August 10, 1977, Records-NWHN, box 2, folder sterilization abuse 1974–1977.
16. Kaiser, "Against Sterilization Policy Here," 26.
17. AVS, "Minutes—Executive Committee Meeting," February 25, 1976, Records-AVS, box 110, folder minutes 1976; CESA, "Structure of Health Care Institutions, 6; Kaiser, "Against Sterilization Policy Here," 26.

18. Elliot, "New York Law Found Failing."

19. "Suit Challenges Curbs on Sterilization of Women," 22.

20. Kaiser, "Against Sterilization Policy Here," 26.

21. Nelson, *Women of Color*, 143; CESA, "Structure of Health Care Institutions," 10.

22. CESA, "Structure of Health Care Institutions," 9.

23. Arrastia, "Suit against the People"; CESA, "Structure of Health Care Institutions," 9; NWHN, "Sterilization Abuse," 28.

24. Shapiro, *Population Control Politics*, 140–141; CESA, "Turning Point in the Struggle to Stop Sterilization Abuse," 4, Records-WEC, box 10, folder 324; Council of the City of New York, Int. No. 1105-A, January 25, 1977, Records-WEC, M471, box 10, folder 324; "New York City Health Dept. Opposes Measure on Sterilization Control," *New York Times*, March 25, 1977.

25. Shapiro, *Population Control Politics*, 142; Nelson, *Women of Color*, 143.

26. Shapiro, *Population Control Politics*, 142.

27. Memo to File, cc: HFP, FSN, EWP, JMBr, Re: PPNYC–Carter Burden Litigation, From: LRR, Date: June 27, 1977, 2, 3, 5, 6, 7, 8, Harriet Pilpel Papers, Sophia Smith Collection, Smith College, Northampton, Mass., box 2, no folder (hereafter cited as Pilpel Papers).

28. Planned Parenthood of New York City, Inc. to Honorable Abraham D. Beame, May 13, 1977, Planned Parenthood Federation of America Records II, Sophia Smith Collection, Smith College, box 38, folder 16 (hereafter cited as Records-PPFA II.)

29. Shapiro, *Population Control Politics*, 153.

30. Meredith Tax, "NOW vs. Sterilization Guidelines," *CARASA News* 2 (November 2, 1978), 3.

31. Karen Stamm and Suzanne Williamson, "The Sterilization Connection," *CARASA News* 3 (March 22, 1979), 22; Karen Stamm, "Update from 'The Sterilization Connection,'" *CARASA News* 3 (April 17, 1979), 11, 19; Shapiro, *Population Control Politics*, 153–154; Planned Parenthood Federation of America, Religious Affairs Committee Meeting, May 25, 1977, 1, Records-PPFA II, box 38, folder 16; "Minilaparotomy Recommended for Most Programs: Simpler and Safer Than Laparoscopic Sterilization," *International Family Planning Digest* 3 (September 1977): 12; McCann and Cole, "Laparoscopy and Minilaparotomy."

32. "Sterilization Loan Program Launched," April 1977, Records-PPFA II, box 67, folder 177. A CESA memo reports the loan fund to be $750,000. See "Report on Phone Conversation with Francine Stein, Administrator, Surgical Services, Loan and Technical Assistance Program IPPF; early July, 1977 with Sandra Sullaway," private papers of Pat Rush, in author's possession; Memo from Francine S. Stein to James J. Marren re: Status of AVS/PPFA Loan and Technical Assistance Program for Budget and Finance Committee Meeting, January 27, 1978, 1, Records-PPFA II, box 67, folder 183; Ruthann Evanoff, "Update from New York City CESA," *CESA News* (March 1978), 5, Records-WEC, box 10, folder 326.

33. Shapiro, *Population Control Politics*, 141–142; CESA, "Structure of Health Care Institutions," 10; CESA, "Organizations and Individuals Endorsing 1105 and Organizations Endorsing Protective Guidelines for Sterilization," Records-WEC, box 10, folder 324.

34. Evanoff, "Update from New York City CESA," 5; Marsha King to CESA, Records-WEC, box 10, folder 321; Endorsements of the "Statement by the Boston Committee to End Sterilization Abuse," Records-WEC, box 10, folder 323.

35. Nelson, *Women of Color*, 19; Meredith Tax, "Fighting Back: A Brief History of CARASA," *CARASA News* 3 (November 1979), 21, 24.

36. Nelson, *Women of Color*, 145.
37. Shapiro, *Population Control Politics*, 154.
38. Karen Stamm, "News," *CARASA News* 2 (April 1978), 13.
39. Rebecca Stanton, "CARASA: Victories and Goals," *CARASA News* 2 (April 6, 1978), 3.
40. "Nadler Bill Debuts in Assembly Health Committee," *CARASA News* 4 (June 1980), 4; "CARASA Action in Review," *CARASA News* 4 (July/August 1980), 5; Kaiser, "Against Sterilization Policy Here," 26.
41. NWHN, "Sterilization Abuse," 32; Shapiro, *Population Control Politics*, 35; "Sterilization Regulations," *CARASA News* 3 (July/August 1979) 5, 7; Ann Teicher and Sue Ritz, "Campaign against Sterilization Abuse," *CARASA News* 3 (July/August 1979), 6–7; Nelson, "From Abortion Rights to Reproductive Freedom," 219–225, 227.
42. Women Against Sterilization Abuse, "For Immediate Release," August 11, 1977, Records-WEC, box 10, folder 326; CESA Western Massachusetts, "Regional Report: Western Massachusetts," 1, 2, 6, Records-WEC, box 10, folder 375; "Chicago CESA," *CESA–Chicago Chapter*, n.d., private papers of Katherine Mallin, in author's possession; Marcy Grant to Katherine Mallin, June 8, 1978, private papers of Katherine Mallin.
43. Paul Wagman, "U.S. Goal: Sterilize Millions of the World's Women," *St. Louis Post Dispatch*, April 22, 1977; CESA, "Documentation for the Ejection of the PIEGO Program from Washington University Medical School," May 1976, Records-WEC, box 11, folder 413; CESA, "Sterilization Abuse Happens Here Or: How Wash. U Contributes to Population Control," Records-WEC, box 11, folder 413.
44. Gutiérrez, "Racial Politics of Reproduction," 254–256.
45. Velez-I, "Se Me Acabo La Cancion," 85; Espino, "Woman Sterilized as Gives Birth," 70, 75.
46. Dreifus, "Sterilizing the Poor," 119.
47. Coalition for the Medical Rights of Women, "Regulations of Informed Consent," January 8, 1977, Records-WEC, box 13, folder 443; "Groups Working in the Ad Hoc Committee," Records-WEC, box 13, folder 443.
48. Coalition for the Medical Rights of Women, "Regulations on Informed Consent for Sterilization"; *California Medical Association v. Lackner*, 124 Cal. App. 3d 28 (1981); "Sterilization Victory!" *Coalition News* (April 1976), 1, Barbara Seaman Papers, Schlesinger Library, Radcliffe College, Cambridge, Mass., box 3, folder 146 (hereafter cited as Seaman Papers); Committee to Defend Reproductive Rights of the Coalition for the Medical Rights of Women to Beverlee A. Myers, Director, Department of Health Services Re: Proposed Changes in Title 22 Division 5 of the California Administrative Code pertaining to Sterilization and Hysterectomy, August 5, 1982, 4, Records-NWHN, box 2, no folder; Sterilization Abuse and Informed Consent Rights Research, Education, and Organizing Project, "Call to Action," January 8, 1977, 1, Records-WEC, box 13, folder 443.
49. Sterilization Abuse and Informed Consent Rights Research, Education, and Organizing Project, "Call to Action," 8; Coalition for the Medical Rights of Women, "Public Hearings on Sterilization Regulations," Records-WEC, box 13, folder 443; Deanne Bunce, "Update on Sterilization Regs," *Coalition News* (August 1977), 4, Charles Deering McCormick Library of Special Collections at Northwestern University, Evanston, Ill.
50. CESA, "Turning Point in the Struggle," 4.
51. Allan Chase, "Counseling Curbs Unwise Sterilization," *Medical Tribune*, September 28, 1977, Records-NWHN, box 2, folder sterilization abuse 1974–1977.
52. *California Medical Association v. Lackner*.

53. Mary Foran, "Where Are the Sterilization Regs Now?" *Coalition News* (October 1977), 1, Records-NWHN, box 2, no folder; *California Medical Association v. Lackner.*
54. *California Medical Association v. Lackner.*
55. R2N2, "Need for Regulations," 7.
56. Ibid.; "State Tells New Sterilization Rules," *Los Angeles Times,* January 16, 1980, Records-NWHN, box 2, folder sterilization abuse 1978–1982; Committee to Defend Reproductive Rights, "Testimony at Public Hearing Re Repeal of State Informed Consent Regulations Governing Sterilization," June 10, 1980, 1, private papers of Pat Rush.
57. Roberta Young and Alice Wolfson to Beverlee Myers, January 21, 1980, Records-NWHN, box 2, folder sterilization abuse 1978–1982, capital in original.
58. Coalition for the Medical Rights of Women, "Rebuttal," 1, 1980, private papers of Pat Rush.
59. Shapiro, *Population Control Politics,* 147; Kathryn Bonfiglio and Ginny Gordon memo to CESA Chapters RE: Regional Conference on Coordinating Anti-Sterilization Abuse Work, March 24, 1978, Records-WEC, box 10, folder 326; Untitled document with update on regional work, Records-WEC, box 10, folder 326; "Statement by Joseph A. Califano, Jr., Secretary of Health, Education and Welfare," *HEW NEWS,* For Immediate Release, Thursday, December 1, 1977, 2–5, Records-WEC, box 11, folder 412.
60. "Statement by Joseph A. Califano, Jr."; 42 FR 6218, *Proposed Restrictions Applicable to Sterilizations Funded by the Department of Health, Education, and Welfare,* December 13, 1977.
61. "Statement by Joseph A. Califano, Jr.," 15–16; Schedule of Regional Hearings, 3, December 21, 1977, Records-WEC, box 11, folder 412; Belita Cowan, Ann Sablosky, Helen Quick, Carol Kolsky, and Mary Fillmore, To Sisters and Colleagues, January 22, 1977, Records-NWHN, box 2, folder network action/letters '77–'80; *HEW News,* For Immediate Release, January 3, 1978, 1, Records-NARAL, box 3, folder sterilization regulations; "Testimony of Native American Solidarity Committee on Proposed Restrictions Applicable to Sterilizations Funded by the Department of Health, Education and Welfare, Delivered by Rita Toll," February 22, 1978, Boston, 1, Records-WEC, box 11, folder 412; Lawrence, "Indian Health Service," 1–2, 80.
62. Adisa Douglas, "Report on the National Conference on Sterilization Abuse, Sponsored by the Interreligious Foundation for Community Organization, as Presented to the Governing Board of the National Council of Churches of Christ in the U.S.A.," November 10, 1977, Records-WEC, box 10, folder 321; Shapiro, *Population Control Politics,* 137.
63. "Comments of the Boston Women's Health Book Collective Regarding the Proposed Rules Governing Federally Funded Sterilizations, Boston Hearings," February 10, 1978, 2, Records-WEC, box 11, folder 412.
64. Karen Mulhauser, "Testimony before Department of Health, Education and Welfare for Public Hearings on Proposed Sterilization Regulations," January 17, 1978, 2, Records-NARAL, box 3, folder sterilization regulations.
65. Tax, "NOW vs. Sterilization Guidelines," 3; Carole Anne Douglas and Janis Kelly, "N.O.W. National Conference," *off our backs* 8 (November 30, 1978), 7; Mulhauser, "Testimony before Department of Health, Education and Welfare," 1.
66. Mulhauser, "Testimony before Department of Health, Education and Welfare," 4; Douglas and Kelly, "N.O.W. National Conference," 7.
67. Meredith Tax, "NOW Resolution," *CARASA News* 2 (November 2, 1978), 2.
68. Chase, "Counseling Curbs Unwise Sterilization"; NWHN, "Why Sterilization Guidelines Are Needed," 4; Elissa Krauss, "Hospital Survey on Sterilization Policies, March 1975," 4, 21, Records-ACLU, box 1898, folder 5.

69. Bogue and Sigelman, *Sterilization Report*, 2.
70. Tax, "NOW vs. Sterilization Guidelines," 3; Douglas and Kelly, "N.O.W. National Conference," 7; Letter to Pamela Horowitz, Esq., October 4, 1978, 1, Records-NWHN, box 2, folder network action/letters '77-'80.
71. Tax, "NOW vs. Sterilization Guidelines," 3; Letter to Pamela Horowitz, 1.
72. Tax, "NOW vs. Sterilization Guidelines," 1.
73. National Commission for the Protection of Human Subjects, "Comment of the National Commission for the Protection of Human Subjects on Proposed Rulemaking Governing Sterilizations Funded by DHEW," March 29, 1978, 3, 8–9, Records-NARAL, box 3, folder sterilization regulations.
74. Rosenbaum, "H.E.W. to Issue New Regulations to Prevent Forced Sterilizations," A20; Joann Ellison Rodgers, "Sterilization: Playing the Waiting Game," *Mademoiselle* (August 1978), 114, Boston Women's Health Book Collective Records, Schlesinger Library, Radcliffe College, Cambridge, Mass., box 7, folder reproductive rights items (hereafter cited as Records-BWHBC.)
75. "A.V.S. Supports Intent of D.H.E.W. Regulations on Voluntary Sterilization," For Release, November 7, 1978, 3, Pilpel Papers.
76. "NMA Supports a 72-Hour Delay from Consent to Sterilization," *Family Practice News* (October 1977), Records-NWHN, box 2, folder sterilization abuse 1974–1977.
77. "Testimony of Sidney M. Wolfe and Ted Bogue, Public Citizen's Health Research Group before HEW Hearings on Proposed Restrictions on Sterilization," January 17, 1978, Records-NWHN, box 2, folder sterilization federal regulations-70s; "Statement of Sidney M. Wolfe, Public Citizen's Health Research Group on Proposed HEW Regulations for Federally Funded Sterilization," November 30, 1977, Records-NWHN, box 2, folder sterilization federal regulations-70s.
78. "Rothchild on Guidelines," 6, Records-NWHN, box 2, no folder; 43 FR 52146, *Sterilizations and Abortions: Federal Financial Participation*, November 8, 1978. The HHS did amend the rules slightly. It liberalized its ban on all contraceptive hysterectomies to allow for two exceptions: physicians were no longer required to inform patients of the consequences of hysterectomy if patients were already sterile or if patients underwent surgery in a life-threatening situation. 46 FR 5003, *Requirements Applicable to Sterilization (Hysterectomies)*, January 19, 1981.
79. Rothman, *Strangers at the Bedside*, 247–251.
80. CESA, "Local Monitoring Project Report," May 1978–April 1979, 1, 3–4, Records-NWHN, box 2, folder sterilization abuse 1978–1982.
81. Bogue and Sigelman, *Sterilization Report*; Sigelman, *Health Research Group Number 4*, 1, 3.
82. Howie Kurtz, "Sterilization Abuse Discovered in Nine States," *Reproductive Rights Newsletter* (Spring 1981), 8.
83. Bogue and Sigelman, *Sterilization Report*, 8, emphasis added.
84. David M. Priver, M.D., "Letter to Tribune," *Medical Tribune*, April 12, 1978, 11.
85. Howie Kurtz, "Some Doctors Are Critical of Sterilization Guidelines," *Washington Star*, June 22, 1980, Records-NWHN, box 2, folder sterilization abuse 1978–1982.
86. Howie Kurtz, "Sterilization Widespread in Maryland," *Washington Star*, June 22, 1980, Records-NWHN, box 2, folder sterilization abuse 1978–1982.
87. Ibid.
88. Ibid.
89. Bogue and Sigelman, *Sterilization Report*, 10.
90. CESA, "Local Monitoring Project Report," 1.

91. The original amendment, passed in 1976, provided federal funding of abortion only in instances in which continuing a pregnancy threatened the woman's life. In 1977 and 1978, Congress passed less restrictive bills that funded abortions when pregnancy endangered the mother's life and in cases of rape or incest. Stephen L. Isaacs, "The Law of Fertility Regulation in the United States: A 1980 Review," *Journal of Family Law* 19 (November 1980): 73; National Lawyers Guild New York Anti-Sexism Committee, *Reproductive Freedom: Speakers Handbook on Abortion Rights and Sterilization Abuse* (New York: National Lawyers Guild New York Anti-Sexism Committee, 1979), 9–11; Binion, "Reproductive Freedom and the Constitution," 15–16; *Beal v. Doe*, 32 U.S. 438; 97 S. Ct. 2366 (1977); *Maher v. Roe*, 432 U.S. 464; 97 S. Ct. 2376 (1977); *Poelker v. Doe*, 432 U.S. 519; 97 S. Ct. 2391 (1977).

92. Mulhauser, "Testimony before Department of Health, Education and Welfare," 1.

93. Low Income Family Aid, "HEW Hearing on Proposed Sterilization Guidelines," February 22, 1978, 3, Records-WEC, box 11, folder 412; "Testimony of the Puerto Rico Solidarity Committee," 3, Records-WEC, box 11, folder 412; Sarah Grusky, "Testimony on Proposed H.E.W. Sterilization Guidelines," February 7, 1978, 4, Records-WEC, box 11, folder 412; Shauna L. Heckert, "Chico Feminist Women's Health Center, DHEW Testimony," 3, box 11, folder 412, Records-WEC; "Testimony of Native American Solidarity Committee," 11; "Testimony of Alice Rothchild, M.D.," on Public Hearings on Proposed HEW Sterilization Regulations, 3, Records-NWHN, box 2, folder sterilization federal regulations 70s.

94. CARASA, *Women Under Attack: Abortion, Sterilization Abuse, and Reproductive Freedom* (New York: CARASA, 1979), 49, 51–52.

95. Low Income Family Aid, "HEW Hearings on Proposed Sterilization Guidelines," 3.

96. "Sterilization Study Confirms the Worst: Reprinted from the Newsletter of the Committee to Defend Reproductive Rights in San Francisco," *CARASA News* 7 (March/April 1983), 13, 17.

97. CARASA, "Principles of Unity," *CARASA News* 4 (January 1980), 3; "R2N2 Principles of Unity," *Reproductive Rights Newsletter* (Summer 1981), 25.

98. Nelson, "From Abortion Rights to Reproductive Freedom," 254–272; "1979 CARASA Conference Speeches: Perspectives for the Future," *CARASA News* 3 (March 22, 1979), 10; Nelson, *Women of Color*, 158, 171.

Chapter 7 — The Endurance of Neo-eugenics

1. Richard Lewis, "OCAW v. American Cyanamid: The Shrinking of the Occupational Health and Safety Act," *University of Pennsylvania Law Review* 133 (1985): 1177; Fran Moira, "Sterilization: Continued Abuse," *off our backs* 10 (November 30, 1980), 7; "Employees Allege Cyanamid Pressured for Sterilization," *Wall Street Journal*, January 3, 1979; Rosalind Pollack Petchesky, *Abortion and Woman's Choice: The State, Sexuality, and Reproductive Freedom* (Boston: Northeastern University Press, 1990), 345; Judith A. Scott, "Keeping Women in Their Place: Exclusionary Policies and Reproduction," in *Double Exposure: Women's Heath Hazards on the Job and at Home*, ed. Wendy Chavkin (New York: Monthly Review Press, 1984), 180.

2. "ACLU Charges Forced Sterilization of Women," *WomenWise* 3 (July 30, 1980), 10; Scott, "Keeping Women in Their Place," 181.

3. *Roe v. Wade*, 410 U.S. 113 (1973).

4. Wendy Chavkin, "Occupational Hazards to Reproduction: A Review Essay and Annotated Bibliography," *Feminist Studies* 5, no. 2 (Summer 1979): 313; "Industrial Sterility," *Newsweek*, August 29, 1977, 60.

5. Chavkin, "Occupational Hazards to Reproduction," 313–314.

6. Solinger, *Wake Up Little Susie*, 42; Levenstein, "Gendered Roots of Modern Urban Poverty," 242–243.

7. Solinger, *Wake Up Little Susie*, 42; Gordon, *Pitied but Not Entitled*, 43–46, 51–52.

8. *Madrigal v. Quilligan*, No. CV 75–2057-JWC, Opinion, Filed June 30, 1978.

9. Roberts, *Killing the Black Body*, 104–106, 118.

10. Nancy Ordover, *American Eugenics: Race, Queer Anatomy, and the Science of Nationalism* (Minneapolis: University of Minnesota Press, 2003), 181–182.

11. Donald Kimelman, "Poverty and Norplant: Can Contraception Reduce the Underclass?" *Philadelphia Inquirer*, December 12, 1990, quoted in Roberts, *Killing the Black Body*, 106.

12. Roberts, *Killing the Black Body*, 108.

13. Daylene K. English, *Unnatural Selections: Eugenics in American Modernism and the Harlem Renaissance* (Chapel Hill: University of North Carolina Press, 2004).

14. David Frankel, Letter to the Editor, *Washington Post*, December 29, 1990, quoted in Roberts, *Killing the Black Body*, 107.

15. Meredith Blake, "Welfare and Coerced Contraception: Morality Implications of State Sponsored Reproductive Control," *University of Louisville Journal of Family Law* 34 (Spring 1995/1996): 5; Roberts, *Killing the Black Body*, 109–110.

16. Ordover, *American Eugenics*, 190, 191; Roberts, *Killing the Black Body*, 108–110; Blake, "Welfare and Coerced Contraception," 5.

17. Ordover, *American Eugenics*, 186.

18. It is unclear what the consequences would be if either person violated the order and procreated. Marc Santora, "Negligent Upstate Couple Is Told Not to Procreate," *New York Times*, May 11, 2004, http://query.nytimes.com/gst/fullpage.html?res=9B0CE1DC133CF932A25756C0A9629C8B63, accessed April 25, 2008. California courts had previously determined that the state could not force a woman to use Norplant.

19. Http://www.projectprevention.org/reasons/statistics.html. This statistic is as of October 15, 2007.

20. Jennifer Mott Johnson, "Reproductive Ability for Sale, Do I Hear $200?: Private Cash-for-Contraception Agreements as an Alternative to Maternal Substance Abuse," *Arizona Law Review* 43 (Spring 2001), www.lexis-nexis.com, accessed April 25, 2008; Nelson, *Women of Color*, 181.

21. Nelson, *Women of Color*, 181; http://www.projectprevention.org/about/new_chapters.html, accessed April 25, 2008; http://www.projectprevention.org/program/howwehelp.html, accessed April 25, 2008.

22. Http://www.cashforbirthcontrol.com/program/faqs.html. The url cashforbirthcontrol.com no longer belongs to CRACK. As of 2004, CRACK's url is www.projectprevention.org, accessed March 1, 2004.

23. Daniello Costell, "Is CRACK Wack?" Salon.com, http://dir.salon.com/story/mwt/feature/2003/04/08/crack/, accessed April 25, 2008.

24. Ibid.

25. Joelle Babula, "Breaking the Cycle," *Las Vegas Review*, March 17, 2001, http://www.projectprevention.org/cause/quotes.html, accessed April 25, 2008.

26. Eric Gershon, "Woman on a Mission," *Hartford Courant*, July 15, 2006; Abigail Goldman, "Making a Choice," *Las Vegas Sun*, February 27, 2007; Gabrielle Glaser, "The Toughest Easy Money an Addict Ever Earned," *Oregonian*, July 12, 2006; Liz Trotta, "Sterilization Group Hit with Charges of Racism," *Washington Times*, January 8, 2003.

Index

abortion, 6, 9, 26, 56, 58, 60, 63, 72, 92,
116–117, 128, 153, 215, 216, 221; boards,
24, 248n39; American Civil Liberties
Union and, 116, 119–120; Black Panthers
and, 179; feminists and, 132, 149–150,
175, 178, 186, 193, 197–198, 205,
211–213; parental consent for, 137–138,
216; policy, 26, 95–96, 117, 118,
137–139, 144, 211–213; spousal consent
for, 137–138; with sterilization, 24,
152–153. *See also* Hyde Amendment;
Roe v. Wade
Acosta, Guadalupe, 112
age/parity policies: 120 rule, 22–24, 50,
114–117, 118, 217; ACOG and, 117–118,
126; Association for Voluntary Sterilization and, 40–41; Operation Lawsuit,
119, 125–126, 128–131, 134, 136,
144–145, 149–150, 184, 186; relation to
forced sterilization, 22–24, 123–124, 166;
relation to voluntary sterilization, 50, 69;
urologists' policies, 55; and women's
roles in society, 24, 215, 216. *See also*
sterilization: hospital restrictions
Agency for International Development
(AID), 69, 194
Aid to Dependent Children (ADC), 75, 77.
See also welfare
Aid to Families with Dependent Children
(AFDC), 75, 77, 95. *See also* welfare
Alabama, 90, 101, 152, 155, 182
American Civil Liberties Union (ACLU):
and forced sterilization, 22, 148, 152,
163; Massachusetts Civil Liberties Union,
134; New York Civil Liberties Union,
126, 132, 195, 197, 210; and Office of
Economic Opportunity sterilization
policy, 96, 247n19; Operation Lawsuit, 6,
22, 114–116, 119–121, *122*, 124, 218;
Reproductive Freedom Project, 80,
119–120, 139, 141, 152–153, 163; sterilization legislation, 79; Texas ACLU,
140–141

American College of Obstetricians and
Gynecologists (ACOG), 23, 35, 117–119,
121, 126–127, 134, 191, 207
American Cyanamid Company, 214–215
American Eugenics Society (AES), 10, 21
American Hospital Association (AHA), 106,
160
American Institute of Family Relations
(AIFR), 10, 21
*American Journal of Obstetrics and
Gynecology*, 24
American Medical Association (AMA), 23,
32, 35
American Public Health Association
(APHA), 35, 118
American Urological Association (AUA),
23, 35, 118
Andrade, Miguel Vega, 87–88, 165
Appalachia, 46–47
Arizona, 62, 152–153
Association for Voluntary Sterilization
(AVS): and childfree lifestyles, 62–63;
and eugenics, 26–29; and family
planning clinics, 42–49; history, 5–6,
10–11, 26–31; insurance coverage of
sterilization, 66–69; letters to, 38–40,
41–42, 59, 62; membership, 28; and
National Welfare Rights Organization,
173–175; and Operation Lawsuit, 23, 87,
115–116, 119–120, *122*, 123–124,
131–132, 144, 218; and physicians,
31–36, 37, 59; and Planned Parenthood,
36, 193–195; and population control
community, 28, 33–34, 37, 47–48; and
pronatalism, 29–30; public relations
campaign, 36–37; service programs,
37–49; sterilization clinics, 64–65,
194–195; and sterilization guidelines, 18,
193–196, 203, 207; sterilization of
persons with mental disabilities, 31, 38.
See also Birthright Inc.; Human
Betterment Association of America;
Sterilization League of New Jersey

About the Author

Rebecca M. Kluchin received her Ph.D. in American history from Carnegie Mellon University. She is an assistant professor of history at California State University, Sacramento.

Available titles in the Critical Issues in Health and Medicine series:

Breinigsville, PA USA
15 February 2011
255621BV00002B/1/P